BIOETHICS AROUND THE GLOBE

BIOETHICS AROUND THE GLOBE

Edited by Catherine Myser

OXFORD
UNIVERSITY PRESS

OXFORD
UNIVERSITY PRESS

Oxford University Press, Inc., publishes works that further Oxford University's objective of excellence in research, scholarship, and education.

Oxford New York
Auckland Cape Town Dar es Salaam Hong Kong Karachi Kuala Lumpur
Madrid Melbourne Mexico City Nairobi New Delhi Shanghai Taipei Toronto

With offices in
Argentina Austria Brazil Chile Czech Republic France Greece Guatemala Hungary Italy
Japan Poland Portugal Singapore South Korea Switzerland Thailand Turkey Ukraine
Vietnam

Published by Oxford University Press, Inc.
198 Madison Avenue, New York, New York 10016

Library of Congress Cataloging-in-Publication Data

Bioethics around the globe / edited by Catherine Myser.
p. ; cm.
Includes bibliographical references.
ISBN 978-0-19-538609-7
1. Bioethics. 2. Bioethics—Developing countries. 3. Globalization. I. Myser, Catherine.
[DNLM: 1. Bioethics. 2. Developing Countries. 3. Internationality. WB 60]
QH332.B51718 2011
174'.957—dc22 2010041917

---

9 8 7 6 5 4 3 2 1

Printed in the United States of America on acid-free paper

This book is dedicated to my father, John T. Myser, Sr., for his 75th birthday. Thank you for teaching ocean magic through Pacific Ocean tidepools and scuba, and for inspiring a lifelong passion for global explorations. You are always at the core of every new adventure I undertake!

CONTENTS

SECTION THREE: *Bioethics as a Means for Negotiating Social,
Regional, and/or National Identity, and Bioethics as Nation-Building*

SECTION FOUR: *Bioethics as a Battleground for Religious and
Political "Culture Wars": The Politics of Bioethics*

ACKNOWLEDGMENTS

First, I would like to acknowledge a key intellectual mentor, Renee C. Fox, PhD. Her brilliant and revelatory work in the sociology of medicine and bioethics has been a continuous inspiration guiding my own intellectual explorations—in and outside the United States—throughout my career. Moreover, her generous and encouraging correspondence over the years has offered invaluable support.

Second, I would like to acknowledge the United States government-sponsored Fulbright international educational exchange program, which has generously awarded me three scholarships to study and teach bioethics and clinical ethics in Sweden and Turkey over the last two decades. Of most recent influence, I would like to acknowledge Fulbright Turkey, especially Sureyya Ersoy and Ulku Inal of the Istanbul branch; my uniquely welcoming Yeditepe University colleagues led by Anthropology Department Chair Akile Gursoy; and my extraordinarily generous Turkish friends and family, Kazim Uzunoglu and Sennur and Gulten Yilmaz; for their invaluable support during my 2004–2005 year as a Fulbright Professor and Senior Scholar in Istanbul. This overseas exchange experience was the pivotal moment enabling me to recognize and begin to explore the "cultural meanings and social functions of bioethics," an unanticipated research topic which uniquely revealed itself in Turkey, additionally stimulating me to commission the broader global study featured in this book. This Fulbright year exemplifies the unique capacity of overseas study, perspectives and re-visioning to reveal and challenge unrecognized assumptions and unconscious academic practices and to evolve one's academic discipline in unexpected and exciting ways, to increase mutual understanding between scholars and nations around the globe and to enrich one's resulting professional service.

Third, I would like to acknowledge Ray DeVries, PhD, for generously sharing his vast international network of social scientists and bioethicists, without which it would have been impossible to locate the scholars possessing the in-depth ethnographic experience and unique lenses required to bring my vision of a comparative anthropology and sociology of bioethics around the globe to life.

I acknowledge these and other invited contributors for their willingness, patience, and ability through proactive and serial edits of their respective chapters to bring my overall vision to life. I similarly acknowledge the multidisciplinary, international peer reviewers who ensured the book's high intellectual standards, including: Tod Chambers, PhD; Subrata Chattopadhyay, MD, PhD; Thomas Eich, PhD; Pam Heatlie, JD; Bruce Jennings, MA; Carlo Leget, PhD; Trudo Lemmens, JD; Betty Wolder Levin, PhD; Kayhan Parsi, JD, PhD; and Maartje Schermer, PhD.

Fourth, I acknowledge my Oxford University Press Editor, Peter Ohlin, for his faith in and support of this project, his assistants Lucy Randall and Molly Wagener for their efficient and collegial support, and production team members at OUP (Susan Lee) & Glyph International (Aparna Shankar).

Last, but in no way least, I acknowledge my family and friends for their love and support throughout this project and all endeavors I undertake.

ABOUT THE AUTHORS

Richard E. Ashcroft is Professor of Bioethics in the School of Law, Queen Mary, University of London. He trained in history and philosophy of science, and has worked mainly on ethical issues in biomedical research, and public health ethics. His current research is in ethics in health promotion, and on the relationship between human rights and bioethics. He is editor in chief of *Principles of Health Care Ethics* (Wiley-Blackwell, 2nd ed. 2007).

Solomon (Solly) R. Benatar. Emeritus Professor of Medicine, Founding Director Bioethics Centre, University of Cape Town, and Professor Dalla Lana School of Public Health & Joint Centre for Bioethics, University of Toronto. *Global Health and Global Health Ethics* was published by Cambridge University Press in 2011.

Björn Bentlage studied Oriental and Islamic studies at the universities of Bochum (Germany) and Alexandria (Egypt) and graduated with a Magister degree in 2007. He is now working at the Martin Luther University in Halle-Wittenberg, Germany while finishing his PhD on legal and social development in contemporary Egypt.

Subrata Chattopadhyay is founder-head and professor of physiology at the College of Medicine and J.N.M. Hospital, West Bengal University of Health Sciences, India. Trained in modern medicine, he pursued his doctoral and post-doctoral studies in molecular biomedical science and passed Erasmus Mundus Master of Bioethics program *magna cum laude*. His current research interests include, among others, spirituality, *dharma*, Eastern worldviews, medicine and ethics, and cross-cultural perspective in global bioethics.

Michael D. Coughlin is a Clinical Ethicist as well as Associate Professor in the Department of Psychiatry and Behavioural Neurosciences at McMaster University, Hamilton, Ontario. Michael trained both in theology (Catholic University of Chile) and in developmental neurobiology (Stanford University) and has 25 years of experience as a clinical ethicist. His neuroscience work has focused on growth factors in neuronal development and his bioethics work has focused on research ethics and on the development and role of the health care ethics consultant.

Raymond De Vries, is Professor in the Center for Bioethics and Social Sciences in Medicine at the University of Michigan Medical School. He is co-editor of *The View from Here: Bioethics and the Social Sciences* (Blackwell, 2007) and is at work on a critical social history of bioethics.

Mary Dixon-Woods is Professor of Medical Sociology at the University of Leicester. She trained in sociology, and has worked on a wide range of issues in the sociology of medicine and medical research. She has a special interest in the sociology of governance, patient safety, and child health. She has published widely in sociological and medical journals. She is also an authority on methods of synthesising different kinds of evidence in health technology assessment.

Thomas Eich is Professor for Islamic Studies at the Asia Africa Institute at Hamburg University in Germany. His publications include "Islam und Bioethik," "Muslim Medical Ethics" (co-edited with Jonathan E. Brockopp) and "Induced miscarriage in early Maliki and Hanafi fiqh," *Islamic Law and Society*, 16 (2009), 302–36.

Andrea Frolic is currently the Clinical & Organizational Ethicist at Hamilton Health Sciences and Associate Professor of Family Medicine at McMaster University. Andrea's academic training includes a BA and MA in Religious Studies and a PhD in Anthropology at Rice University in Houston, Texas, along with a fellowship in Clinical Ethics from the University of Texas, MD Anderson Cancer Center. She contributes to the development of standards for health care ethics through participation on national taskforces in both the U.S. and Canada. Andrea's research interests focus on team ethics consultation, end of life care, narrative ethics and the intersection of ethics and health policy.

Fred Gifford is Professor and Associate Chair of Philosophy, Faculty Associate in the Center for Ethics and Humanities in the Life Sciences, and Director of the graduate specialization in Ethics and Development at Michigan State University. He has led for several years a study abroad program on bioethics in Costa Rica.

Rob Irvine is an Associate of the Centre for Values, Ethics and Law in Medicine (VELIM), the Medical Faculty, University of Sydney. He has interests in the sociology of and sociology in bioethics, cultural and moral politics of bioethics and bioethical topics, and the social, moral and political issues that surround human-animal relations. Recent research and publications have focussed upon the political condition of bioethics and environmental bioethics. He has an honours degree in sociology and a PhD in sociology from the University of Edinburgh. He has taught sociology and ethics at the University of Newcastle and the Community Health and Research Training Unit (CHRTU), University of Western Australia. Before joining the CHRTU he was a Research Fellow at the Abt. Für Mediziniche Soziologie, Albert Ludwigs' Universität, Freiburg im Breisgau.

Bruce Jennings is Director of Bioethics at the Center for Humans and Nature and is editor of its electronic journal, *Minding Nature*. He teaches at the Yale University School of Public Health and New York Medical College. He is Senior Consultant and an elected Fellow at The Hastings Center, where he served as Executive Director from 1991–1999. A political scientist by training, he has written extensively on bioethics and public policy issues.

Bernard Keating teaches Catholic biomedical ethics and bioethics in faculties of Pharmacie and Médecine Dentaire at Laval University in Québec City, Canada. His most recent work is on the ethics of research, ethical problems related to the development and commercialization of drugs, and on the nourishment and artificial hydration of patients in a permanent vegetative state.

Ian Kerridge is Director and Associate Professor in Bioethics at the Centre for Values, Ethics and the Law in Medicine at the University of Sydney and Staff Haematologist/Bone Marrow Transplant physician at Westmead Hospital, Sydney, Australia. He has published widely in ethics and medicine and is the author of over 100 papers in peer-reviewed journals and five textbooks of ethics, most recently *Ethics and Law for the Health Professions* (Federation Press, 2009).

Paul A. Komesaroff is a physician, medical researcher and philosopher at Monash University in Melbourne, Australia. He is Director of the Monash Centre for Ethics in Medicine and Society, Executive Director of Global Reconciliation, Ethics Convener of the Royal Australasian College of Physicians and Chair of the Australian Health and Development Alliance. He is Chair of the Editorial Board of the *Journal of Bioethical Inquiry* and author of more than 300 articles in science, ethics and philosophy and twelve books, including *Experiments in Love and Death* (2008), *Pathways to Reconciliation: Theory and Practice* (2008) and *Objectivity, Science and Society* (2008).

Miguel Kottow is Full Professor at the Universidad de Chile and is currently lecturing at the School of Public Health of Universidad de Chile, and is affiliated to the Universidad Diego Portales as member of its Research Ethics Committees. He is the author of 5 books, numerous articles, contributions to anthologies on bioethics and related subjects. He is a member of 8 international editorial boards. His current main interests include fundamentals of bioethics and public health bioethics.

Francis Masiye received a Bachelor of Philosophy in Ethics from the Pontifical Urbaniana University in Rome through his studies at the Salvatorian Institute of Philosophy and Theology in Tanzania. In 2004, he pursued a Master of Philosophy (M.Phil.) at the University of Malawi Chancellor College and he later joined the

University of Malawi College of Medicine as an Assistant Research Officer for the Wellcome Trust Bioethics Research Project. He also coordinated a WHO-Global Forum for Health Research Policy Study in Malawi and has participated in various research consultancies with the Malawi National AIDS Commission, Concern Universal and the Malawi-Liverpool-Wellcome Trust. In 2006, Mr. Masiye attended a Fogarty Fellowship Program in Bioethics and Research Ethics at the Johns Hopkins Bloomberg School of Public Health in Baltimore, USA. He has also been trained as a Clinical Research Associate (CRA) and Clinical Trial Inspector by Kendle South Africa and Ashdown Clinical Research Organization in the UK and Malawi. Currently, he is serving as a Compliance Officer for the College of Medicine Research and Ethics Committee (COMREC) in the University of Malawi. He also serves as a Research Associate for the Community Health Division at the University Of Malawi College Of Medicine. He has published several articles in bioethics and research ethics in the *Malawi Medical Journal*, the Springer and the *British Medical Journal*. His main research interests are in Research Ethics (informed consent, disclosure & justice), Public Health and Medical Anthropology or African Anthropology. His scholarly interests are in Bioethics, Research Ethics, Public Health, Medical Anthropology (African Anthropology) and Clinical Trial Monitoring.

Joseph Mfutso-Bengo is a full professor of Bioethics. He holds a diploma in Philosophy from ICS Balaka. He did Fogarty funded post-doctoral fellowship in research ethics at Johns Hopkins University in the USA. He obtained a Master of Arts with majors in Theology and Philosophy from University of Innsbruck in Austria and Doctor of Theology from University of Regensburg in Germany with special interests in practical theology, canon law and ethics. Prof J Mfutso-Bengo conducts empirical research in bioethics. His areas of interest and publications address medical ethics, public health ethics, clinical research ethics, ethics of genetics and social justice. He is the chair of the College of Medicine Research and Ethics Committee and co-chair of the National Health Science Committee respectively. He is also the Director of the Center of Bioethics for Southern and Eastern Africa. He is the Head of Community Health Department at the College of Medicine university of Malawi. He speaks German, English and Chichewa.

Jonathan D. Moreno is the David and Lyn Silfen University Professor of Ethics and Professor of Medical Ethics and of History and Sociology of Science at the university of Pennsylvania. He holds a courtesy appointment as Professor of Philosophy. He is also a Senior Fellow at the Center for American Progress in Washington, DC, where he edits the magazine *Science Progress* (www.scienceprogress.org). He was a member of President Barack Obama's transition team for the Department of Health and Human Services.

Kristina Orfali, a graduate from the Ecole Normale Supérieure, received her PhD from the Ecole des Hautes Etudes en Sciences Sociales in France. She is an Associate Clinical Professor of Bioethics in Pediatrics at Columbia University and a Faculty Associate at the Center for Bioethics and the Institute for Social and Economic Research and Policy (ISERP). She has published work in a cross-cultural perspective on patients hospital experiences, on clinician and family decision making in life and death contexts. Her more recent work focuses on ethical dilemmas and international variations in medical prognosis. She is the co-editor of *The View from Here, Bioethics and Social Sciences* (2007) and of "*Who is my Genetic Parent? Donor Anonymity and Assisted Reproduction: a Cross-Cultural Perspective*" (2011). Trained as a sociologist in France, Kristina Orfali has been an Assistant Professor in Medicine and Assistant Director at the MacLean Center for Clinical Ethics at the University of Chicago and Directeur de Recherche at the CNRS in France.

Qiu Renzong was born in Suzhou, China and is Emeritus Professor of the Institute of Philosophy and Honorary Director of the Centre for Applied Ethics, Chinese Academy of Social Sciences. He is also Professor and Chair of the Academic Committee at the Department of Social Sciences and the Humanities/Center for Bioethics of Peking Union Medical College. He is Vice-President of the National Ethics Committee of the Ministry of Health in China and Member of the UNAIDS Reference Group on AIDS and Human Rights. He was the 2002 Winner of the World Network of Technology Awards in Ethics, and 2009 Laureate of the UNESCO Avicenna Prize of Ethics of Science.

Ana Rodríguez is a professor at the Escuela de Filosofía at Universidad Nacional de Costa Rica. She co-founded and presently chairs its Masters Program in Bioethics. She specializes in applied ethics and philosophy of science, and she has been an active member of several bioethics committees.

Leslie Rott, is a sociology PhD candidate currently working on her dissertation at the University of Michigan. Her research interests fall into the areas of bioethics, the body, disability, medical sociology, the use of medical technologies, qualitative methodology, and stigma.

Moisés Russo lectures in bioethics at Universidad Diego Portales in Chile. He is a Medical Doctor with an MA in Bioethics from the Erasmus Mundus Program and an MA in Applied Economics from Georgetown University/ILADES. He is currently a Radiation Oncology resident at Instituto de Radiomedicina in Santiago.

Bob Simpson is Professor of Anthropology at Durham University. His work has focused particularly on the encounter between new biotechnologies and local systems of values and beliefs in South Asia. His recent research has focused on the place of bioethics in international collaborations in biomedical science.

Anton A. van Niekerk is Chair of the Philosophy Department and Director of the Center for Applied Ethics at Stellenbosch University, South Africa. He has published widely in the field of bioethics, particularly about HIV/AIDS in Africa. He is a director of the International Association of Bioethics.

INTRODUCTION

FIRST STEPS TOWARD A COMPARATIVE ANTHROPOLOGY AND SOCIOLOGY OF GLOBALIZING BIOETHICS

REFLECTING ON THE CULTURAL MEANINGS AND SOCIAL FUNCTIONS OF BIOETHICS

Catherine Myser

The development, professionalization, and institutionalization of contemporary "bioethics" began almost four decades ago in the United States, and has since then rooted and sprouted by fits and starts all around the globe. Increasingly, the theories, practices, and institutions of United States bioethics have been "exported" to other developed countries. Either directly or through these other developed countries, bioethics has also been exported to increasing numbers of developing countries, often within a paradigm of building "ethics capacity." In these additional developed and developing countries, bioethics has undergone further transformations, whether consciously or unconsciously; e.g., as local cultural features have been incorporated, or are vying for influence. All these social and cultural processes have occurred so rapidly, and perhaps so unthinkingly, that there has not been adequate time and opportunity for self-reflection, self-study, self-critique, and even self-correction of bioethics where required. Perhaps we in the field operate under the specious assumption that exporting "ethics" can only be good, at least on balance. In any case, I believe the time is right in the development of the field for some "customs checks" on all sides of the national borders in question, exploring what is intentionally or unintentionally being developed and exported or imported, any unintended (negative) effects of exporting or importing "nonnative" species of bioethics into other countries, and relevant "local" developments or transformations that are taking place, whether noticed or unnoticed, outside or even inside the countries in question.

This book thus aims to explore, identify, and analyze the evolution, cultural meanings, and social functions of bioethics theories, practices, and institutions around the globe, including developed and developing countries, and thus provide a rich basis for comparison of "older" and "newer" bioethics programs and institutions. As such, it is basically an anthropology and sociology of globalizing bioethics as currently understood and applied around the globe. Such cultural meanings and social functions of bioethics have not been subjected to adequate—especially empirical—exploration on a national or international basis. Accordingly, this book—recognizing that bioethics is contingent on, for example, nation, society, culture, economics, politics, religion, and history—aims to provide an exploration of these varying fields, and the overall field of bioethics (not presuming to define "bioethics" homogenously in advance, but allowing for national and international variations to emerge) as an essential step to advance, and transform as appropriate, the development of national and international bioethics. Such self-study, and any necessary self-critiques and self-corrections it invites based on the data gathered, are crucial for bioethics as it continues to develop and disseminate around the globe.

The exploration being undertaken in this book project is especially important if bioethics genuinely seeks to serve each society in which it operates, rather than imposing unexamined and perhaps inappropriate values, ideologies, theories, and practices. Indeed, as various contributors to this proposed volume will reveal, there may be more hidden curricula and unintended values operating than we realize in the cultural construction and social functions of bioethics, especially in rapidly globalizing bioethics. Topics include government agendas (e.g., nation-building, national identity formation, nationalism); agendas of powerful associated professions (e.g., medicine, law); theological/religious agendas; agendas of competing political groups and ideologies; economic, commercial, and/or corporate agendas; external actors (e.g., United States, United Kingdom, and/or global funders); and/or other cultural and social agendas consciously or unconsciously advanced or contested by bioethics work in particular countries, based on their unique history, politics, and culture. Bioethics may thus unwittingly be advancing ideologies, power structures, and institutions that in the end undermine the ethics enterprise and overall social justice—in particular countries and generally around the globe—despite its best intentions.

For one compelling example, my ethnography of bioethics in Turkey[1] reveals that one social function of bioethics in Turkey—as constructed by secularist social elites in schools of medicine—is to advance secularizing, democratizing,

1. This ethnography was completed as a Fulbright professor and senior scholar in Istanbul, Turkey (2004–2005), building on my earlier ethnographies of Turkish bioethics conducted in Istanbul, Ankara and Urfa, Turkey (2002).

and modernizing (i.e., nation-building) movements also at work in Turkish society. Some relevant insights of Turkish medical anthropologist Akile Gursoy offer support for my findings. After noting that "medicine throughout the contemporary world is associated with state control, social authority, and power," Gursoy argues that "the first and fiercest battles over the establishment of secularism, the roots of nationalism, and the abolishment of the *shar-ia* [Islamic religious law] was fought through the establishment of modern medicine in Ottoman society . . . From its inception . . . modern medicine in Turkey . . . alongside the army and school of political science [was] intermingled with the processes of . . . Westernization, nationalism, secularism, and atheism."[2] A secular Islamic republic since the 1920s, Turkey has struggled to reconcile tensions between secular, modern, and democratic values, and Islamic values, throughout that history. Accordingly, this tension similarly operates in the microcosm of Turkish bioethics which is uniformly located within its medical schools. This results in counterintuitive repression of any Islamic bioethics in Turkey, despite its being a majority Muslim country. One key ethical question is thus whether a secular bioethics—crafted by intellectual and social elites, and adapting Anglo-American bioethics theories and practice already an awkward fit with Turkey's sociocultural context—can adequately serve Turkey's Muslim majority population.

On the other hand, bioethics is no doubt doing significant good around the globe, and the empirical study being undertaken in this book can also highlight bioethics theories, practices, and institutions that might be rendered yet more effective. Thus, in the end, this book aims at more self-reflective bioethics theorizing, practices, and institutions, as well as better and more effective service around the globe, ever more attuned to relevant sociocultural factors and processes.

The book is divided into four sections, considering nine developing countries (and yet more in the "missionary bioethics" chapter) and five developed countries, explicitly seeking to give voice to more developing countries which are currently underrepresented in international bioethics discussions and publications. A single book cannot really offer a "representative" sample of countries, but this book offers a regionally well balanced sample—including Africa (2), Asia (3), Australia (1), Europe (3), the Middle East (1), North America (2), and South and Central America (2)—and in some cases offering interesting side by side comparison of differing countries in a geographic region. As no single bioethics scholar or team of bioethics scholars possesses the knowledge of all regions and countries under consideration, this collection draws on the expertise of a broadly multidisciplinary group of experts who collectively possess such empirical knowledge and experience. This includes individuals or small teams of coauthors

2. Akile Gursoy, Beyond the Orthodox: Heresy in Medicine and the Social Sciences From a Cross-Cultural Perspective. *Social Science and Medicine* 43:5 (1996), pp. 580, 592–593.

commissioned for this project from among: (a) bioethics scholars native to a particular country; or (b) nonnative social scientists or other bioethics scholars with in-depth ethnographic or other relevant knowledge of a particular country. Accordingly, one secondary aim of this book is to reflect and improve interdisciplinarity in and around "the field" of bioethics—incorporating the theoretical insights and methodological innovations of humanities, social science, science, health care, and other disciplines—all of which can provide intellectual leadership at the borderlands of bioethical questions. Therefore, the core disciplinary training of each contributor is noted in the summary of each chapter in this introduction.

Globalizing Western Bioethics: Some Perils and Pitfalls of "Missionary Bioethics" and Ethics "Capacity Building" in the Developing World and the East

Section One addresses some perils and pitfalls of exporting Western bioethics—i.e., Anglo-American and Western European bioethics—into developing countries, especially Eastern countries.

For example, in Chapter 1, sociologists DeVries and Rott use the analogy of "missionary" bioethics, and share examples from DeVries' empirical research among scholars from the developing world receiving bioethics training in Europe, to highlight some of the unwitting harms of exporting "the gospel" of good clinical and research ethics theory and practice into the developing world, despite "noble intent" to protect patients and research subjects. They argue that Western bioethicists have followed a similar shift to that taken by religious missionaries, from imported to indigenous "evangelization," and are currently attempting "indigenization" (bringing citizens from developing countries to the West to train them to import the missionary message back into their own local cultures). They do so both to cope with "the export problem" of Western bioethics as it collides with local, non-Western ethical systems and to avoid "colonial abuses." However, DeVries and Rott reveal the weaknesses of such an approach from the perspective of developing world scholars themselves; e.g., questionable motivations as well as specific problems and misfits of Western ethics models and "issues." DeVries and Rott's core message for globalizing bioethics is that an imbalance in power and influence between "missionary" bioethics trainers and "missionized" developing world trainees diminishes a two-way flow of information among equals that might mutually enrich Western and non-Western bioethics, and also enhance the social relevance of bioethics around the globe.

Chapter 2, authored by physician/physiologist Chattopadhyay (who completed his bioethics MA in the European training program that DeVries ethnographically studied), offers an excellent example of the crucial insights that an

Eastern insider can offer to improve Western and Eastern bioethics alike. First, he reminds us that multifaith, multilingual, and multicultural societies—commonplace in the era of globalization—comprise multiple "realities," all of which pose myriad intracultural and crosscultural challenges for the development of a more culturally competent national and international bioethics. With refreshing self-criticism, he features his own country as a "Pandora's box of intricate issues" for a "U.S.-born Western bioethics headquartered in Paris" and for nascent Eastern bioethics in the "pan-Indian reality," highlighting unique developing world challenges such as "colonized minds" and pervasive political, medical profession, and health sector corruption. He offers a similarly honest and hard-hitting appraisal of the myopia, dissonance, and "neocolonial moral imperialism" of Western bioethics—e.g., the UNESCO Universal Declaration on Bioethics and Human Rights—as a "transgenic [alien] culture" out of which intended "good" may instead come "evil," and suggests many sophisticated and useful corrections from his Eastern worldview.

In Chapter 3, anthropologist Simpson explores significant cultural, institutional, and economic impediments affecting bioethics "capacity building" in Sri Lanka (many of which overlap with the complex realities and challenges Chattopadhyay highlights in India), e.g., the "serious paradox" and ongoing "colonizing power" of entrenched westernized European and Anglophone biomedicine and Western Hippocratic medical ethics. Simpson suggests that both marginalize indigenous medical and value systems, and thus make it important to "reach back" to more ancient Eastern traditions to rediscover more applicable values and beliefs. In addressing the question of whence a more suitable "Asian ethics" might derive, Simpson provides a subtle and concrete analysis and argument that building bioethics capacity from "the blueprints of an international bioethics . . . shaped to fit the contingencies of local circumstance" is more an "irregular process of improvisation and irregularity [than] an exercise in neat and perpendicular architecture." This is particularly true, he says, as varied internal and external professional, financial, and cultural stakeholders vie for influence on a backdrop of Sri Lanka's "brutal and traumatic . . . cataclysms" of ethnic, religious, and civil strife, and resultant militarization of society, "rendering 'culture' far from homogenous and harmonious but complex, conflicted, and contested" and making democratic representation in bioethics particularly fraught.

A Robust Range of Sociocultural Interests and Forces Shaping Bioethics Around the Globe: Cultural Meanings and Social Functions of Bioethics

Section Two highlights a robust range of sociocultural interests and forces currently shaping bioethics around the globe.

For example, in Chapter 4, sociologist Orfali suggests that in French bioethics there is: (a) a strong "rhetoric of nationalization" (Paillet, 1999); (b) a "self-appointed [universalizing] mission;" and (c) explicit opposition to the "outside forces" of U.S. and "Anglo-Saxon" bioethics values (especially "autonomy") and models—making *nationalization, universalization*, and *opposition* to Anglo-American bioethics three key social functions of French bioethics. The major players shaping French bioethics, with effectively no input from its lay public, are: (a) its centralized state, trusted in the Jacobin tradition as the appropriate "defender of the public good" which will implement core French values such as "human dignity" and "solidarity," albeit with abstract accountability to "mankind and future generations" rather than to individual patients and families in "bedside ethics"; and (b) a strongly paternalistic medical profession, highly trusted by society to take "*ethical responsibility*" for decisions—even those with admitted "eugenic" implications—construed as part of its *medical* expertise and mandate. Any development of bioethicists, or associated "professionalization" of bioethics, is therefore rejected in French bioethics, maintaining the decision-making authority of French political and medical elites, and ideally also influencing international bioethics, e.g., in UNESCO declarations similarly emphasizing "human dignity" and "solidarity," and in UNESCO initiatives assisting the creation of permanent National Bioethics Commissions based on the pioneering French model. According to Orfali, these core French cultural values (rather than the Catholic Church as others speculate) cause more "grandiose questions [such] as the impact of science, research, technology, and medicine on the human being and the future of mankind"—encountered in, for example, prenatal testing, embryo research, assisted reproduction, surrogate mothers, neonatal care, human genetics, cloning, eugenics, transplantation/commodification of human bodies, and end-of-life care—to attain heightened cultural meaning and thus "bioethical" prominence in France.

In Chapter 5, U.K. philosopher Ashcroft and sociologist Dixon-Woods similarly oppose treating the historically, socioculturally, and legally contingent "U.S. version" of bioethics as normative for defining bioethics itself, or for assessing the quality and degree of bioethics development in other countries. They offer an initial sociology of U.K. bioethics as a "complex, newly emerging social phenomenon," describing its emergence, forms, and purposes as being controlled and shaped by actors other than bioethicists. Unlike in France, bioethics in the United Kingdom is "reasonably well established as an academic field"; however, U.K. bioethicists remain "relatively marginal" as a resource to solve "real life" bioethics problems in clinics and the British polity. Key players in U.K. bioethics are, rather, its medical profession (viewed with significant skepticism by other professionals and the public); its "consultative" state; and various "activist" laypersons and civil society associations such as patients' groups, medical charities, and conservative Christian groups, all vying for influence through appeals to "ethics" (although often framed in different language). As for the medical profession's initial claims to the "ethical character" of individual practitioners and the corporate body of medicine—already seen by some as a strategic maneuver to secure occupational autonomy and status, exclusive practice rights, and market monopolization—they are further undermined by various medical treatment "scandals," leading to an increased government role in "disaster management" and external regulation of medicine's professional ethics to "protect public safety." Ashcroft and Dixon-Woods highlight the "importance of the NHS as a public service, administered by central government and accountable to parliament and the electorate" as a key lens and infrastructure through which ethics issues are recast as "political problems" and "systems failures," marginalizing "medical ethics tropes" and calling instead for "regulatory" solutions. They also suggest that the attendant "consultation culture" of the British state uniquely legitimizes public activists, public opinion, and "public consultation" in the U.K. setting (in stark contrast with French bioethics as described by Orfali), instead of "ethical expertise"—which may suffer from generalized mistrust of professional expertise following professional ethics scandals in medicine—or "ethical argumentation."

Political scientist Jennings turns our attention from Western Europe to Central and Eastern Europe in Chapter 6. He offers a unique exploration of the emergence and social functions of bioethics born in the West—where it serves a key moral and legal function of bridling the new power and "alleviating the danger" of new science and medicine—being "exported" and "reborn in the East . . . behind what was once the Iron Curtain" in Central and Eastern Europe. There, Jennings asserts, it serves as "a discourse with which to affirm and contest power, equality, individual and group identity, knowledge, duty and trust." He supports his argument by outlining: (1) historical, sociocultural and economic factors impeding bioethics development during the Soviet period, yet allowing bioethics to "blossom" with the discrediting of communism; (2) the ambivalence of Central European bioethics toward "neoliberal values" and a free market society; and (3) Central European bioethics as a possible "Third Way" discursive space for social ethics "between capitalism (resisting its most extreme forms) and communism (rejecting its past ethic of communistic utilitarianism)." Given that Jennings explicitly credits over 100 colleagues from, e.g., Russia, Hungary, Poland, the Czech Republic, Slovakia, and Lithuania for sharing their own histories and perspectives (between 1988–1995) regarding the important role of bioethics reforms in "[building their respective] new societies," this chapter serves as another example of some (positive and negative) lessons that "Eastern" European bioethics can offer "Western" European and Anglo-American bioethics.

Shifting our focus to South and Central America, Chilean public health doctor and sociologist Kottow and physician/bioethicist Russo argue in Chapter 7 that Latin American nations share "fairly uniform" historical and sociocultural common features that directly shape Latin American bioethics. These include: (a) ongoing "neocolonial conditions" as the effects of 250 years of Spanish and Portuguese conquest and colonization; (b) sustained social and political influence of a Catholic Church which "took part in [this] conquest" through "strong missionary activity," and continues public service and inculcation of its values through excellent schools, universities, and hospitals; (c) "economic dependence on foreign capital, know-how, and marketing," reproducing "the colonial situation of a periphery [producing] for the benefit of a foreign economic power" (e.g., present-day "imported research protocols" advancing pharmaceutical interests and following "external ethics committee evaluations [that are] often insensible to local ethical needs"); and (d) "undaunted socioeconomic inequities." They argue that such features directly lead Chilean mainstream bioethics to attribute cultural and ethical prominence to priority setting, allocation and rationing of scarce resources, justice and social protections addressing inequities and disparities (including disparities multiplied by external funders like the World Bank while they advance their own political interests, e.g., privatizing medicine)—whereas the "deeper advocacy" should be for universal health care access that does not accept such inequities. They also argue that Chilean secular bioethics must take on the social function of contesting the "immutable principles [of] an outspoken and very influential . . . religious orthodoxy" (e.g., limitations of patient autonomy to refuse any life-sustaining treatments based on "sanctity of life" claims) which are directly influenced by European Catholic bioethics and "the traditional principlism of [the American Catholic university] Georgetown." However, they also indicate that Chilean traditional society and conservative media, neither of which "take pains to ensure pluralism," and conservative universities as well as bioethics programs with "fervent and highly vocal religious commitment," preclude a young and insufficiently powered Chilean bioethics from: "revising [cultural and] moral values," effectively advocating for disempowered minorities, and effectively defending "liberal bioethics stances." This leads Kottow and Russo to advocate for secular representation in civil society as an "urgent need"—the prime model being the "grassroots procedure of the Oregon (USA) model"—to engage a broader representation of the Chilean population in public deliberation, and to promote democratic education and consensus as "essential to ensure fairness and legitimacy" in Chilean bioethics.

In Chapter 8, philosophers Gifford and Rodriguez reflect on whether emerging Costa Rican bioethics will derive its ultimate identity in relation to bioethics in other countries, e.g., Chile, Brazil, and/or Spain—creating a "distinctive

Latin American bioethics"—or in relation to the United States, or even "*sui generis.*" They highlight "background factors" at work in Costa Rica, and shared by other Latin American countries, including: (a) the "considerable" influence of the Roman Catholic church on public opinion and policy (as in Chile); (b) a "culture of secrecy and corruption" in government and medicine, leading, for example, to "closed door" health policy and reforms; (c) the entrenched power and political interests of a "strongly paternalistic" medical profession that also resists critique; (d) a general "culture of trust in (especially medical) authority" and resulting failure to question authority; (e) all exacerbated by "the general unempowered position of the average Costa Rican" (e.g., lacking any legal recourse such as malpractice suits) and a cultural tendency favoring agreement and nonconfrontation.[3] The role of international financial institutions such as the World Bank and International Monetary Fund, enacting their own agendas to privatize government agencies and reduce public spending, is highlighted, as it is in Chile. However, here the "covert privatization" of Costa Rica's highly regarded public health service ("the Caja")—previously "based on the principles of universality, equality and solidarity," and now shifting in favor of the "values of competition and profit"—are directly linked to the overlapping interests of the medical profession. Primary care doctors, possessing a different worldview committed to public health, preventive care, and primary care, suggest that a key social function of Costa Rican bioethics is "counteracting this new [for-profit medical] model," leading Gifford and Rodriguez to conclude that Costa Rican bioethics may evolve differently depending on which set of cultural and professional principles and values wins out. Equally disturbing, Gifford and Rodriguez state that research ethics oversight in Costa Rica is similarly "privatized" and "for profit" in key respects, with bioethics and regulation often regarded as "an improper imposition [hindering] research," making conflicts of interest especially prominent in internationally funded human-subjects research there. The above conditions have coalesced at the same time that Costa Rican bioethics is "generating its self-consciousness." Gifford and Rodriguez suggest that such conditions are therefore directly shaping what issues are perceived as "crucial" for bioethics education and research (and by whom and why); what internal or external cultural and political interests "bioethics expertise" will ultimately serve (acknowledging competing agendas and attendant risks of "cooptation" of bioethics); what disciplines will accordingly emerge as core for the training and work of

3. It is worth noting (regarding points b, c, and d) that Costa Rica's non-physician authors are much more sensitive than Chile's physician authors to the role of the medical profession as both a negative force and possible positive force (at least via primary health doctors) to the development and functioning of bioethics in Latin America.

bioethics "experts"; and what social functions (e.g., critical discussion and adequate oversight versus "mere rubber stamp," or challenging authority versus providing "public relations" support) Costa Rican bioethics will adopt.

Philosopher van Niekerk and physician Benatar turn our attention to African bioethics, suggesting in Chapter 9 that South African bioethics originates in its initial phases as "[spill]over" from British and European academic institutions—as a result of its colonial past—serving the primary social function of "humanizing" medicine and society. However, they argue that South African bioethics gradually, and in parallel with the intensifying liberation struggle against apartheid, becomes "linked to more indigenous concerns," and increasingly takes on social functions advancing local social, political, and humanitarian concerns. They highlight: (a) the apartheid state as a "repressive, authoritarian society" under which public and professional debates on ethics are limited; and (b) the death of Steve Biko as a "reprehensible moral aberration" yet very significant turning point, as two key factors contributing to the indigenization of South African bioethics and leading it to function—in partnership with human rights and its concomitant ideology of [Western] liberal individualism—not only as an academic enterprise but as "a motive . . . for social action [and] resistance to tyranny." One core critique targets the World Bank and the IMF (like Latin American bioethics). Yet in Africa such "imperialist economic and ideological powers" and their specific "adverse effects of covert economic apartheid" are regarded as justifications for an emerging social function of South African bioethics to "unmask" and contest such actions of international institutions in the developing world. An additional target is the "big business" of human-subjects research carried out by multinational conglomerates in developing countries, with van Niekerk and Benatar issuing the caveat that bioethics has a special responsibility not to be "hijacked" by associated "commercial, profit-seeking agendas" (e.g., in related research ethics capacity building), and should furthermore "promote justice" in the distribution of research benefits to include developing country nations whose peoples serve as research subjects. Lastly, van Niekerk and Benatar admit that the current incarnation of South African bioethics presently lacks the anthropological skills and cultural knowledge to refract its Western-inspired bioethics through "the lens of African culture"—and, in some instances (e.g., HIV/AIDS safe-sex education), faces deeply entrenched suspicion by traditional black Africans as itself having "underlying motives of imperialist educators," e.g., "interfering with procreation."

In Chapter 10, philosophers Mfutso-Bengo and Masiye offer a more traditional African lens on African bioethics—featuring bioethics in their native Malawi—that van Niekerk and Benatar felt unable to offer regarding Western-influenced South African bioethics. They assert that—from Malawi's earliest creation myths, through liberation struggles against British colonialism, and finally in internecine battles for "human dignity, human rights [and] democracy"—ethics and bioethics have served social functions of resolving human conflicts and fighting core injustices and atrocities. A Roman Catholic Pastoral Letter of 1992 is singled out as motivating and supporting the popular mass movement dismantling a 30 year dictatorship—and attendant "massive social, political, and economic injustices"—and leading directly to the creation of "a new democratic era" enshrined in law. However, this redefining and "birth of Christian ethics" is also seen to undermine Malawian "cultural integrity . . . identity . . . dignity [and] indigenous values, traditions and morals," leading Mfutso-Bengo and Masiye to champion "African *ubuntu/uMunthu* ethical theory and bioethics" to take on the key social function of restoring and preserving" this "national cultural heritage" and urging medical students to apply it in their medical practice. They describe the cultural meanings of this "communalistic" African Bantu bioethics—with its relational concepts of humanism, personhood, and "interdependence [transcending] self-determination"—and contrast it directly with individualistic Western bioethics, especially autonomy and its application in narrowly construed informed consent practices. Such practices are, they argue, regarded as foreign and antithetical to African thought, with "individualistic tendencies [and] selfish behavior among Africans" being "looked down upon" and thus "actively discouraged in general among traditional Africans." Mfutso-Bengo and Masiye hasten to add that they do not advocate, e.g., "dumping . . . first-person informed consent" as a crucial safeguard against exploitation of individuals, but rather advocate that "Western bioethics in Africa" must be more broadly contextualized "in the light of ubuntu/uMunthu" as a "precious gift" from Africa and "unique paradigm . . . advancing [interdependent] human development and welfare."

Philosopher Qiu Renzong states in Chapter 11 that the birth and growth of bioethics in China is a "progressive process" stimulated by the Chinese government's policy of "reform and openness." With increasing cultural valuation of nation-building, development, and international competition in accordance with globalization, Chinese bioethics takes on the social function of "[speeding] up China's modernization," albeit with the "essential integrity" to temper the push from some in medicine and government to "[surge] ahead without constraints . . . to catch up" with international developments. Accordingly, Qiu argues that Chinese bioethics is not only a graft transplanted from outside by Western scholars, but rather finds "fertile soil" in China responding to perceived urgent local and national needs, enabling bioethics to "[establish] its root deeply . . . and [grow] its stem, branches and leaves [in] Chinese air." In particular, the globalization of research is described as transforming China into "a very energetic laboratory [surpassing India as the largest clinicopharmacological trials base] in the process of economic growth, scientific research, [and] social development... making innovation in every area of life (including bioethics and research ethics) a necessity." As in many other countries featured in this section, "disastrous [market-oriented] reforms" of the healthcare sector, the end of public aid, "erosion of medical professionalism" and concomitant public mistrust of "wolves in white" due to increasing conflicts of interest (e.g., physician self-interest versus altruism), increased "defensive medicine" with the medical profession aided by the legal profession, and profit pursuits of pharmaceutical companies are all highlighted as "formidable" forces in China. All are seen to require bioethics oversight and regulation to protect increasingly vulnerable rights and interests of patients and human subjects. A specific cultural question that Qiu believes underlies the institutionalization of bioethics in China and Asia (both comprising "a wide diversity of cultures") is balancing: (a) the "major premises" of "[shared] universal values" and concepts (e.g., informed consent) associated with Western international bioethics; and (b) the "minor premises" of traditional culture (e.g., the "monistic, gradualist, and relational" Confucian concept of personhood) that might beneficially be incorporated. Qiu offers an intriguing "reconciliation approach" for assimilating the positive elements of native culture as "peripheral" elements to tailor "core" international ethical guidelines for effective and respectful application in China, using informed consent theory and "family/community involvement" practice as an illustration, to achieve a "harmonized, as well as diversified" Confucian approach.

Bioethics as a Means of Negotiating Social, Regional, and/or National Identity, and Bioethics as Nation-Building

Section Three focuses a lens on one key "social function" of bioethics around the globe; i.e., serving as a means of negotiating social, regional, and/or national identities, and bioethics as nation-building.

For example, in Chapter 12, anthropologist Frolic, neurobiologist Coughlin, and theologian Keating argue that Canadian bioethics is preoccupied with questions of national identity, which have unique cultural meaning in Canada. Anxiety over what defines a Canadian and what makes Canada unique as a nation is fueled by perceived external and internal challenges to a coherent national identity. These challenges include: American popular culture and political influence; Québec nationalism; increased non-European immigration alongside multiculturalism as public policy; weak federalism; regional economic disparities; urban versus rural cultures; and a highly fractured political landscape. Accordingly, as in several other countries featured in Section Two, Canadians define themselves and their bioethics as "not American," and sometimes also as "not French."

Therefore, Canadian bioethics reflects and refracts the country's preoccupation with national identity and nation-building, which informs both its official discourse and informal practice. In other words, one key social function of Canadian bioethics is to advance nationalist discourse and nation-building. Frolic et al. intriguingly contrast this to countries (e.g., again some featured in Section Two) that seek through their national bioethics work to advance "globalizing," "homogenizing," or "universalizing" projects. Frolic et al. also discuss tensions between nationalism and a competing commitment to diversity and inclusion, and between bioethics as an academic/professional field and bioethics as an advocacy vehicle in Canadian public policy. This chapter thus provides one fascinating case study of the relationships between bioethics and the project and pitfalls of nation-building, raising crucial questions about the influence of history, culture, and politics on the enterprise of bioethics.

In Chapter 13, Middle East studies scholars Thomas Eich and Björn Bentlage argue that, although Egyptian bioethics is just beginning to emerge as a discipline in its own right, bioethics functions as *the* place for Egyptians to freely negotiate their values and vision of Egyptian society, as a means of negotiating and shaping Egyptian identity. As in many other Muslim-majority countries, bioethics is considered a branch of the ethical reasoning inherent to Islamic law; accordingly, the fundamental referential framework for defining Egyptian identity is Islam. However, negotiating Egyptian identity as an Islamic identity is not described in a neat binary of Islam versus the West. Rather, it is about asserting Egyptian Islamic identity in the face of strong influences and challenges from Western countries (including western NGOs which are often suspected of having hidden "Westernization" agendas, among other international relations, conferences, and declarations with secular and rights-oriented frameworks), as well as Saudi Arabia (e.g., contesting the "Saudification" of Egyptian Islamic identity). Eich and Bentlage identify the key actors in the field of Egyptian bioethics across a spectrum of government religious actors, government nonreligious actors, non-Egyptian actors (e.g., UNESCO's bioethics program in the region), and the media. They feature two short case studies, both relating to sexual mores and the role of women in Egyptian society, revealing a heightened cultural meaning and emphasis on, for example, how to control female sexuality in and through Egyptian bioethics. These case studies illustrate interactions of the described actors and show how bioethical debates in Egypt—situated in their wider sociopolitical context to glean their deeper implications—quickly develop into negotiations of Egyptian identity at large, revealing friction in Egyptian society toward "Western" international and scientific standards on one side, and notions labeled "Islamic" and often identified with Saudi Arabian influences on the other side.

Bioethics as a Battleground for Religious and/or Political "Culture Wars": The Politics of Bioethics

Lastly, Section Four offers a consideration of bioethics as a battleground for religious and political "culture wars."

Sociologist Irvine and physician/philosophers Kerridge and Komesaroff assert in Chapter 14 that at no time in its history has bioethics been above the political struggle for power and influence in the public marketplace of ideas, highlighting Australian bioethics as an example. The politics they have in mind is fourfold. First, bioethics functions as a political mode of discourse in the public struggle for discursive hegemony, with bioethicists vying for dominance for their particular theories and methods as the best or most legitimate knowledge. Given the "central fact" of religious discourse, institutions, and their significant general power and influence in Australian society, often assisted by its federal and state governments (e.g., to secure privileged places on consultative and law reform committees), Irvine et al. portray secular bioethics itself as being founded as a "counterpoint" new discipline emphasizing rational and correct reasoning over inherited custom, with key associated social and epistemological functions. Core targets include: biotechnological innovations assigned heightened cultural meaning, for example, reproduction and beginning of life issues; especially those with powers perceived as "transgressive" or "threatening" to moral agents and the social order; and challenging the authority and dominance of medical science (here aided by grassroots movements such as feminist, patients' rights, and consumerist). Second, unlike in the United States (where they see bioethicists to express misgivings over the politicization of bioethics), Irvine et al. describe key institutions such as the Australasian Bioethics Association as purposely moving bioethics discourse beyond philosophical or theological inquiry, and connecting bioethics democratically to political activity, for example, advancing moral/political discourse and taking up definite political projects within the organization. Third, bioethics functions socially and politically as an arena of intense conflict and struggle for certain interests, linking ethical awareness with political conviction and social action (e.g., Australian and New Zealand bioethicists publically challenging the Australian federal government's policies on detaining refugees). Fourth, to which the bulk of their analysis is dedicated, bioethics functions as a political field through which the Christian right competes against secular science and bioethics, and liberal ideology, in overt "culture wars," seeking to amplify religious doctrines, traditional family values and ethics, and the social (Christian) order that the Christian right perceives to be "under siege" in Australian society and politics, with human embryonic stem cells featured as an exemplary case.

In Chapter 15, political scientist Jennings and philosopher Moreno similarly regard bioethics in the United States as "contested [political] terrain," in this case for competing visions of American liberalism ("autonomy liberalism" versus "identity liberalism"). They argue that bioethics grows out of, and indeed is unimaginable without, an open society; i.e., one that is respectful of individual rights and interests, dedicated to reasonable compromise and mutual accommodation, and optimistic about individual privacy, free choice, equal opportunity, and liberty ordered by law. They additionally assert that, in accordance with the U.S. belief in moral progress, a key social function of U.S. bioethics is to be an agent of such progress—a moral sensibility well suited to its origins in the progressive and consumerist "new liberalism" of the 1960s and 1970s, entailing social functions like scrutinizing dehumanizing effects and alleviating dangers associated with biomedical technology, and attacking medical authoritarianism and paternalism. Jennings and Moreno also argue that U.S. bioethics has become a new discipline and profession so rapidly and successfully because of its ideological service to mainstream (post-Vietnam War) American liberalism's public philosophy, advancing the social ideal of the self-sovereign individual, and controlling but not challenging fundamentally—thus accommodating—structures of power in capitalist medicine and biotechnology. Currently, however, Jennings and Moreno believe there are two conflicting American liberalisms vying for influence in and through U.S. bioethics. These are "autonomy liberalism" which embraces autonomy as the fundamental *universal* feature of humankind conveying human identity sui generis, and "identity liberalism" which respects identity adhering in difference rather than universality—developed in response to social science, feminist, and ethnic critiques of individualism—which accordingly more highly values tolerance, mutual respect, and social cooperation. According to Jennings and Moreno, identity liberalism moves U.S. bioethics away from its disciplinary center of gravity in analytic moral philosophy, and instead toward critical legal theory, postmodern social sciences, feminism, and disability studies, spawning a "new left." Bioethics influenced by "autonomy liberalism" thus attracts a culture war backlash by "new right" conservative thinkers, as well as by conservative religious groups, both of whom seek to appropriate bioethics. Using examples such as the Terry Schiavo case, human stem cell research and mammalian cloning, and George W. Bush's Presidential Bioethics Council, Jennings and Moreno describe how this "new right" has taken up the domain of bioethics to gain more policymaking influence and drive the social conversation about ethics and biotechnology in the United States, thus sweeping up bioethics into national partisan politics. They also describe how progressive thinkers, previously slow to grasp the right's embrace of bioethics, are increasing their own strategies to contest the right in and through U.S. bioethics.

I am privileged to offer in this volume these fascinating examples and first steps toward a more comprehensive comparative anthropology and sociology of globalizing bioethics. Based on these examples, I invite readers similarly to apply the unique lens that I commissioned the contributors in this volume to apply—considering the evolution, cultural meanings, and social functions of bioethics—further to interrogate whether the contingent sociocultural factors and ideologies revealed to be shaping "bioethics" in their own or other countries truly advance or undermine the bioethical enterprise and avowed social justice goals. At the very least, it is vital to be more conscious of such realities and their possible negative or positive, and intended or unintended consequences, so the contributions we seek to offer in and through bioethics theories, practices, and institutions indeed benefit all those whom we seek to serve.

1

GLOBALIZING WESTERN BIOETHICS

Some Perils and Pitfalls of "Missionary Bioethics" and Ethics "Capacity Building" in the Developing World and "Eastern" World

1

BIOETHICS AS MISSIONARY WORK

THE EXPORT OF WESTERN ETHICS TO DEVELOPING COUNTRIES

Raymond De Vries and Leslie Rott

Introduction

Like the Christian missionaries from Europe and North America that preceded them, bioethicists are intent on bringing the gospel—the "good news"—to those in the developing world. The missionary gospel is the New Testament story of salvation offered by the death and resurrection of Jesus Christ; the gospel of bioethics is "good clinical practice," the Belmont Report,[1] and the Declaration of Helsinki.[2] Both missionaries and bioethicists may object to this comparison. Missionaries will point out that they are devoted to a *spiritual* task, not to the secular work of developing regulations and guidelines for the practice of medicine and medical research. For their part, bioethicists will likely resent being described with a term associated—in their minds, at least—with those who destroyed local cultures and paved the way for colonial abuses. These objections are, of course, based on stereotypes. Not all missionaries are tools of imperialistic nations, and most do far more than care for the souls of those they minister to; while bioethicists help create and write regulations, their ultimate goal is to protect patients and research subjects from harm and exploitation.

In spite of the consternation it may cause bioethicists and missionaries, the metaphor of missionary work is useful for understanding the place of bioethics in the developing world. Lessons learned from the failures and successes of missionary efforts illuminate (and suggest solutions for) the cultural and social problems encountered by those in the West who wish to share the good news of bioethics. For instance,

---

1. Available at: http://www.hhs.gov/ohrp/humansubjects/guidance/belmont.htm.

2. Current version available at: http://www.wma.net/en/30publications/10policies/b3/index.html

it is clear that bioethicists have followed—consciously or unconsciously—one important example from the missionary movement: the shift from imported to indigenous evangelization.[3] Beginning in the mid-nineteenth century and throughout the twentieth century, missionaries faced resistance from their host countries. In some places, most notably China, missionaries were expelled; in other places, missionaries were increasingly regarded as colonialists. Mission organizations responded to this turn of events with the notion of "indigenization." No longer would missionaries from the West be exported to other countries. Instead, citizens from those countries would be brought to the West and trained to situate the missionary message in the local culture. This meant translating the gospel into local languages, using local organizational forms in the creation of churches, and adapting local customs to the teaching of the gospel. Over time, indigenization came to be called "contextualization," and it was described as an effort to protect, and be relevant in, local culture.

Although they do not use the term, those in the West who wish to bring the benefit of bioethics to the developing world have seen the value of indigenization. Indigenization is a solution to what Solomon (2006) describes as the "export problem" of Western bioethics—a problem that is unavoidable when bioethics, a creation of Western culture, collides with the systems of ethics found in local, non-Western cultures.[4] Pursuing the indigenization solution, bioethicists from the developing world are currently being trained in the United States (via the National Institutes of Health Fogarty International Center[5]), Europe (via the Erasmus Mundus Masters program in bioethics[6]), and the United Kingdom (via The Wellcome Trust[7]). Having learned the language and logic of Western bioethics, trainees return to their home countries to spread the "gospel" (Solomon, 2006).

What do we know about the "success" of the indigenization of bioethics? Research addressing and/or evaluating these specific training programs has been scant, and the descriptions and evaluations that do exist tend to be programmatic

---

3. See http://www.gameo.org/encyclopedia/contents/I54ME.html for a brief description of the indigenization movement in mission work from a Mennonite point of view.

4. Solomon (2006, p. 337) outlines three different forms of the export problem: temporal, local, and personal.

5. See http://www.fic.nih.gov/programs/training_grants/bioethics/overview.htm.

6. See http://med.kuleuven.be/education/Bioethics/index.html.

7. See http://www.wellcome.ac.uk/Funding/Medical-humanities/Grants/Biomedical-ethics/index.htm.

(i.e., "Did we meet the goals of the funder?") rather than critical and reflective ("Have our bioethics programs helped local norms and values to be realized?").[8]

From Noble Intent to Unwitting Harm

The use the metaphor of missionary work makes visible interesting similarities in the work of missionaries and bioethicists. For the most part, the desire to spread the gospel begins with noble intent—the goal is to bring the benefits of developments in one part of the world to another part of the world where those benefits are not experienced or understood. Those benefits may be eschatological or existential, but in either case, the motivation is to proffer aid and share lessons learned. But, as we have seen in some of the transactions between missionaries/ bioethicists and the people they serve, noble intent is not sufficient to bring good results. An imbalance in power between would-be helpers and those to be helped creates a one-way flow of influence from "missionaries" to "locals" that not only diminishes the possibility of mutual enrichment, but also creates the possibility of unwitting harm.

A recent evaluation of a research ethics training workshop at a Nigerian university implicitly illustrates the problem of one-way flow of influence (Ajuwon & Kass, 2008). The authors begin their report by noting that "training in research ethics affords scientists, especially those from developing countries, the opportunity to contribute to ever increasing international debates on ethical issues. . ." (p. 2). Indeed, "international debates on ethical issues" *should* be informed by insights of those in the developing world. But just a few pages later, we learn what the program actually accomplished: "Post-training improvements were found in participants' knowledge of the principles of research, the application of these principles, the international regulations, and the operations of an IRB" (p. 8). Measured by its own evaluation metric, this program was focused on teaching Nigerians the wisdom of Western bioethics ("principles, the international regulations, and the operations of an IRB"), not on seeking wisdom from the traditions of Nigeria.

Arguing from a natural law perspective, Boyle (2006, p. 321) points out: "fragmentation of the pursuits of health around the world implies that no authority within any health care or biomedical community such as a medical association or expert group [can] qualify as having global bioethical authority. . . [U]ntil the

8. See Ajuwon & Kass, 2008; Benatar, 2004; Benatar, 2005; Benatar & Landman, 2006; Benatar, Daar, & Singer, 2005; Ezeome & Marshall, 2008; Hyder, Harrison, Kass & Maman, 2007; Kass, Hyder, Ajuwon, Appiah-Poku, Barsdorf et al., 2007; Marshall, 2005; Marshall & Koenig, 2004; Raja & Singer, 2004; Rotimi, Leppert, Matsuda, Zeng, Zhang et al., & International HapMap Consortium, 2007.

world is much more integrated and unified, there will be no properly bioethical legislature or Supreme Court for the whole world." We know that religious, legal, psychological, historical, and ethical differences have an impact on bioethical views both within and between countries (Bayertz, 2006) but, as we shall see, this seemingly obvious fact gets lost in many ethics training programs in developing countries. Benatar (2005), a bioethicist from South Africa, chides those from the West who would "improve" the ethics of countries in the developing world:

> What should be avoided is the previous colonial mentality of wanting to study and improve others while oblivious of the need to address the more sophisticated and covert faults of Western researchers' own societies. The desire to improve the behavior of others should also be associated with awareness that one's own exemplary moral behavior might be more effective in promoting ethical behavior and respect for human rights than [. . .] attempts to change the cultural attitudes of others while neglecting our own adverse cultural attitudes.

The Inside View of Indigenization: Bioethicists-in-Training Speak

In order to better understand what bioethicists from the developing world are learning, the first author conducted interviews with 21 trainees at a European-based bioethics program.[9] The program was intended for those working in bioethics in countries outside the European Union, and nearly all students were from the developing world.[10] These interviews, which lasted between one and one-and-a-half hours each, revealed several important things about efforts to indigenize bioethics. We discuss here three of these: (1) problems with the sources of, and models of, ethical reasoning; (2) a lack of fit between the ethical issues taught in classes and the ethical problems in the students' home countries; and (3) the motivation(s) for establishing Western bioethics in the developing world.

Sources and Models of Ethical Reasoning

A majority of the students in this training program came from parts of the world where Christianity was not the dominant religion. And yet, here in Europe,

9. The research was reviewed by the research ethics committee at the Katholiek Universiteit, Leuven, and deemed exempt.

10. Two students out of a cohort of 25 were from North America; one student was working in Africa, but was a citizen of an EU country.

reasoning about ethical issues is deeply rooted in the Christian tradition and Christian scholarship of the West. Students were aware of this, and felt a degree of disconnect with their own histories. A student from China pointed out:

> "... if I want to accept all of the theologies and, too, the methods for the bioethics for Chinese people, it's a little bit difficult ... in China, we have different religions ... and very few people believe in God ... they are not Christian ... so they have no sort of knowledge about Christian history, about Jesus, so you know, a lot of bioethics, methods, and theories came from Jesus ..."

Another said:

> "... [in lectures] there's some link to the Christian, yeah, I don't understand it because [as] a Buddhist, I have no God. Why do we have to put a lot of faith in God? ..."

He did go on to suggest that there was some value to what he was learning, even though it was outside his tradition: "I have some cultural conflict here, but I think that's interesting, [it] gives me an opportunity to see something in a new light ..."

Apart from the religious and philosophical sources of ethics, students also admitted that much of their own exposure to ethics and bioethics came from the West. This is to be expected, given that the overwhelming majority of published knowledge about ethics—in books, reference works, and on the Internet—comes from Europe and North America. Asked where they learned what they knew about bioethics before they enrolled in the training programs, nearly all mentioned Western sources:

> "... of course electronic journals. Search by Internet ... .the *Encyclopedia of Bioethics* [in English]"
>
> "... we get most of the readings literature from Western, from America, yes, from American journals ..."
>
> "... from the Internet, mainly"

One student, asked to help organize research ethics committees in her home country, talked about how she used American materials to train herself and would-be committee members:

> "I was looking on different training materials, mainly from National Institutes of Health, so, and then the most well-known universities in the U.S. ... So I went through there because they have online courses for their

researchers; so I pass several courses, I have a couple of certificates, just online created certificates . . ."

As one student pointed out, training in the Western way of bioethics is "interesting," but the model of ethical reasoning that is almost universally taught—principlism—is not an easy fit in most developing countries. Based on the well-known four principles—autonomy, beneficence, nonmaleficence, and justice—principlism is easily taught and applied to a wide variety of ethical dilemmas, at least in societies where these principles fit seamlessly with cultural values. In fact, it can be argued that the four principles are sufficiently abstract that they can float above, and yet account for, the peculiarities of culture. For example, regardless of our cultural differences, we can all agree that nonmaleficence is a good thing—but we must hasten to add that what you and I call "harm" may vary. The same can be said of autonomy: in the United States, autonomy is conceived in a radically individualist manner, but in other cultures we can adjust the idea to incorporate more familial and communal ideas of autonomy. In the atomistic United States, a free and independent individual should (must?) determine her care, whereas in more communal societies, autonomous decisions occur in consultation with, or by decision of, recognized authorities.

Pushed too far in this direction, however, the principles become meaningless. Can we really speak of autonomy if a treatment decision for an adult woman is made by others? In their study on issues of informed consent and health workers in developing countries, Hyder and Wali (2006) suggest that "some have argued that certain principles of individual informed consent may not be in keeping with the cultural norms and practices in developing countries," such as having a tribal leader speak for the entire village (p. 34).[11] Dawson and Kass (2005)[12] have also suggested that the practice of IRBs in the United States requiring written consent is impossible in some developing countries where literacy rates are low (see also Molyneux, Wassenaar, Peshu & Marsh, 2005). Marshall (2008) has suggested that "researchers must be committed to developing culturally appropriate strategies for obtaining and documenting informed consent" (p. 207).

Looking specifically at Nigeria, Ezeome and Marshall (2008) suggest that the influences of family, gender roles, respect for elders, religion, availability of money for healthcare, and illiteracy are all factors that inhibit the process of obtaining informed consent from patients and/or research participants. Further, they

11. Coincidentally, such communication with leaders is often the only way to gain access to a community (Hyder & Wali, 2006).

12. They differentiate between three types of consent paradigms; "regulatory," "community," and "individual."

suggest that "a greater problem is presented by those whose beliefs about health and illness are inconsistent with Western medicine" (p. 9).

Bioethics students from the developing world saw several problems with the principlist approach they were learning. Not surprisingly, the principle of autonomy was identified as most problematic. Many of the students saw a disjuncture between their cultural values and the individualism implicit in autonomy. A student from a Muslim country noted: "... in [Islam] ... justice [is more important] than autonomy ... Islam said first your neighborhood ... not first yourself."

Another discussed a Buddhist view:

> "... [an author I am reading] argues that in Buddhism you have no concept of autonomy.... She said that the central concept is compassion, and it emphasized paternalism. So for myself, this is what I think for myself, compassionate paternalism, it's not that bad."

From India:

> "[In rural India] their idea of autonomy is totally different, like they're not, even for signing our hospital admission sheet, it is not a patient or immediate person, it is ... the family [that] was signing for that patient, even for admission, even for taking out of the hospital, it's not the patient who is signing ... we are not thinking the autonomy of the person, we are thinking about the collective autonomy of the whole family."

A cultural lack of fit is not the only problem with the principles. A student from the Philippines astutely noted that the structure of health care there—in particular, the power of physicians—would make difficult the realization of patient autonomy:

> "... you know, one of the things that we will be encountering when we go back [to the Philippines] as trained bioethicists will be, by and large, the medical science. I mean, the medical practice there is still very paternalistic, and as I said ... they would be threatened by us; I mean the doctors, the medical people. You know, I cannot remember a malpractice suit against any doctor which [was] won."

A student from India pointed out that autonomy is meaningless when patients have no power:

> "... principlism did not answer many questions for me ... [In India] people cannot exercise their autonomy ... so what do you do with just

giving them autonomy? . . . It's incomplete, yeah, it's a useful principle no doubt, but it's not practical [in India] . . . Unless you empower people to exercise their autonomy, autonomy has no meaning."

A physician from India summarized the frustration of many students with the emphasis on Western ways of ethical reasoning:

> "In the history of medical ethics, for example, the reference point is Hippocrates' Oath, as if no code of medical ethics really existed in other systems of medicine, or before Hippocrates. How many bioethicists really know and even care to know that ancient India and China had elaborate systems of medicine and medical ethics before Hippocrates? [And] you must be kidding if you discuss here Buddha or Confucius or Shankara, or even Gandhi for that matter! And, there are professors who have 'one-size-fits-all' type of one set of 'principles,' and they want us to master that aerobatic art of balancing the 'principles' in beating off the worst kind of ethical malaise."

Ethical Issues Here and There

Training in bioethics typically involves review of ethical theories (described above) and in-depth discussion of critical ethical issues. These discussions offer the opportunity to apply ethical theory to real-life situations, and allow students to practice the move from the theoretical to the applied. What are the ethical issues covered in coursework of students from the developing world? Here are three course descriptions from the curriculum of the students who were interviewed:

Ethics of Reproductive Technologies: The aim of this course is to familiarize participants with an ethical approach of assisted reproduction. The goal is not only to essentially inform the participants about the latest developments and challenges in this area of medicine, but also to help them develop a critical and ethical clarification of this subject. This course works from an interdisciplinary (theological, legal, psychological, medical) perspective.

Ethical Theories and Methods of Ethics: The aim of this course is to analyze the major philosophical and theological approaches to ethics, including deontology and utilitarianism. Participants will get acquainted with the personalist traditions in fundamental ethics and its consequences in different areas of applied ethics. The most common methods to evaluate bioethical issues will be analyzed. Ethical arguments will be analyzed and assumptions underlying a debate will be evaluated. Students will also be confronted with the importance of the narrative context, and with moral leadership.

Human Genetics and Medical Technology: The course aims to educate participants on a range of ethical subjects that currently are the focus of debate in genetics. Teaching will focus on the moral problems generated by the Human Genome Project, as well as the ethical boundaries in the clinical application of new knowledge in, for example, genetic counseling, genetic screening, gene therapy, and cloning. The implications of scientific progress for the image of the human being, as well as for modern culture, will also be studied.

This curriculum is not atypical. Review of the course requirements for those in the Johns Hopkins Fogarty African Bioethics Training Program reveals a few more relevant-sounding titles—for example, there is a "Short Course in International Research Ethics"—but course content is equally skewed toward Western ideas. The description of the International Research Ethics course reads: "Introduce trainees to the major principles and theories of Western bioethics, to U.S. and international guidelines that govern human participants research" (Hyder, Harrison, Kass & Maman, 2007, p. 677). In their evaluation of the Hopkins African Bioethics Training Program, Hyder, Harrison, Kass, & Maman (2007) suggest it has been empowering to students but, significantly, they also indicate that the training is still too Western-centric, lacking in curricula more appropriate to developing countries (pp. 675, 682; see also Marshall & Koenig, 2004).

In our interviews, students in the European program noticed this lack of fit:

> " . . . here [in Europe] we learn in the class [about the most recent] developments . . . [things] we hardly get [in India] . . . In confrontation with the culture, [in] confrontation with the religion, how [will these technologies be seen]? Because we want to preserve our culture, we want to preserve the purity, it is easy to destroy that, as Spanish did in the Philippines; [that] we don't want . . ."

At one point, students from the program approached the faculty about making the coursework more relevant to conditions in their home countries. As one student explains, they were rebuffed:

> ". . . would you like to know what was a surprising thing for me? That when we were talking about adjusting this program to the need not just to talk about the [European] situation, but a little bit wider, and people from

India were highly interested to talk about HIV... the reaction was, 'but we are a *European* course.' (emphasis added)

Students also felt that the assigned readings were not aligned with what they would need to know when they returned home. One student talked about the need to learn the basics, even if she did not know "who Levinas is:"

"... for me, it is sometimes too much, too many terms, not the right context, and I will prefer to debate, to talk, to share something like that, because it is the way I learn better, rather than just to have a philosopher who is using a very specific language."

Along the same lines, another student commented:

"I'm not a native speaker of English so when I'm reading a text... I can be lost somewhere, and also there are materials that I don't like, I mean [when] I'm done I understood what it is about, my question is 'but was it a waste of time?'"

Why Teach Western Bioethics to Students from the Developing World?

Given the lack of fit between the content of training programs in bioethics, and the bioethical situation and needs of countries in the developing world, it is reasonable to ask "Why do these programs exist?" The answer to that question is not simple. In our search for an answer, we look to both what we learned from students and to campaigns by for-profit organizations marketing their clinical trial services. In her explanation of the difference between medical ethics and bioethics, a student from India reveals an important motivation for the export of Western bioethics (emphasis added):

"Medical ethics was something like the ethics related to clinical care and the doctor, how we should be with patients and all that. That was what we were taught in medical school... *But now because research is coming in a big way, especially with a lot of international collaborations, the U.S. ethos of bioethics is coming in a big way.*"

A cursory search of the Internet shows that this student understands the current situation. As Petryna (2005) has pointed out, the number of clinical trials in the developing world has grown markedly over the past 15 years, as pharmaceutical companies search for "naïve bodies" (bodies that are not under the influence of several drugs, as is the case in many Western nations), and more favorable ethical environments.

The FDANews, a private organization that describes itself as a "premier provider of domestic and international regulatory, legislative, and business news and information for executives in industries regulated by the U.S. Food and Drug Administration" (http://www.fdanews.com/about), regularly offers seminars on how to conduct drug trials in the developing world. This one, offered in January 2009, is typical (http://www.fdanews.com/conference/detail?eventId=2678):

> **Conducting Clinical Trials in Developing Countries:**
> **Boots-on-the Ground Strategies to Maintain Compliance**
> ... you can ensure your trial goes smoothly by benefiting from a 'boots-on-the-ground' view of how to manage the compliance aspects of running clinical trials in developing countries. Learn more than just what the regulations say—but how they translate in real life.
>
> In this 90-minute audioconference, internationally recognized expert **Mark Barnes** of Huron Consulting will detail the latest legal and compliance pitfalls facing drug and device sponsors, CROs and research sites conducting clinical trials in developing countries. As a frequent traveler to these nations, Mark not only knows the international law and GCP requirements but also the local customs, regional compliance issues and legal landmines that can trip up clinical trial operators.
>
> **Sign up** your entire team to listen in and learn:
>
> - The regulatory challenges in planning and conducting clinical trials in the developing world
> - How to plan for optimal subject recruitment and retention
> - The challenges of clinical and research recordkeeping and data management
> - How to select sites and collaborators
> - How to set up, train and support community advisory boards and local IRBs or research ethics committees...

Students are aware of the need for better bioethics in the developing world. In their comments on the coming of the pharmaceutical industry to their countries, they demonstrate a mix of motives for learning the ways of Western bioethics: to protect the subjects of research, and to encourage economic development. This student from China was typical:

> "No, just now, [we have] no formal [research ethics] committees [in China], no, so it's a big problem. I think I like to come here and learn more

knowledge about this field, I want to do some work in this field ... at least I can help to organize the bioethical review communities in my universities, for our country ... I know doctors, they do some clinical trials, they have no approval ... they didn't do the informed consent ... they didn't have the review ... [from] the research review committees, so it's a big problem, they do some trials, it's not good."

She goes on to discuss the director's enthusiasm for having European-trained bioethicists in China:

"... my director, director of our institute, he's very good person and he has a lot of ideas for the future development, and when he learned [that] I got [a] scholarship, and of the European community, and I can come to European countries to learn bioethics, he [was] very excited. He said, 'ahh it's good, it's good for you and also for our institutions. I know in Europe the bioethics have a very good ... they pay a lot of attention in this field and they have a lot of knowledge in this field and I think you can learn a lot of things there.'"

Similarly, a student from an Eastern European country noted:

"... we have several IRBs registered, just because let's say our genetics center, probably 7, 8, 10 years ago, [was] became interested to work with some French organization and they, one of the requirements was: 'where was your IRB?' So these people started to work on that ..."

Students also recognize the personal benefits of becoming a bioethics expert. A student from India pointed out: "... in business ethics there are many experts already available, but not in bioethics so if I do it in bioethics, I'll be more relevant (laughs) ..."

Conclusion: Beyond Missionary Bioethics

Our intent here is to highlight the similarities in the dissemination of the missionary gospel and the bioethics gospel. While we do not want to suggest that bioethics is a kind of religion, we should acknowledge there *are* those who see undeniable links between bioethics and religion. Bioethics in the West can be seen as a secularizing movement,[13] but it is fair to say that the theories and

13. De Vries and Conrad (1998, p. 240) claim that bioethics emerged as a response to the needs of a secularized society: "Because secularized society lacks a foundation for ethical

concepts that animate Western bioethical reasoning trace their roots to Judaism and Christianity. Erickson (2006, p. xi) goes a step further. He claims that *all* reasoning—about ethics or any other topic—is inextricably tied to religion:

> ... the intimacy of religion with culture, and culture with methods of reflection and inquiry, [suggests that] ... intellectual investigation itself will have a religious dimension to it as well, whether unwitting, more cognizantly devotional, or in the service of some other dynamic or end.

Erickson's surmise may be debated, but it does underscore the fundamental problem of missionizing bioethics: How can the essential ideas and goals of bioethics be realized in varied cultural and social environments?

We are not alone in our concern about the direction of developing world bioethics. McGinnis (2007, p. 401) explicitly compares the indigenization movement in Christian missions with a similar trend in efforts to promote human rights. He concludes that "secular missionaries" have a lot to learn:

> ... an essential ingredient in the missionary strategy of evangelization is conspicuously absent in contemporary programs of development, democratization, or peace-building. In particular, the extensive efforts devoted by Protestant missionaries to the translation of their Biblical message into local languages and symbolic repertoires bear little resemblance to efforts to transplant Western ideals of universal human rights, or the institutional templates of democratic governance, first developed in the United States and Western Europe.

In their discussion of the value of a "bioethics from below," Rennie and Mupenda (2008) suggest that "bioethics research and scholarship [revolves] around issues that, while fascinating and important, currently affect only a small minority of the world's population" and argue for a move away from "a '90/10' gap, i.e., a situation where 90% of discussions on bioethics in the literature and the popular media may revolve around issues affecting 10% of the world's population." They conclude with this interesting comment on the value of *two-way communication* between Western bioethics and bioethics in the developing world:

> ... greater attention to ethical issues arising from biomedical research, clinical practice and public health interventions 'far away' might have a

---

decision-making, moral dilemmas, once readily solved with reference to a faith tradition, now require the articulation of non-religious solutions."

> positive effect on bioethics 'closer to home,' potentially expanding the horizons of the field and enhancing its social relevance.

We agree. The current model of missionizing bioethics needs to be improved, allowing for a two-way conversation among equals. Bioethicists in the United States and Europe can learn a great deal from the ethical traditions of countries in the developing world, just as bioethicists in those countries can learn from the traditions of the West. Like Christian missionaries who discovered new things about God by listening to those they hoped to convert, bioethicists will learn new things about ethics by listening to their students from the developing world.[14]

Although we are critical of the current mode of the spreading of Western bioethics to third-world countries, we recognize that constructive conversations about bioethics require a shared understanding of the cultural similarities and differences that shape ethical ideas and practices. Reflecting on the possibility of a global bioethics, Engelhardt (2006, p. 40) explains:

> . . . global bioethics can at best provide a thin moral framework, a space within which individual and moral communities can peaceably pursue divergent understandings of morality and bioethics within limited democracies and within a global market. Such a global bioethics cannot provide a content-full understanding of the right, the good, virtue, or human flourishing. Content will have to be found within particular moral communities and the moralities and bioethics they sustain.

The way forward is suggested by a group of students at the University of Malawi, College of Medicine, that created Medical Rights Watch (MRW) in an effort to close the gap between what they learned and what was, in fact, useful to members of the cultures from which they came. Using dramatic performance, conferences, and public meetings and demonstrations, MRW is committed to educating the public and to getting "basic bioethics to the attention of all key health decision makers at all levels [. . .] transforming the health system into one that effectively applies justice, beneficence and autonomy" (Divala & Mabedi, 2008). Their success, and the success of any effort at missionary bioethics, should be judged by the degree to which the conversations it creates enrich the moral practices of both the missionary and the missionized.

---

14. Two chapters in this volume (by Chattopadhyay and Simpson) examine how Western cultural dominance has influenced the shape of medical ethics in India and Sri Lanka.

References

Ajuwon, A., & Kass, N. (2008). Outcome of a research ethics training workshop among clinicians and scientists in a Nigerian university. *BMC Medical Ethics*. n.p.

Bayertz, K. (2006). Struggling for consensus and living without it: The construction of a common European bioethics. In H. Tristram Engelhardt, Jr (ed.) *Global Bioethics: The Collapse of Consensus* (pp. 207–237). Salem, MA: M & M Scrivener Press.

Benatar, S. (2004). Towards progress in resolving dilemmas in international research Ethics. *Journal of Law, Medicine, & Ethics*. 32 (4): 574–582.

Benatar, S. (2005). Achieving gold standards in ethics and human rights in medical practice. *PloS Medicine*, 2 (8): e260.

Benatar, S., & Landman, W. (2006). Bioethics in South Africa. *Cambridge Quarterly of Healthcare Ethics*. 15 (3): 238–247.

Benatar, S., Daar, A., & Singer, P. (2005). Global health challenges: The need for an expanded discourse on bioethics. *PloS Medicine*. 2 (7): e143.

Boyle, J. (2006). The bioethics of global biomedicine: A natural law reflection. In H. Tristram Engelhardt, Jr (ed.) *Global Bioethics: The Collapse of Consensus* (pp. 300–334). Salem: M & M Scrivener Press.

Chattopadhyay, S. (2011). Facing up to the hard problems: Western bioethics in the eastern land of India. Chapter 2 in this volume.

Dawson, L., & Kass, N. (2005). Views of US researchers about informed consent in international collaborative research. *Social Science & Medicine*. 61 (2005): 1211–1222.

De Vries, R., & Conrad, P. (1998). Why bioethics needs sociology. In Raymond De Vries and Janardan Subedi (eds.), *Bioethics and Society: Sociological Investigations of the Bioethical Enterprise* (pp. 233–257). Englewood Cliffs, NJ: Prentice-Hall.

Divala, T., & Mabedi, C. (2008). Bringing ethics to the vulnerable: The journey of the Medical Rights Watch (MRW) in Malawi. Poster Presentation, Annual HRPP Conference 2008; Orlando, FLA.

Engelhardt Jr., TH. (2006). The search for a global morality: Bioethics, the culture wars, and moral diversity. In H. Tristram Engelhardt, Jr. (ed.) *Global Bioethics: The Collapse of Consensus* (pp. 18–49). Salem, MA: M & M Scrivener Press.

Erickson, S. (2006). Forward. In H. Tristram Engelhardt, Jr (ed.) *Global Bioethics: The Collapse of Consensus* (pp. vii–xii). Salem, MA: M & M Scrivener Press.

Ezeome, E., & Marshall, P. (2008). Informed consent practices in Nigeria. *Developing World Bioethics*.

Hyder, A., & Wali, S. (2006). Informed consent and collaborative research: Perspectives from the developing world. *Developing World Bioethics*. 6 (1): 33–40.

Hyder, A., Harrison, R., Kass, N., & Maman, S. (2007). A case study of research ethics capacity development in Africa. *Academic Medicine*. 82 (7): 675–683.

Kass, N., Hyder, A., Ajuwon, A., Appiah-Poku, J., Barsdorf, N., et al. (2007). The structure and function of research ethics committees in Africa: A case study, *PloS Medicine*. 4 (1): e3.

Marshall, P. (2005). Human rights, cultural pluralism, and international health research. *Theory of Medical Bioethics*. 26 (6): 529–557.

Marshall, P. (2008). "Cultural competence" and informed consent in international health research. *Cambridge Quarterly of Healthcare Ethics*. 17 (2): 206–215.

Marshall, P., & Koenig, B. (2004). Accounting for culture in a globalized bioethics. *Journal of Law, Medicine, & Ethics*. 32 (2): 252–266.

McGinnis, M.D. (2007). From self-reliant churches to self-governing communities: comparing the indigenization of Christianity and democracy in sub-Saharan Africa. *Cambridge Review of International Affairs*. 20 (3): 401–416.

Molyneux, C., Wassenaar, D., Peshu, N., & Marsh, K. (2005). "Even if they ask you to stand by a tree all day, you will have to do it (laughter)...!" Community voices on the notion and practice of informed consent for biomedical research in developing countries. *Social Science & Medicine*. 61 (2): 443–454.

Petryna, A. (2005). Ethical variability: Drug development and globalizing clinical trials. *American Ethnologist*. 32 (2): 183–197.

Raja, A., & Singer, P. (2004). Transatlantic divide in publication of content relevant to developing countries. *British Medical Journal*. 2004 (329): 1429–1430.

Rennie, S. & Mupenda, B. (2008). Living apart together: reflections on bioethics, global inequality and social justice. *Philosophy, Ethics, and Humanities in Medicine* 2008, 3:25 (http://www.peh-med.com/content/3/1/25).

Rotimi, C., Leppert, M., Matsuda, I., Zeng, C., Zhang, H., et al., & International HapMap Consortium. (2007). Community engagement and informed consent in the international HapMap Project. *Community Genetics*. 10: 186–198.

Simpson, R. (2011). Capacity building in developing world bioethics: Perspectives on biomedicine and biomedical ethics in contemporary Sri Lanka. Chapter 3 in this volume.

Solomon, D. (2006). Domestic disarray and imperial ambition: Contemporary applied ethics and the prospects for global bioethics. In H. Tristram Engelhardt, Jr (ed.) *Global Bioethics: The Collapse of Consensus* (pp. 335–361). Salem, MA: M & M Scrivener Press.

2 FACING UP TO THE HARD PROBLEMS: WESTERN BIOETHICS IN THE EASTERN LAND OF INDIA

Subrata Chattopadhyay

Introduction

"Oh, East is East, and West is West, and never the twain shall meet," wrote Rudyard Kipling, the India-born English poet, in "The Ballad of East and West."[1] Euphemism aside, this poetic expression captures the essence of problems that arise when diverse cultural traditions share a common world. In the era of globalization, multifaith, multilingual, multicultural societies are commonplace. And, East meets West—as do North and South—in cross-cultural international bioethics. Not surprisingly, a myriad of conceptual, methodological, and analytic issues arise as U.S.-born Western bioethics[2] travels abroad and reaches the Eastern land. India's checkered past and uneven present give rise to a number of important questions, in the context of bioethics, that defy easy answers. How does ethics, a branch of Western philosophy, relate to *dharma*[3] or Eastern philosophical systems and worldviews? Is Western secular bioethics sensitive to the moral aspirations and needs of Indian people? How does an individual-centered, rights-based bioethics resonate with the ethos of traditional Indian societies? Can bioethics—a product of and value check on Western biomedicine—be applied to Ayurveda[4] or, for that matter, any other indigenous traditional system of medicine? Does bioethics exist in India anyway?

---

1. Rudyard Kipling (1865–1936) was born in Bombay (presently Mumbai) when India was under British rule. He was a very popular writer in English prose and poetry in the late nineteenth and early twentieth centuries. To his credit, he is the first English-language author to receive the Nobel Prize for Literature, in 1907. George Orwell criticized Kipling as a "prophet of British imperialism."

2. That mainstream bioethics is *Western*—has a strong accent of the West—is no new discovery. See Carrese and Rhodes, 1995; Alora and Lumitao, 2001; Myser, 2007; Chattopadhyay and De Vries, 2008.

3. See glossary on *dharma*.

4. See glossary on Ayurveda.

Many are the questions but few are the answers, especially to the satisfaction of all.

Bioethics in India is, to say the least, a complex and difficult terrain where even angels may fear to tread. Any discussion of "U.S.-born Western bioethics headquartered in Paris" in the Indian scenario may open up a Pandora's box of intricate issues—some of which remain unresolved, others inadequately addressed, and a few even untouched. Worse, attempts to address these issues run the risk of generating more heat than light. This precarious situation notwithstanding, addressing all this is not only relevant to Indian needs, but may also significantly contribute to an enriched understanding of a more locally sensitive and globally responsive international bioethics.

Part of the complexity that Western bioethics poses for India arises from the country's ancient but living spiritual/cultural tradition, and rich diversity of continental character.[5] India is, in the truest sense, a continent within a country, with enormous linguistic, cultural, and genetic diversity, which is second only to the continent of Africa.[6] The country is home to more than a billion people with diverse languages, ethnic groups, religious faiths, cultures, and political ideologies.[7] Coexistence of multiple realms of reality—ugly, bad, good, and divine—in a "land of contrasts" may not only evoke a sense of wonder but also appear to many as paradox or living puzzle. Cases in point are numerous; a few may suffice to illustrate the point of bioethical relevance. The *Kumbh Mela*[8]—"the world's largest congregation of devotees"—and the red-flag marching procession on "anti-imperialism day" are both parts of the Indian reality. The country is at once home to growing number of millionaires[9] and the largest number of poor people in the world.[10] India's healthcare system offers quality medical care at competitive prices to wealthy foreigners, while the country's own poor receive

---

5. The "unity in diversity" has been considered as the "most significant characteristic of Indian civilization."

6. See India in the U.S. Library of Congress–Federal Research Division Country Profile, December 2004.

7. According to the Indian census, 22 languages out of a list of 114 are officially recognized and spoken by one million or more people. The Indian population consists of Indo-Aryan (72%), Dravidian (25%), Mongoloid and other (3%). Hindus comprise approximately 80%, Muslims about 13%, Christians 2.3%, Sikhs 1.9%, Buddhists 0.8%, Jains 0.4%, with others, including Zoroastrianism and Judaism, about 0.6% of the Indian population.

8. Holy pilgrimage of the Hindus, believed to have begun thousands of years ago.

9. According to the 12th Annual World Wealth Report, 2008, issued by brokerage firm Merrill Lynch and consultancy firm Capgemini, the number of millionaires in India increased by 22.7% in 2007.

10. See Kurian, 2007.

only second-rate medical care, if any is available at all. One may find that there are, in reality, several *Indias* co-inhabiting and unequally sharing attention within the geography of present-day India. Any exploration of the cultural meanings and social functions of bioethics in India needs to reflect, represent, and address the issues pertaining to this pan-Indian reality. In discussing bioethics in India, however, it can be easy to be oblivious to the concerns and issues of the other *Indias,* while earnestly dealing with those of one. This chapter attempts to briefly sketch Indian history pertinent to bioethics, and address how ethics has been construed and lived in that sociocultural perspective, and what counts as bioethics appearing in a unique Indian context. Last but not least, the special problems and challenges that bioethics faces in the Indian reality are presented.

India: Ancient and Living Cultural Tradition with Multiple Realms of Reality

Much of the Indian subcontinental past is in the process of being reframed in the light of decolonized, open-minded inquiry, and the present is in flux due to contemporary new developments. Nonetheless, a brief sojourn through India's past may help better understand her rich context, in which diverse issues of bioethical significance arise. Early human settlement of Mehrgarh (7000 BC–2600 BC) is considered to be a precursor of a large urban civilization that emerged in the Indus Valley around 3300 BC.[11] Interestingly, the important Neolithic site of Mehrgarh came up with the oldest evidence of dental surgery.[12] The architectural design of the city of Harappa in the Indus Valley civilization shows well-planned roads, the world's first sanitation system, and a water supply system that reveals an appreciation and concern for public health.[13] It is from the sixth century BC onward—the age coinciding with the life of Buddha (566 BC–486 BC)—that the main lines of India's history appeared to emerge from under the veil of antiquity. The Maurya Empire of the fourth and third centuries BC reached its zenith under King Asoka (304 BC–232 BC). In pursuance of the Buddhist principle of compassion, Asoka made provisions for medical treatment of humans as well as

---

11. Mehrgarh was discovered in 1975 by excavation initiated by a French team of archeologists. Mehrgarh is presently situated in Pakistan. See http://www.guimet.fr/Indus-and-Mehrgarh-archaeological.

12. See Coppa A et al., 2006.

13. See Kumar D, 2001. The Indus Valley civilization developed along the river valleys of the Indus, Ravi, and Sutlej in present-day Pakistan and the northwest part of India. Harappa and Mohenjo-daro are two largest urban settlements of the Indus Valley civilization.

animals throughout his kingdom.[14] The Golden Age, ushered in by the Gupta dynasty (fourth to sixth centuries AD), witnessed spectacular advances in Indian mathematics, astronomy, and medicine.[15] Foreign invasions—nothing new to India's history, for her abundance of material wealth—continued later, with Arab incursions starting in the eighth century and Turkic in the twelfth, followed by those of European traders beginning in the late fifteenth century. Beginning in the early eighteenth century, India was gradually annexed by the British East India Company, and subsequently colonized by the United Kingdom from the mid-nineteenth century forward.[16] Both nonviolent and armed resistance were instrumental to India's independence in 1947 when, in the aftermath of World War II, undivided India—at the end of British colonial rule, and amidst the bloodshed of communal riot—was divided into India and the smaller Muslim state of Pakistan.[17]

Politically, India is a democratic secular republic consisting of 28 states and 7 union territories. India's parliamentary democratic system—however imperfect it might be—has given the country a form of relative stability still elusive in her neighbors in South Asia. After following a state-planned socialist model of development for four decades (1951–1990), India started economic reforms and initiated trade and investment liberalization in 1991. Subsequently, the country exhibited higher economic growth and, with more than 8% GDP growth rate achieved in last couple of years, India experienced an "economic boom." This prosperity, however, had limited reach and came with a price tag of increasing inequality. Thus, "economic boom" notwithstanding, India accounts for about 35% of the poor and 40% of the illiterates in the world, and the ratio of urban to rural income more than doubled during the last two decades, sharply increasing urban–rural income inequality.[18] Further, India ranks 67th among a list of 84 developing and restructuring countries in the 2010 Global Hunger Index;

---

14. Asoka's empire spanned a territory from present-day Pakistan, Afghanistan, and parts of Iran in the west, to the present-day Bangladesh in the east.

15. See Basham, 1954.

16. It is stated that India remained among three largest economies of the world until the early eighteenth century. When the British left India in 1947, the country was one of the poorest in the world—just the opposite of when the British and other European traders arrived.

17. The 1971 war between India and Pakistan resulted in formation of Bangladesh out of East Pakistan.

18. In contrast to the prosperity of large and medium cities, rural areas face economic stagnation and serious agrarian problems that have resulted in farmers' suicides. See Kurian NJ, 2007, for increasing economic and social disparities and their implications for India.

the situation of hunger remains "alarming" in India.[19] Therefore, questions arise about India's "economic boom" and whether it is an illusory sheen of prosperity in a country still plagued by extremes of poverty and wealth. The disparate nature of India's socioeconomic status, like other aspects of Indian experience, may mimic multiple realms of existential reality.

Western Bioethics Visits India

How does ethics—a branch of Western philosophy—relate to *dharma,* or Eastern philosophical systems and worldviews? What does ethics mean, and how is it construed in the Indian context? How can the concepts, principles, and language of an individual-centered, rights-based, mainstream secular bioethics resonate with the ethos of traditional Indian societies?

The word *ethics* is translated, synonymously used, and understood as *niti*[20] in Sanskrit and other Indian languages. Historically, *niti* has been intertwined with and culturally embedded in the concept, idea, and lived experience of *dharma.*[21] The relationship of ethics (as a branch of Western philosophy) and Hinduism (as Hindu-*dharma* or *sanatana dharma* was understood and construed by the Western scholars) has drawn significant attention from researchers seeking to comprehend "Hindu ethics." The very nature of *sanatana dharma,* including its non-monolithic multiform character, not surprisingly poses formidable challenges to Western scholars and their Indian counterparts, who seek to understand and analyze *niti* and *dharma* using the tools and concepts of Western philosophical systems.[22] The theory of right, as well as the theory of good—applicable to people of diverse backgrounds—have been harmoniously synthesized in *sanatana dharma* which, understandably, is inclusive of and broader than ethics. Notably, *sanatana dharma* does recognize multiple aspects of the reality; it glorifies the

19. The Hunger Index measures hunger on three leading indicators and combines them into one index. The three indicators are prevalence of child malnutrition, rates of child mortality, and the proportion of people who are calorie deficient. See 2010 Report of the International Food Policy Research Institute http://timesofindia.indiatimes.com/india/More-hungry-in-India-than-in-Sudan/articleshow/6733033.cms

20. See glossary on *niti.*

21. See glossary on *dharma.* Four major world "religions"—*sanatana dharma*, Buddha-*dharma*, Jain-*dharma* and Sikh-*dharma* (respectively known as Hinduism, Buddhism, Jainism, and Sikhism in the English-speaking world)—originated in the Indian subcontinent. Others religions, such as Zoroastrianism, Judaism, Christianity, and Islam reached the Indian land in the first millennium CE. Significantly, India accepted and assimilated these diverse faiths and practices that also shaped and contributed to her rich culture.

22. This approach fails to comprehend "ethics" in the context of *dharma* or Hindu/Indian philosophy. See Dhand, 2002.

"ideal" but makes room for the "permissible" in ethical conduct, envisions codes of ethics "in general" but also takes cognizance of "particular" contexts, and appreciates commonality while valuing the unique individuality of humans. All human beings, according to *sanatana dharma*, are, at a higher plane, children of the Immortal Bliss and potentially divine; however, it does not necessarily mean all human beings are "equal," as—at a lower plane—their *guna* (qualities, characteristics)[23] and *karma* (thoughts, words, actions)[24] are different. Ideals of individual and collective life are embodied in *dharma* guided by the *satguru* (the Master),[25] in pursuit of the principle of "live and let live." Explicit declared belief in the existence of God is not an obligatory requirement for all concerned—even "atheism" is also considered valid, given the paradigm—in Hindu philosophical worldviews.[26]

When Western concepts, ideas, and languages as used in contemporary mainstream bioethics are uncritically applied to and used in the Indian context, not only do they fail to capture the fine grains of the cultural and moral landscape, they also contribute to creating a "transgenic" culture alien to the land. In the Eastern worldview, there are no segregated, airtight compartments of religion, philosophy, spirituality, ethics, and science. Knowledge is whole, Truth is One,[27] and in the relational nature of life, the goal is synthesis and harmony rather than analysis, division, and compartmentalization. Thus, a person's "personal" ethics can not be divorced from his/her "professional" ethics. It is extremely difficult to conceive an idea of bioethics in India in isolation from the notion of morality in individual and collective life. Moreover, in traditional Indian cultures, the notion of duty *(kartabya)* is of paramount importance and has been held in high regard in both ethics *(niti)* and *dharma*. One's *dharma* determines his or her ethics, which is manifested as duty. It won't be too much of an exaggeration to say that outside conference rooms and academic circles, it is very hard, if not impossible, to imagine a locally sensitive Indian bioethics worth its name devoid of any idea of *dharma*.[28]

---

23. See glossary on *guna*.

24. See glossary on *karma*.

25. See glossary on *satguru*.

26. See Chatterjee & Datta, 1968.

27. The *Rig-Veda* says, *Ekam sat, vipra bahudha vadanti*—"Truth is One, sages call it by various names."

28. The same is true for other countries like Nepal, Sri Lanka, or Thailand, where *dharma* has been intertwined with local culture. In their work on end-of-life care in Thailand, Stonington and Ratanakul (2006) came to similar conclusions. See Stonington & Ratanakul, 2006.

Part of the problem that Western bioethics poses for India is that bioethics—in the Western humanist tradition—is focused on "rights." Underemphasized in bioethics is the fact that a "right" unaccompanied by a "duty" makes little, if any, sense, thus making rights-based Western bioethics something distant, alien, and discordant with the ethos of traditional India. Furthermore, when the notion of "duty-free human rights" permeates and virtually replaces ethics in public space, it creates a moral vacuum in the Indian psyche that allows for neglecting duty and, not surprisingly may lead to bolstering a narrow self-interest incongruent with social responsibility and duty toward the vulnerable.

The language commonly used in contemporary mainstream bioethics may also appear dissonant in the Indian context. There is deep-rooted faith in the existence and transmigration of the *atman* (soul or spirit) in India. There can be death of this physical body, or physical life, but no death of the *atman*, which can neither die nor be killed.[29] Thus, the notion of "end of life" seems to be a misnomer that does not resonate well with the deeply rooted belief in "life after death" held by many Indians.

In Eastern philosophical systems and spiritual worldviews, an individual is embedded in the web of relationships—an "I" does not exist in isolation—a person is rooted in family and community and, in the philosophical sense, is a member of larger expanding circles of country, the whole of humanity, and the cosmos. In general, family is the source of identity, strength, support, hope, and an important factor in decision-making processes including health care. Therefore, limiting an individual within the strict confines of ego-boundary and human rights is an inappropriate and narrow-minded approach to grapple with the reality—an onslaught to the matrix of relationships in which the individual is enmeshed—and thus an assault to the ethos of family, community, and culture.[30]

The Universal Declaration on Bioethics and Human Rights, as promulgated by UNESCO in 2005,[31] perhaps offers an example of how, albeit paradoxically, out of "good" cometh "evil." This declaration signals an era in which ethics and human rights share a common vocabulary, and their distinctions, hitherto believed, become blurred. One of the "principles" in this declaration says, "The interests and welfare of the individual should have priority over the sole interest of science or society." This article not only contradicts the moral values of India's cultural traditions, it also questions the foundations of the Eastern

29. The *Bhagavad Gita (2:20)* says, *Na hanyate, hanyamane sarire*—"The soul is not slain when the body is slain."

30. See Chattopadhyay & Simon, 2008.

31. See UNESCO, 2005. Universal Declaration on Bioethics and Human Rights.

religious/spiritual worldviews. With due respect for the intent of this proclamation, questions arise regarding its claims to "universality." Furthermore, from the perspective of billions of people who badly need public health measures, the idea that the interests and welfare of the individual should have priority over the interests of family or society is an absurd, if not dangerous, proposition. Taken at face value, it makes the whole public health enterprise—as a result of multisectoral initiatives, at considerable cost—untenable on ethical grounds. Interestingly, this declaration—perhaps to balance the individualist obsession—has included articles on solidarity, respect for cultural diversity, and pluralism, which may not mean much in the face of a "tyranny" of individual autonomy.

Medical Plurality and Bioethics

Does bioethics apply to Ayurveda and other healing traditions, or only to modern biomedicine?

Bioethics emerged in late 1960s and early 1970s in the United States as a cultural product of and check on value-free, objective, modern medical science. Assembled in the North American and European cultural context from raw materials of Western moral philosophy, U.S.-born Western bioethics pays scant, if any, attention to other traditional systems of medicine and codes of ethics therein.[32] This posed few problems when bioethics was confined to white[33] Western societies, but as bioethics has moved into other cultures—inside and outside of the Western world—it faces the challenge of diverse cultures with healing traditions other than biomedicine.

In ancient times, India developed her indigenous system of medicine, Ayurveda.[34] Modern biomedicine was introduced into India by the British

---

32. Any discussion of the history of medical ethics almost invariably begins with the Oath of Hippocrates in bioethics literature. A.R. Jonsen writes, in *A Short History of Medical Ethics,* that the oath in *Charaka Samhita,* in Ayurveda, surpasses the Hippocratic oath in both "eloquence and moral idealism" (Jonsen, 2000). Questions may be raised: Where in bioethics discourse are the references to the two most ancient but living systems of medicine—Ayurveda and ancient Chinese medicine—and their medical ethics? See Chattopadhyay and De Vries, 2008.

33. See Myser, 2007.

34. See glossary on Ayurveda. For a brief review of medical practice and ethics in ancient India, see Bhagwati, 1997. Ayurveda is now included in the broad category of complementary and alternative medicine (CAM) in the West. These systems of medicine offer a person with illness a critical connection with life-enhancing cosmic forces. This vital energy takes myriad of forms: a "spiritual vital essence" in homeopathy, "innate" in chiropractic, the flow of "qi" in acupuncture, and "psychic" or "astral" energies in New Age healing practices. It seems that the integral worldview of faith and reason—grossly absent in modern biomedicine—resonates well with the values, beliefs, and philosophical outlooks of a large number of people.

colonialists in early nineteenth century.[35] With English as the medium of instruction, the colonial policy of science education—segregated from *local* culture, science, and medicine—was established that deliberately wanted the indigenous systems of knowledge to die a natural and neglected death.[36] The statutory body of modern medicine, its education system, and "alien" milieu, all served to create and replicate the "core culture of imperialism" during colonial times.[37] Sadly, the colonial legacy of segregation and neglect toward Ayurveda continued in India even after the end of British era.[38] However, lack of colonizer's patronage notwithstanding, Ayurveda and other systems of medicine[39] did not die a natural death in India, but rather survived and persisted, possibly because these healing traditions were embedded in the country's cultural/moral world of life and health. Interestingly, of late, there has been an appreciable change in attitude, from outright rejection to humble appreciation, toward traditional indigenous or complementary and alternative systems of medicine (CAM) in the West.[40] Incorporation, if not assimilation, of Ayurveda and other healing traditions and indigenous systems of medicine within the domain of Western bioethics raises interesting questions regarding bioethics discourse.

The ethos of mainstream Western bioethics is predominantly nonreligious in nature. The distinction and separation of religion and spirituality from Western medical science, though deeply influential, is a *local,* not a universal, phenomenon. For example, there is no difference between Navajo religion and

---

35. The first school of modern medicine was founded by the British in Calcutta (now Kolkata) in 1835, followed by several other schools in different parts of the Indian subcontinent. Interestingly, Ayurveda and modern medicine were both taught initially in Sanskrit for the medical education of native Indians. This policy was overruled later. See Kumar, 2006.

36. It is noteworthy that ancient "Indian surgeons were expert in repair of noses, ears, and lips. In this respect Indian surgery remained ahead of European until the 18th century, when the surgeons of the East Indian Company were not ashamed to learn the art of rhinoplasty from the Indians" (Basham, 1954). As early as in the sixth century BC, Ayurvedic physicians had knowledge of about 39 medicinal plants for treatment of 30 disease entities (Saha, 1999).

37. See Kumar, 2006.

38. See Banerjee, 1979.

39. India practices "medical plurality" or diverse systems of medicine, although modern Western medicine (popularly known as *allopathy*) is the predominant one. Apart from Ayurveda, other systems of medicine that are practiced in India include *Unani-Tibb* (Greco-Arabic system) and Homeopathy.

40. Many U.S. medical schools now offer courses on CAM as part of their training of medical graduates. CAM is also part of medical education and practice in developing countries with better health indices, like Cuba and Sri Lanka. Moreover, scientific research on different modalities of CAM has further expanded the horizon of existing knowledge about the human body, health, and disease.

Navajo medicine.[41] Like Navajo medicine, Ayurveda also did not develop a chasm between faith and empirical science as found in modern biomedicine. Can Western secular bioethics accommodate, for example, physician prayer for the patient, or a "justified paternalism" of doctors serving patients in the most unselfish and compassionate manner? It is questionable how and whether the conceptual framework of mainstream Western secular bioethics can relate to Ayurveda or other healing traditions of the world, and be sensitive and responsive to world's multiform systems of medicine.[42]

Bioethics in an Unethical Setting

Can any bioethics worth the name flourish in an *unethical* setting?

Perhaps the most serious ethical crisis that faces medicine and undermines the cause of ethics in Indian medicine and science is created by the unethical setting—the dampening "ethical climate"—of the state and its social institutions.[43] Corruption is undeniably an all-pervasive part of contemporary Indian reality, and the health sector is no exception. India regrettably ranks 87th on a list of 178 countries in the corruption perception index.[44] Reports of gross professional misconduct, academic dishonesty, abuse of power, and corruption are

---

41. R.C. Begay (2003) writes about the American Indian healing tradition: "As an American Indian, I am aware of an entirely different tradition of healing that never split from spirit world. There is no difference, for example, between Navajo religion and Navajo medicine. American Indian medicine consists of spoken prayers, songs that are prayers, rituals, and instruments of prayer. Even herbal medicine comes with prayers for a person's spirit. It is interesting to me that modern providers have recently 'discovered' holistic medicine. It is something like the way Columbus 'discovered' America." See Begay, 2003.

42. This question needs to be addressed in many countries that have, for historical reasons, "medical plurality" or diverse healing traditions. Regarding appropriateness of use of Western bioethical theories and methods within and outside of the Western world, see Carrese & Rhodes, 1995; Alora & Lumitao, 2001; Stonington & Ratanakul, 2006; Myser, 2007; Chattopadhyay & Simon, 2008.

43. The moral decay and corruption that already afflicted the political milieu of India has slowly permeated other arenas, including the medical system. True, for many Indian physicians medicine is still a vocation, a calling to serve the needy and vulnerable in resource-poor settings; the ethos of the medical establishment, however, has unquestionably changed for the worse in recent decades.

44. This composite index is based on 13 independent surveys. It scores countries on a scale from zero to ten, with zero indicating highest level of perceived corruption and ten indicating no corruption whatsoever." India scores 3.3 out of 10. Denmark, New Zealand and Singapore top the list with 9.3 scores. See the Transparency Report 2010, http://www.transparency.org/policy_research/surveys_indices/cpi/2010/results

commonplace in Indian medicine.[45] Unfortunately, the statutory bodies and professional organizations of biomedicine lost their moral compass, and lack the positive will to regulate unscrupulous activities and nurture the ethical practice of medicine.

What difference does this "culture of corruption" make for the cause of bioethics in India? First of all, it not only makes old problems worse, it also creates new problems—and sustains both. Corruption traps millions of people in poverty, and perpetuates existing income and health inequality. India's healthcare system is dominated by the private sector. Corruption in the health sector drains existing resources, makes access to health care more difficult, increases treatment costs, contributes to ill health in vicious cycles, and further reduces income ability, thus perpetuating the nexus of poverty and illness. Moreover, this culture of corruption creates fertile ground for "kidney bazaars" and "female feticide," and keeps these "illegal" businesses sustainable and thriving, with the poor and women as unfortunate victims.[46] In this background of the unethical setting of a morally compromised medical establishment, "outsourcing" of clinical trials to India[47] is bound to raise serious concerns among the conscientious. In the social reality of poverty, exploitation, and corruption, clinical trials—unless strictly regulated—are potential sources of harm to the exploited poor subjects, who are often recruited as "voluntary" participants with little knowledge or genuine practice of "informed consent."[48] On the other side, the Indian government has been promoting "medical tourism" as an emerging area for economic growth. As India excels in providing quality healthcare at much cheaper prices to overseas tourists, the medical tourism industry is projected to be the major engine of economic development after information technology. Medical tourism is forecast to become a $2.3 billion business by 2012.[49] The policy of giving incentives for

---

45. See Gitanjali, 2004; Sharma, 2001. The extent of moral degeneration and abuse of power can be gauged by the facts that the president of the Medical Council of India (MCI—the Indian equivalent of the U.K. General Medical Council) was arrested for corruption and debarred from practicing medicine in 2010. The irony is that this tainted doctor was the president-elect of the World Medical Association in 2009.

46. Members of the medical community are, undoubtedly, part of and participants in these "illegal" businesses, which continue undercover. See the Voice of America report, "Illegal Human Kidney Trade Thrives in India," http://www.voanews.com/english/archive/2008-02/2008-02-14-voa18.cfm, and Jafarey et al., 2007. See the report, "Female Foeticide Persists in India Despite Law," http://www.merinews.com/catFull.jsp?articleID=124946.

47. See Nundy & Gulhati, 2005.

48. In 2005, the Ministry of Health and Family Welfare, Government of India, amended Schedule Y of the Drugs and Cosmetics Rules, permitting concurrent Phase II or Phase III clinical trials in India. Not surprisingly, there has been a sharp increase in clinical trials since the amendment of Schedule Y. See Srinivasan & Loff, 2006.

49. See Medical Tourism, http://india.gov.in/overseas/visit_india/medical_india.php.

the establishment of institutions offering high-quality medical care to eligible "consumers" while neglecting state-run medical facilities for the general population can hardly be justified.

Filling the Moral Gaps—Toward a Bioethics in India

Does bioethics really exist, as an entity to reckon with, in India? If not, in what ways are bioethical concerns then addressed?

As Indian medicine witnessed erosion of its moral values, perpetuated by the apathy and inaction of statutory bodies and professional associations, moral resistance came from the disenchanted within the medical community. A group of conscientious doctors formed the "Forum for Medical Ethics Society" in the early 1990s to focus attention on the need for ethical norms and practices in health care. This society started publishing the journal *Medical Ethics* in 1993, which has continued as the *Indian Journal of Medical Ethics* since 2004. This quarterly open-access journal probably serves as the only open forum available for regular discussions on healthcare ethics with special reference to the problems of India.[50] Importantly, the journal also served as a launching pad for the organization of three national bioethics conferences held in the recent past.[51] Earlier, an International Bioethics Workshop on "Bioethical management of biogeoresources" was held at the University of Madras (in 1997), and came out with a "Chennai Statement on Bioethics."[52] The recommendations of that workshop-cum-seminar included, among others, introduction of bioethics teaching, formation of an Indian society of bioethics, and publication of an Indian journal dedicated to the cause of bioethics. More a decade or so since the Chennai statement, the teaching and learning of bioethics is still largely absent in the Indian medical education system, and an Indian society of bioethics is yet to be made functional. There is no university chair or department of bioethics in colleges and higher institutions. Interestingly, although bioethics—as a recognized academic or professional entity—is still in a nascent stage of formation, bioethical concerns have been addressed by a number of quarters, including state agencies and grassroots organizations.

50. *Indian Journal of Medical Ethics*, http://www.issuesinmedicalethics.org

51. The theme of the first National Bioethics Conference, held at Mumbai in 2005, was "Ethical Challenges inHealth Care: Global Context, Indian Reality," and for the second National Bioethics Conference, held atBangalore in 2007, the theme was "Moral and Ethical Imperatives of Healthcare Technologies." The theme of the third National Bioethics Conference, held at New Delhi in 2010, was "Governance of healthcare: ethics, equity and justice."

52. See Azariah, Azariah, & Macer, 1998.

Bioethics from the Top—When Bureaucracy Features Ethics

The Indian Council for Medical Research (ICMR), "the apex body in India for the formulation, coordination and promotion of biomedical research," has been involved with formulating ethical guidelines for biomedical research, bioethics training, providing ethics consultation, maintaining a database, and coordinating international collaboration on bioethics.[53] In 1980, it came up with a policy statement on "ethical considerations involved in research on human subjects." Subsequently revised and updated twice, in 2000 and 2006, this policy statement became the "ethical guidelines for biomedical research on human participants"[54] and was submitted to the Ministry of Health and Family Welfare to empower the document with legal status. The ICMR also reportedly prepared draft national guidelines on stem cell research and therapy, safety assessment of derived GM foods, and bio-banking in India. Having received a training grant from the U.S. National Institutes of Health, the ICMR initiated a centrally coordinated bioethics training program that organized several training workshops and educational events.[55]

In 1998, the National Academy of Sciences in India organized an "International Bioethics Symposium on Human Genome Research: Emerging Ethical, Legal Social and Economic Issues." Acting upon the recommendations of this symposium, the Department of Biotechnology, Government of India, established a National Bioethics Committee, which subsequently issued a document on "Ethical Policies on the Human Genome, Genetic Research and Services."[56]

These government-sponsored activities, although much needed in the Indian reality, hardly offer any public space to informed citizens, including philosophers, theologians, social scientists, activists, and others, to contribute to bioethics in India and are, unfortunately, bureaucratic in nature. There is little doubt that the state-sponsored bio-*ethics*—with its top-down approach, limited participation, and little, if any, transparency—might better be characterized as bio-*bureaucracy*.

53. See Bio-Medical Ethics, ICMR, http://icmr.nic.in/human_ethics.htm.

54. See Ethical guidelines for biomedical research on human participants http://icmr.nic.in/ethical_guidelines.pdf.

55. See Bioethics education for India, http://icmr.nic.in/bioethics/cc_biothics/index.html.

56. See Tandon, 2005. In India, no official national bioethics commission exists that addresses ethical problems pertaining to science and society, engages in deliberations, and advises the government or public.

Bioethics from Abroad: The Emperor's New Clothes

Ayurveda is a second-class citizen in her own land; modern medicine is perhaps best described as "glorified" moneymaking enterprise. To make matters worse, there is no place for religion/spirituality/philosophy/ethics/history/humanities in the medical curriculum followed by Indian colleges of modern biomedicine.[57] Not surprisingly, many bioethicists in India have been trained abroad, notably through the National Institutes of Health in the United States, and the Erasmus Mundus Master of Bioethics program sponsored by the European Commission.[58]

Many of these efforts, although well-intentioned, risk inadvertently being "quasi-colonizing" in nature. Programs in which a select group of international students get to learn the American or European mantra of "universal" ethical principles, with some fine touches of multicultural liberalism, are somewhat problematic. Given that colonial science and biomedicine contributed to creating an alien culture of "colonized minds," and the Indian medical establishment is apathetic if not hostile to Ayurveda and other traditional medical systems, the possibility and danger of creating a "neocolonial moral imperialism" as a result of spreading bioethics—whether in the form of theories, policies, practices, or institutions—cannot be ruled out.

Bioethics from the Bottom Up: Human Rights Come to Rescue Ethics

In a country that was subjugated to "alien" rule for about 900 years, where crimes against humanity were committed numerous times, it is not surprising that the force of "human rights" would permeate ethics discourse, more so in a society marked by injustice and abuse of power. The social and political upheavals of the late 1960s and early 1970s touched upon the health arena, and subsequently the People's Health Movement was born, with the theme of "health as a fundamental right."[59] This health movement put forth health concerns and other social issues of the poor and vulnerable, largely invisible and voiceless, to make them a more visible section of society in the public agenda.

---

57. Moreover, the Indian education system, reflecting the rigid disciplinary boundaries of a past colonial era, hardly offers any opportunity for pursuing interdisciplinary studies and research, as in bioethics. See Chattopadhyay, 2008.

58. Following the Universal Declaration on Bioethics and Human Rights in 2005, UNESCO has been involved in planning and organizing a "core curriculum" in bioethics.

59. See Jan Swasthya Abhiyan—People's Health Movement, http://phm-india.org/.

Since the days of Ayurveda pioneers, physicians have been held in high regard in traditional Indian cultures, and historically have played an important role in decision-making processes in health care. This did not create problems until the doctor–patient relationship assumed a very different character in the era of growing commercialization of medicine. In a significant development in 1992, the purview of the Consumer Protection Act of 1986 was expanded to include paid medical service, in order to regulate medical malpractice.[60] It is noteworthy that this move to offer patients a mechanism for redress of grievances was opposed by the Indian medical establishment.

As social and consumer rights spilled into the health front, and brought with them issues pertaining to bioethics, the women's rights movement also addressed health and other social issues faced more particularly by women. Notably, this played an important role in the campaigns for banning sex selection of the fetus to prevent female feticide,[61] and protection of women from domestic violence.

Bioethics in Another World: Religious Organizations and Service

India is constitutionally secular, with provision of "freedom to practice religion" with specific protection for minority religions. In the land of *dharma,* historically, religion and spirituality have played significant roles in health and medical care. Philanthropic organizations of religious faiths have established a number of healthcare institutions, and many of them offer quality service at a very affordable price, if not free of charge, to their serving population. The ethics of compassion and caring service they practice lies on a different wavelength, and perhaps outside the margins of academic and professional bioethics discourse. There is hardly any involvement of philosophers, theologians, or religious personalities in state-sponsored or human-rights-inspired bioethics initiatives in India.[62]

---

60. See Nagral, 1992.

61. Recently, Google and Microsoft have pulled their ads from the websites for gender-selection products and techniques, as these are illegal in India. See http://www.medicalnewstoday.com/articles/122269.php.

62. It is noteworthy that members of a particular religious community are, however, "used" when it is felt their mediation would help a health program; e.g., members of the Muslim community were made mediators for convincing sections of the community about the benefits of the polio immunization program.

The Easy and Hard Problems for Bioethics in India

Few will argue with the claim that bioethical issues, concerns, and problems in India are diverse and plentiful. The list of broad themes is potentially long: ethics of economic development; environmental degradation; population control, hunger, poverty, income and health inequality; addressing the menace of corruption; resource prioritization for preventive/curative/palliative medicine; public health ethics in the control of communicable and noncommunicable diseases; protection of human subjects in organ transplants and clinical trials; ethical guidelines for research in science and clinical medicine; formation of a national bioethics commission and institutional ethics committees; designing a bioethics curriculum sensitive to the Indian context; effective regulatory mechanisms to ensure compliance with ethical guidelines, and so on, so forth. Each of these issues and problems deserves serious attention and needs to be addressed. Practically speaking, the areas of intervention range from Ayurveda to arsenic poisoning of underground water, from "organ bazaars" to organic farming, and from torture to terrorism. Nonetheless, some problems appear to be easier to solve than others. It may be useful to divide the problems of bioethics in India into "easy" and "hard" categories.[63]

The "easy" problems of bioethics are those whose definition and resolution involve some sincere initiative and active "political will," and that are likely to come up with visibly tangible results. Examples of "easy" problems include, among others, formation of a national bioethics commission and institutional ethics committees at multiple levels; formulating ethical guidelines in frontier areas of research like stem cells or nanotechnology, and for protection of human subjects in clinical trials; introducing a bioethics curriculum as part of education, etc. The "hard" problems are those which demand multisectoral and multidisciplinary approaches—beyond "political will"—to given bioethical problems, and implementation of any formulated ethical policies and guidelines to the "on the ground" realities of multifaith, multilingual, multicultural Indian societies. This also includes addressing historically unresolved issues like reconciling the relationship of Western moral philosophy with *dharma*, the dominant sociopolitical/economic/moral constructs such as "development" and "civilization,"[64] and use of these multiform constructs within and outside the Western world in the era of globalization. The easy problems are "easy" because we have clear ideas how to address the problems in order to solve them. The "hard" problems are hard

63. I am thankful to Professor David Chalmers for this idea of "easy" and "hard" problems that he put forward in consciousness research. See http://consc.net/papers/facing.html.

64. Gandhi was asked by a reporter: "Mr. Gandhi, what do you think of Western civilization?" Gandhi replied, "I think it would be a good idea!"

because they resist solutions offered by any single-track, linear approach that defines bioethical problems in terms of the concepts, methods, tools, and languages of mainstream Western secular bioethics. These problems challenge us to question concepts, ideas, beliefs, and value systems held by so many for so long—it is no easy job.

There is no Indian bioethics for Indian people in the pan-Indian context at the moment. What we have is, at best, bioethics-related activities in Indian territory that are shaped by various key agents, forces, and ideologies, including the influence of Western power centers and the agendas *they* set for the Indian audience.[65] Few would contest the idea that it is unfair to use and impose, either consciously or inadvertently, the dominant sociocultural/moral constructs of white Western bioethics—with theories, methods, and languages based on its own worldviews, cultural ethos, and norms—and to override the values and goals of non-Western cultures and societies. In other words, to put it bluntly—exporting Western "moral imperialism" is *unethical.* At the same time, it is no less inappropriate not to engage in meaningful initiatives where bioethics can play an important role in making a positive difference in the lives of individuals and communities.

The challenge for bioethicists within (and outside) India in the twenty-first century is to think hard with an open mind and explore the possibility of finding the moral equivalent of "unity in diversity"—exploring a common ground of morality amidst multiple realms of existential reality, while acknowledging and respecting diversity.

The journey is not easy, but certainly worth undertaking and potentially rewarding.

Acknowledgment

This paper is dedicated to Sri Sri Thakur Anukulachandra (1888–1969), who founded *Satsang* ("Holy Gathering," or the Association for Life and Growth) as a mission to unite people of diverse faiths, languages, nationalities, and cultures on the basis of the integral philosophy of Being and Becoming, while nurturing their unique individuality.

---

65. How is it decided whether female feticide, or HIV/AIDS, or polio eradication, or any other issue, for that matter, would be the subject of a public health campaign in a state at a given period of time? Not too rarely, this is decided according to the priorities set by the international agencies. Regarding ethical issues surrounding the polio eradication program, see Paul & Dawson, 2005.

Glossary

Ayurveda Commonly known as the Hindu or Indian traditional system of medicine. Derived from two Sanskrit words—*ayus,* meaning life, and *veda*, meaning knowledge. Ayurveda is believed to originate from the *Atharvaveda.*

Atharvaveda The last of the four *Vedas,* also known as "the fourth *Veda.*" The three other *Vedas* are *Rig-Veda, Sama-Veda, And Yajur-Veda.*

dharma The word is derived from the Sanskrit root *dhri,* meaning to uphold, support, sustain, nurture. Thus, *dharma* is what upholds and nurtures life, or Beings; practically, *dharma* may be considered as the ideal-centric way of harmonious life in the principle of "live and let live." In absence of any appropriate English word for *dharma,* "religion" is often used as a synonym, although "spirituality" would be a better (but imprecise) substitute.

sanatana dharma *Sanatana*=eternal, time immemorial; *sanatana dharma* literally means "eternal way of life and growth." *Sanatana dharma* is more commonly known as Hindu-*dharma* or "Hinduism" in the English speaking world. Buddha-*dharma*=Buddhism; Jaina-*dharma*=Jainism; Sikh-*dharma*=Sikhism. Buddhism, Jainism, and Sikhism may be considered as grown-up children of the same mother, *sanatana dharma.*

guna Qualities, characteristics, attributes.

karma Acts, which include thoughts, words, and actions. This word is derived from the Sanskrit root *kri* (to act). *Karma* also means the effects or consequences of past acts—performed earlier, either in this life or previous one(s)—on one's present or future condition. The doctrine of *karma* has a very important role in *sanatana dharma* and in all her streams, particularly Buddha-*dharma.*

kartabya Duty. Derived from the *Sanskrit* root *kri* (to act), this word literally means "what ought to be done."

niti Ethics, morality. The word also refers to ethical values, principles, rules, or policy.

satguru The Master who guides from darkness of ignorance to light of knowledge in human life.

Veda The most ancient sacred texts known to mankind. The *Vedas* are considered to be the fountainhead of *sanatana dharma.* This Sanskrit word is derived from the root *vid* (to know); thus, the *Vedas* also mean the body of knowledge.

References

Alora AT, Lumitao JM (eds.). (2001). *Beyond a Western Bioethics: Voices from the Developing World.* Washington: Georgetown University Press.

Azariah J, Azariah H, Macer D, Eubios Ethics Institute. (1998). Bioethics in India. Proceedings of the International Bioethics Workshop in Madras: Bioethical Management of Biogeoresources, Jan. 16–19, 1997. University of Madras. Chennai. Christchurch, NZ: Eubios Ethics Institute.

Banerjee D. (1979). Place of the indigenous and the Western systems of medicine in the health services of India. *International Journal of Health Services.* 9: 511–519.

Basham AL. (1954). *The Wonder that was India.* London: Sidwick and Jackson.

Begay RC. (2003). Science and Spirituality. *American Journal of Public Health.* 93: 363.

Bhagwati SN. (1967). Ethics, Morality and Practice of Medicine in Ancient India. *Child's Nervous System.* 13: 428–434.

Carrese JA, Rhodes LA. (1995). Western bioethics on the Navajo reservation: Benefit or harm? *Journal of American Medical Association.* 274: 826–829.

Chatterjee S, Datta DM. (1968). *An Introduction to Indian Philosophy.* Calcutta: Calcutta University.

Chattopadhyay S. (2008). An Earnest Appeal: We Need Spirituality in Medical Education. In Macer D. (ed.). *Asia–Pacific Perspective in Bioethics Education.* Bangkok: RUSHAP UNESCO.

Chattopadhyay S, De Vries R. (2008). Bioethical concerns are global, bioethics is Western. *Eubios Journal of Asian and International Bioethics.* 18: 106–109.

Chattopadhyay S, Simon A. (2008). East meets West: cross-cultural perspective in end-of-life decision making from Indian and German viewpoints. *Medicine Health Care and Philosophy.* 11: 165–174.

Coppa A, Bondioli L, Cucina A, Frayer DW, Jarrige C, Jarrige JF, Quivron G, Rossi M, Vidale M, Macchiarelli R. (2006). Palaeontology: early Neolithic tradition of dentistry. *Nature.* 440: 755–756.

Dhand A. (2002). The dharma of ethics, the ethics of dharma – Quizzing the ideals of Hinduism. *Journal of Religious Ethics.* 30: 347–372.

Gitanjali B. (2004). Academic dishonesty in Indian medical colleges. *Journal of Postgraduate Medicine.* 50: 281–284.

Jafarey A, Thomas G, Ahmad A, Srinivasan S. (2007). Asia's organ farms. *Indian Journal of Medical Ethics.* 4: 52–53.

Jonsen AR. (2000). *A Short History of Medical Ethics.* New York: Oxford University Press.

Kumar D. (2006). *Science and the Raj. A Study of British India.* (2nd edition.) New Delhi: Oxford University Press.

Kumar D. (2001). *Disease and Medicine in India.* Indian History Congress. New Delhi: Tulika.

Kurian NJ. (2007). Widening economic & social disparities: Implications for India. *Indian Journal of Medical Research.* 126: 374–380.

Myser C. (2007). White normativity in United States bioethics: A call and method for more pluralist and democratic standards and policies. In Eckenwiler & Cohen, eds. *The Ethics of Bioethics* (pp. 241–259) Johns Hopkins University Press.

Nagral S. (1992). The Consumer Protection Act. *Journal of Postgraduate Medicine.* 38: 214–215.

Nundy S, Gulhati C.M. (2005). A new colonialism?—Conducting clinical trials in India. *New England Journal of Medicine.* 352: 1633–1636.

Paul Y, Dawson A. (2005). Some ethical issues arising from polio eradication programmes in India. *Bioethics.* 19: 393–406.

Saha M. (1999). *History of Indian Medicine based on Vedic Literature Satapatha Brahmana*. Calcutta: The Asiatic Society.

Sharma DC. (2001). President of Indian medical council found guilty of corruption. *Lancet*. 358: 1882.

Srinivasan S, Loff B. (2006). Medical research in India. *Lancet*. 367: 1962–1964.

Stonington S, Ratanakul P. (2006). Is there a global bioethics? End-of-life in Thailand and the case for local difference. *PLoS Med* 3: e439.

Tandon PN. (2005). Bioethics: an emerging discipline. *Indian Journal of Medical Research*. 121: 1–4.

UNESCO. (2005). The Universal Declaration on Bioethics and Human Rights. Paris: UNESCO. http://unesdoc.unesco.org/images/0014/001461/146180e.pdf

3 CAPACITY BUILDING IN DEVELOPING WORLD BIOETHICS

PERSPECTIVES ON BIOMEDICINE AND BIOMEDICAL ETHICS IN CONTEMPORARY SRI LANKA

Bob Simpson

In 2005, a Universal Declaration on Bioethics and Human Rights was adopted at the UNESCO General Conference. The Declaration resolves to set out "a foundation for humanity's response to the ever-increasing dilemmas and controversies that science and technology present for humankind and the environment." The document is an important milestone for those engaged in the task of setting global standards to combat the abuses and injustices that scientific advance might bring. Moreover, it is one of the primary mechanisms for going beyond the standard setting of earlier declarations, in that it attempts to "add value" by encouraging the building of capacity in bioethics (Langlois, 2008; Ten Have, 2006). By encouraging networking, transfer of resources and information, the creation of databases, and providing support for the development of ethics committees, it is hoped that greater receptivity will be fostered to the ideas and values that underpin the project of bioethics in general, and the UNESCO Declaration in particular. However, as many of those attempting to realize these declarations on the ground have pointed out, such aspirations have little effect unless the capacity exists to put them into practice (Benatar & Singer, 2000; Singer & Benatar, 2001: 747; Bhutta, 2002). To this end, local initiatives are now being facilitated and supported through a plethora of international networks working toward reducing the perceived inadequacies in bioethical competence.

My aim in this essay is to provide a brief account of precisely this process of engagement in Sri Lanka, and the patterns of acceptance and resistance that contain and shape the impetus to build capacity in this and similar settings.[1] In what follows, I draw on research carried out

---

1. The research was funded as part of a Wellcome Trust Fellowship under the Medicine in Society Programme (Biomedical Ethics GR067110AIA), enabling

into the reception of new reproductive and genetic technologies between 2000 and 2003 (Simpson, 2005a and 2005b). This work considered issues of infertility and the new technologies (Simpson, 2003), genetic testing and its relation to abortion policies (Simpson et al., 2003, Simpson, 2007), and gamete donation and its relation to organ donation practices (Simpson, 2005b). In the course of this research, it became apparent that there were a number of other bioethical "hot-spots" developing for Sri Lankans. Many of these were linked to the absence of an infrastructure to provide protection for human subjects in biomedical research. Concern was regularly expressed, by professionals and lay people alike, about subjects' exposure to exploitation and abuse, and this has resulted in considerable efforts to strengthen ethical review procedures (Dissanayake, Lanerolle, & Mendis, 2006, Simpson, 2001, Sumathipala & Siribaddana, 2003). The areas to which these efforts have been directed include: collaboration and the danger of unequal relationships with foreign partners, especially in clinical trials; weak informed consent procedures, which might lead to patients/research participants experiencing harm, especially in a context where medical paternalism is deeply engrained; commercial exploitation of doctors and patients by drug companies, through inducements and inappropriate advertising; badly conducted clinical trials; weak protocols for data collection and storage; poorly regulated transactions in human organs and tissue.

It is not my purpose in this essay to consider these bioethical hot-spots in detail. My objective here is to draw attention to the place of local beliefs, values, and institutional structures in the encounter between global biomedicine and the demand for bioethics that it brings in its wake. To achieve this objective will require a brief overview of historical, social, and political dimensions of biomedicine in Sri Lanka.

A Brief Social History of Biomedicine in Sri Lanka[2]

The tradition of biomedicine is very firmly established in Sri Lanka. The Civil Medical Department of the British colonial administration was first established

---

me to carry out four and a half months of fieldwork in Sri Lanka. A one-month pilot field trip in summer 2000 was funded by the Nuffield Foundation (Social Sciences Small Grants Scheme).

2. The "Democratic Socialist Republic" of Sri Lanka is an island of some 20 million people. The main ethnic groups are Sinhalese (74%), Tamils (19%), and Moors (7%), with smaller groups, such as Malays and Burghers, accounting for less than 1%. In terms of religious affiliation, the main groupings are Buddhist (69.3%), Hindu (15.5%), Moslem (7.6%), and Roman Catholic (6.9%). The largest communities within Sri Lankan society at present are Sinhala Buddhists (approximately 69% of the population) and Tamil Hindus (approximately 15%). In relation to other countries in the South Asian region, Sri Lanka has a favorable per capita GDP (US $829)

as a department, separate from the one dealing with the occupying military forces, in 1858. Although aimed specifically at the control of smallpox, the creation of a department to address the health needs of the local population, as distinct from the needs of the colonizers, marked an important step on the road to a national health service (Uragoda, 1987:81). The Colombo Medical School, opened in 1870, is the second oldest in Asia and has a distinguished tradition of providing biomedical education to the local population. Yet, even today, the medical profession preserves a strong sense of identity modeled upon the structures that took root during the British colonial period. The Anglicization of medicine was, and continues to be, reinforced by the use of English in medical (and other professional) education. The language issue remains a source of tension, as the majority of the population receive primary and secondary education in their mother tongue (Sinhala or Tamil), but then have to take their medical degrees in English. Furthermore, an entrenched Anglophone biomedicine has had the effect of marginalizing indigenous systems of medicine. As Pieris notes, in the nineteenth century, discussions regarding the development of a medical school identified one of its aims as being to "send out well-educated young men to open up the dispensaries of the Island and to diffuse a knowledge of European medicine among the poorer classes of the community and (thereby) in time supersede the ignorant *vedarala*" (cited in Pieris, 2001:17). Such attitudes became well established and continue to manifest among some contemporary practitioners of biomedicine. For much of its history, then, the medical profession has not only been highly Westernized, English-speaking, and of high status, but also one that was cut off from the beliefs and values about health and illness held by the majority of the population.

In recent times, other factors have come to shape the culture of biomedical practice in Sri Lanka. One of the most important of these has been an inexorable shift toward deregulation and an open market economy. Following the election in 1977 of a right-wing government with an agenda for fundamental market reform and economic liberalization, the private sector has come to play an increasingly important role in health care, raising concerns that it might even displace the state as the key provider of health services. In 1978, for example, doctors were for the first time allowed to engage in private practice in addition to their government responsibilities, a development that spurred a spectacular growth in private healthcare provision, particularly in tertiary care. More recently, the import of equipment to private medical institutions has been greatly accelerated by the

and a very high rate of literacy (estimated to be over 90%). Since independence from British colonial rule in 1948, Sri Lanka has been able to develop and maintain a free national health service with reasonable access across the island.

granting of duty-free concessions. The result of these and other developments has been an overall trend toward high-quality private medicine. In contrast, the public sector, which to date has provided free health care at the point of need, has fallen far behind the private sector in some fields.[3] Sri Lanka has limited resources with which to combat the widespread poverty and underdevelopment that is a fundamental cause of poor health, and the state is rapidly becoming a residual provider, catering for the large numbers of people who are unable to afford private care. The government sector has been further undermined, particularly in primary care provision, as pressures from the World Bank and other international financial institutions bring change to earlier patterns of welfare expenditure (Jayasinghe, 2002:6–7).[4]

Under these circumstances, the consolidation and expansion of biomedicine continues to proceed apace. However, for many doctors and their patients the acceleration in scope and complexity of medical treatments brings with it an ambivalence. Versatility in biomedicine is undoubtedly a source of power, *kudos,* and a firm link with global systems that betoken modernity and development. Yet, the embrace is often a resentful one. There is a deep concern that doctors, who were once "gods amidst men" (*Daily News*, *Readers' Mail*, March 1, 2003) have now fallen prey to the market and become selfish money grubbers who have turned their backs on compassion and social responsibility. The growing numbers of medical negligence cases further evidences this trend in recent years.[5] In the very recent past, the idea of prosecuting such cases would have been simply unthinkable. Likewise, uncritical acceptance and imitation of everything that emerges from the West is no longer acceptable. The record of foreign governments and multinationals, particularly where pharmaceuticals are concerned, has prompted a more sober evaluation of the costs and benefits of what is on offer, and a good deal of self-critical examination of the medical profession, in the post-independence period (see for example Dharmasiri, 1997, for a particularly caustic critique).

3. Notwithstanding these trends, Sri Lanka is often cited as a nation that has been able to achieve improvements in the health of its population that are disproportionate to the state of the economy (Nuffield Council on Bioethics, 2002:20). With health expenditure running at only 3% of GDP (compared with 7.1% in Japan and 5.2% in India), Sri Lanka still maintains a comparatively high level of life expectancy for the region (65 for males and 73 for females), and also maintains a relatively high ratio of doctors and nurses to the general population (36.5 doctors and 102.7 nurses/10^5 of the population).

4. For example, see details of the World Bank sponsored Health Sector Development Project. Available at: http://www.hsdp.lk:8181/index.jsp (accessed 20th September 2008).

5. The first and most celebrated of these was the case of De Soysa versus Arseculeratne (Gooneratne, 2005).

Trends in Biomedical Ethics

Implicit in the emergence of a more critical evaluation of the benefits of medical science has been a parallel debate about the appropriateness of Western biomedical ethics, and from where a more appropriate ethics might be derived. To date, the development of medical ethics in Sri Lanka has been strongly influenced by the Western Hippocratic tradition, and subsequently incorporated values and orientations found in canonical documents such as the Nuremberg Code and the Helsinki Declaration (Babapulle, 1992). However, as Arseculeratne (1999) has pointed out, this creates a serious paradox. Doctors versed in Western medical ethics practice on a population that is predominantly Asian in ethos and outlook, and the doctors, to a large extent, are ignorant of indigenous traditions of healing and medical ethics; as he put it in a lecture given in November 2002, they remain "Asian in blood and English in morals, intellect, and attitude."

This sense of mismatch between the ethical values that underpin the western biomedical tradition and the reality of local circumstance has led to growing disenchantment. The question that some doctors are now beginning to pose is not so much "what have we gained by engagement with Western medicine and the ethics that come with it?" but "what have we lost?" As in the West, there is a fear that the ever-accelerating embrace of new technologies and treatments takes place without appropriate structures of accountability and regulation in place. The image is a familiar one: society and its democratic institutions are somehow left behind, struggling to get a hand on the tail of runaway medical and scientific progress. However, in the developing world the problem has additional dimensions. The development of biomedical ethics in the West is premised on certain assumptions about affluence, stability and the toleration of pluralism. Conversely, in circumstances where there is widespread poverty, and crises over the management of pluralism, resulting in war and heightened militarization, capacity in biomedical ethics will follow distinct contours. For example, if biomedical ethics discourse and practice remain with the elites of the medical world, who in turn restrict their practice to a wealthy, Westernized clientele, then capacity building offers little by way of challenge. Here, the continuities between, say, London and Colombo, when it comes to what is available for paying customers, should not be underestimated. However, the more capacity extends beyond this affluent veneer and into the harsh realities of Third World living, then the more trenchant are the calls for a biomedical ethics that is both relevant and appropriate.[6] Debates begin

---

6. Cf. Garrafa and do Prado who, speaking from a Brazilian perspective, have sought to make this point even more explicit by calling for a "hard" bioethics, presumably in contrast to a "soft" bioethics, which they see as currently being diffused from northern countries (Garrafa & do Prado, 2002).

to emerge about how local perspectives might be meaningfully incorporated into rapidly diffusing models of hegemonic virtue. Indeed, the question is being asked as to whether there is a culturally distinct Asian bioethic (De Castro, 1999; Qui, 2004). The essence of such an ethic is summarized by Pellagrino as being "less dialectical, logical or linguistic in character, less analytical, more synthetic, or more sensitive to family or community consensus than to individual autonomy, more virtue-based than principle based" (Pellagrino, 1992). In other words, the tendency to medicalize society at every turn is countered by other voices seeking to socialize medicine. In Sri Lanka, as in many other developing world contexts, there is a push among some intellectuals, doctors, and medical scientists to move away from an ethics that relies on rules, analysis, and intellection, toward one that is more experiential and oriented to practical results. In Sri Lanka, it is argued that this kind of ethics lies closer to the epistemological orientations of Asian religious and philosophical traditions in general, and Theravāda Buddhism in particular (Premasiri, 1996; cited in Arseculeratne, 1999).

The idea of a culturally appropriate biomedical ethics thus necessarily involves attempts to reach back into traditions that were previously denigrated and subordinated. Thus, for example, at the WONCA (World Organisation of National Colleges and Academies of Family Medicine) conference held in Colombo in 2002, a session dealing with "human rights, heritage and values in family practice" concluded with a slide showing an ancient saying: "*rajakam naetnam vedakam*," which was translated as "if you cannot be a king be a doctor." Linking doctors with the glorious beneficence of the ancient kings was clearly an attempt to remind doctors of the nobility and honor that is attached to their profession. However, for an audience of Western-trained family doctors, it is significant that the "doctor" referred to in the quotation was never an allopathic doctor, but a practitioner of the older tradition of Ayurvedic medicine. The Ayurvedic physician, or *vedarala,* is, for many Sinhalese, a venerated figure, highly respected for his or her commitment to healing, and the epitome of compassion, kindness, and generosity (Nichter & Nordstrom, 1989). For the *vedarala,* medical ethics was never something separate that needed to be acquired as an accoutrement to their technical mastery, but was wholly integral to their practice. Yet, at a time when the idealized image of the *vedarala* is often used by a critical public as the means to highlight the shortcomings of biomedical doctors, it is interesting to note that doctors themselves seek to align their values and attitudes with those of this more ancient tradition. Similarly, references by doctors to canonical texts such as the Bhagavadgita (2500 BC), the Ayurvedic treatises of Susruta and Charaka (c. 800 BC), and the chronicles of medieval Sinhalese history, such as the Mahawamsa (461–479 AD), in the context of medical ethics, serve to link their own practice to an Eastern tradition, while at the same time pointing out that these traditions are of far greater antiquity than those that underpin biomedical ethics in the West.

In contemporary Sri Lanka, linking current medical practice with values, attitudes, and orientations that connect with traditions that are authentic and legitimate, in that they are to be found beneath the heavy overlay of science, medicine, and ethics brought by the colonizers, is a laudable aspiration. However, in practice it is rather less straightforward, given the highly conflicted notions of just what constitutes authenticity and legitimacy in postcolonial and neocolonial settings. The management of genealogies of knowledge, even in the field of ethics, is a fraught activity in the fractured and pluralist setting of Sri Lanka at the beginning of the twenty-first century. Thus, when there is talk about cultural differences that need to be respected and treated with sensitivity in the evolving discourse of biomedical ethics, one is inclined to ask: Which culture, and which differences? Assumptions made, for example, in documents such as the Nuffield Council on Bioethics (2002)—that there is a unitary and global system of biomedical ethics that encounters cultural units that, while different on the outside are, in a quaintly functionalist sort of way, uniform and consistent on the inside—are deeply problematic. At a time when biomedical ethics appears to have begun to take on board the significance of *inter*national cultural differences, it is appropriate to draw attention to the importance of *intra*national cultural differences, also. For the majority of Sri Lankans, who are Sinhalese and Buddhist, the logical place to begin to build a locally informed response to Western biomedical ethics is out of Buddhism's own tradition of virtue-based, consequentialist ethical analysis. However, there are other traditions—Hindu, Christian, and Moslem—and other positions—secular, humanist, and rationalist—that render "culture" far from homogenous and harmonious, but complex, conflicted, and contested. Under such circumstances, "building capacity" is not an exercise in neat and perpendicular architecture, but a more irregular process of improvisation and irregularity as the blueprints of an international bioethics are shaped to fit the contingencies of local circumstance.[7] In the next section I turn to a consideration of some of the ways in which these contingencies have influenced the development of bioethics in Sri Lanka.

Biomedical Ethics in a Hot Climate

Sri Lanka is a country that has lived through much brutal and traumatic civil unrest. From the early 1980s until it's bloody conclusion in 2009 the government

7. See Arseculeratne et al., 2008, for a more comprehensive account of the dialogue that has emerged around the issues of "indigenous bioethics."

of Sri Lanka was pitted against a ruthless and determined campaign by the LTTE (Liberation Tigers of Tamil Elam), who wished to secure a separate state in the north of the Island. In the late 1980s the country also experienced violent convulsions as educated but disenchanted rural Sinhala youth began a Marxist-cum-nationalist-inspired insurrection, which resulted in widespread civil disorder. Estimates vary but as many as 100,000 people may have been killed during these bouts of ethnic and civil strife. As a result of these two cataclysms, militarization of society has increased, and human rights and democracy itself have all been weakened (Hasbullah & Morrison, 2004; Winslow & Woost, 2004). Under such conditions, confidence in the benevolent operation of power and authority has been severely shaken.

It is into this volatile mix that the idea of bioethics has been progressively introduced and consolidated. In recent years, considerable efforts are being made to develop local capacity by supporting existing ethical review bodies and developing new ones (Dissanayake, Lanerolle & Mendis, 2006). Awareness of ethical issues features more prominently as part of university medical curricula. Bioethics is also communicated to the wider community through NGOs such as the Forum for Research and Development (also see Sumathipala & Siribaddana, 2003). Local initiatives are being facilitated and supported through participation in international networks, such as the Forum for Ethical Review Committees in Asia and the Western Pacific (FERCAP), the Strategic Initiative for Developing Capacity in Ethical Review (SIDCER), and the Global Forum on Bioethics in Research (GFBR).

Thus, local efforts to build capacity proceed apace and, on the face of it, appear consistent with international models and expectations. There is what might be described as a modernist aspiration to establish collectively agreed and widely shared codes, guidelines, and protocols indicating how to proceed when confronted with the difficult choices engendered by rapid advances in biomedical technology and research. In practice, however, the attempts to govern, regulate, oversee, advise, and offer judgment, which come as part and parcel of the bioethical enterprise, are received in particular ways in a society that is currently experiencing high levels of militarization and a preoccupation with security, surveillance, and control. Attempts at a systematic institutionalization of ethics in Sri Lanka must thus engage with the internal disputes and conflicts that characterize most aspects of social and political life. The aspiration to improve the quality of research through effective review, or to provide guidance on contentious issues of biomedical advance, unfolds through multiple claims to authority when it comes to evaluation, approval, and monitoring.

The establishment of a Forum for Ethical Review Committees in Sri Lanka (FERCSL) has gone a considerable way toward providing a context (in the form of a website), documentation (in the form of standardized application forms), and training, which can bring together those with an interest in promoting bioethics in general, and ethical review of research in particular. However, these efforts are still largely upward facing rather than downward acting; they speak more to an imagined international audience than to vulnerable citizens and subjects that are in need of protection. Rivalry exists between universities and, in certain respects, bioethics becomes another arena in which to express these rivalries. For example, questions are frequently raised about the competence and composition of different committees.

These contests of authority, although minor in the scale of things, are an important characteristic of the "third space" that opens up with the global interplay of culture, technologies, and ethics in developing world contexts. They were made evident in a series of discussions about the regulation of new reproductive and genetic technologies that took place with doctors and clinicians during fieldwork carried out in 2000 and 2002–2003.[8] Genetics and Assisted Reproductive Technologies (ARTs) were both fields in which there was little or no local regulatory framework at that time and which were deemed ripe for a "national" response of some kind (Simpson, 2001).[9] The ease with which these technologies are transferred, coupled with their potential to generate complex ethical, legal, and social questions, raised concerns within the medical profession that little was being done to oversee their proliferation.

The first concern is what might be thought of as the problem of representation. The emergence of a transnational biomedical ethics is built upon a broadly secular and rationalistic aspiration, in which ethical review is constituted as an extension of democratic representation. For example, the WHO's "Operational Guidelines for Ethics Committees that Review Biomedical Research" suggests that ethics committees should be "multi-disciplinary and multi-sectoral in composition, including relevant scientific expertise, a balanced age and gender distribution, and laypersons representing the interests and concerns of the community" (WHO, 2000). Those with whom I spoke readily acknowledged that there should be community representation in the regulation of the new technologies. However, "community," in the

---

8. The discussion here refers specifically to the question of regulating new biotechnologies, and lies outside a discussion of research ethics per se. At the time of writing, I am engaged in a project that deals specifically with research ethics and international collaboration in Sri Lanka (International Science and Bioethics Collaborations funded by the ESRC RES-062-23—0215)

9. Under the auspices of the National Science and Technology Commission, an expert working group drew up a set of preliminary guidelines in 2003 (NASTEC, 2003). This document has formed the basis for the establishment of dedicated guidelines to deal with advances in genetics and reproductive medicine, respectively. The working group also recommended the establishment of ethics committees at national level to oversee each of these fields.

context of major ethnic tensions, often equates with representation from major religious groupings. While carrying local practice beyond Western models of medical humanism and into the realms of what has been described as an *Asian bioethic* is a desirable objective, suspicions and concerns were voiced about the involvement of representatives of religious groups in fora set up to consider ethical questions. In particular, there was anxiety that such involvement could bring the divisive and destructive assertion of religious fundamentalisms into play.

The desire to keep medicine unified and secular was keenly felt by those who were only too aware of the physical consequences of communal conflict. The trick would appear to be one of constructing frameworks for ethical review that are secular enough to allow rational dialogue to proceed, but open enough to give the impression of inclusive representation. However, the accommodation of "cultural sensitivity" into a local ethical awareness is a fraught activity. Buddhism, as the religion of the majority community, presents particular problems in this regard. On the one hand, there is a nationalist valorization of Buddhism. In its more extreme forms it has been argued that Buddhism provides an important focal point for resistance to hegemonic globalization (Wickremasinghe, 2001:150). As such, Buddhism is enlisted by some as part of a populist, anti-development, anti-Western-science discourse that seeks to challenge the preoccupation that doctors have with Western models of progress and development. In the context of technological development, there is also a countervailing tendency that threatens to bring conflict between Buddhism and other religions. For some Buddhists, claims are made to the effect that the membrane that separates science from religion is altogether more permeable than with other religions. Absence of divinity, rejection of creationism, belief in rebirth, and a highly rationalistic analysis of phenomenal existence lead to Buddhism being identified with science in a way that other religions are not (Kirtisinghe, 1984; Simpson, 2009; Verhoeven, 2001). Indeed, the radical insistence by some Buddhists on a scientific rationalism as the grounds for knowledge is used to bring their religion into a powerful alignment with biomedicine. This is the case for many medical practitioners who happen to be Buddhist. The place of Buddhist representation in the institutionalization of ethics is thus doubly problematic: For some, there are concerns that it could provide an unhelpful brake on progress, but for others the worry is that it might propel acceptance of new developments in ways that people from other religious communities find troubling and offensive. For example, although reproductive cloning is outlawed in many parts of the world, surveys regarding the attitudes of doctors and medical students to these techniques suggest a surprisingly high level of acceptance, with 40% of doctors and 25% of students prepared to countenance such techniques (Simpson et al., 2005). In a society as pluralistically complex as Sri Lanka, then, the idea that "culture" might be easily and unproblematically woven into the business of ethical oversight and review is far-fetched, to say the least. In attempts to instantiate something like a collective view by means of an ethics committee, the sensitivities that surround questions of ethnicity, religion, class, and caste in the wider society, are rarely far from the surface and must necessarily be navigated with great skill.

A second theme concerns the relationship between the processes of ethical regulation, and the larger field of political relations within which it is located. As suggested earlier, authority and power in Sri Lanka do not currently operate easily in the abstract realms of "civil society," but do so through conduits of relationship and shared personal and professional history. As many of my informants pointed out, they work in a "small world" in which people are precisely mapped in terms of their status, allegiances, and affinities. Concerns about "cronyism" and undue political interference in the conduct of decision-making are common, along with a certain despondency that honest attempts to realize procedures that are fair, transparent, and robust are all too often confounded as decisions made, or guidelines agreed, meet with limited compliance across the sector. Indeed, the problem of how to move beyond mere rhetoric and give regulation and review "teeth" was a recurrent theme in discussions. Influence over the private sector was a particular source of anxiety in this regard, with some doctors expressing extreme pessimism that any meaningful regulation of the new technologies was possible at all, as long as the private sector was so much in the ascendant. It was as if a two-tier morality was in operation, in which the public sector was subject to close scrutiny, whereas the private sector could operate more or less unfettered. Under such circumstances, doubts were expressed as to whether the currently developing capacity in bioethics would improve rights, protection, and care for citizens in line with its rhetorical claims.

Finally, medical practitioners and researchers are themselves uneasy in negotiating the new insights that an engagement with bioethics brings. Making doctors in Sri Lanka entails induction into rigid professional hierarchies, and the inculcation of authority and confidence. However, the attention now being drawn to biomedical ethics, as opposed to a medical ethics that rarely strays beyond the bedside or the surgery, means a step into unfamiliar terrain. A certain kind of reflexivity and transparency is demanded by the current ethical paradigm shift. Doctors must make their practices explicit in ways that they have not done before, and there may well be disruption to established hierarchies and networks, as well as resistance and obfuscation. At the outset, they have to acknowledge that, in any move to socialize medicine, answers are not clear and authoritative; there is ignorance and limited capacity within the medical profession when it comes to dealing with such issues. Just as capacity building involves forming new publics, it also entails creating new kinds of medical practitioners—and, not least, ones who are comfortable sloughing off professional identities that are rooted in an earlier colonial era.

Conclusion

This essay has been concerned with the spread of ideas and values. The spread or diffusion in question follows a familiar gradient: north to south, "developed" to "developing," urban to rural, scientifically proficient to scientifically lagging (Watson et al., 2003) and, as in other areas of development endeavor such as health, education, human rights, and civil society, it is driven by an aspiration to raise awareness, empower, and democratize through the dissemination of knowledge and a devolution of responsibilities and decision making. The shift, from centralized power and paternalism to more distributed models of governance and control, is integral to the quest for global justice in health and development. Yet, there are cultural, institutional, and economic impediments to the spread of ideas and values; for those who wish to promote them, it is often the case that those who would benefit most from this vision of progress are invariably those who are least well equipped and most unprepared to embrace it. It is in recognition of this problem that the notion of capacity building has increasingly been brought into play when discussing transfer strategies. Rooted in the language of physics and electricity, capacity is defined in the Oxford English Dictionary as "holding power, receiving power." Its use in the context of strategies for development of one kind or another introduces an important conceptual shift: It is not adequate merely to communicate ideas and values; the conditions for their reception and retention must also be in place, which in turn gives rise to the idea of capacity that must be built if power of some kind is to be realized. For ideas and values to be received and held, other things have to be in place, such as training, institutional templates, legal frameworks, models of governance, and the resources to create an irreversible and sustainable shift in practice.

What I hope to have illustrated by focusing on the issue of capacity building in bioethics in general, and in Sri Lanka in particular, are some of the ways in which the benevolent push of those who would wish to see improvements in the capacity of developing world countries to respond to global biomedical advances is met by the complex contingencies of local circumstance. The contribution of social sciences at this meeting point is crucial. Just as global declarations are of limited value without the capacity to receive and hold the ideas they contain, capacity building will in itself remain a largely rhetorical exercise if it is not accompanied by detailed analyses of the specific contexts. In the Sri Lankan setting, the current fragility of democracy, and the extent of militarization, give the development of bioethics capacity a particular shape and direction. Against this backdrop, the institutionalization of biomedical ethics tends to be about the consolidation of connections with the international networks that operate above, and with limited penetrance into, the day-to-day contexts that lie below. Indeed, far from the unifying and consolidating intentions of the global bioethics movement, the drive to build capacity may simply fall into the more widespread propensity to fission and fragmentation that besets much social and political activity in Sri Lankan society. To fully characterize these processes is a complex and engaging task, and I, and others in this volume, have merely scraped its surface. The development of a clearer account of capacity in context is a key objective, if bioethics is to achieve the ambitious and transformative potential promised in its current declarations.

Glossary

Ayurveda a South Asian system of medical treatments based on the idea that imbalances in the three humors of the body (wind, bile, and phlegm) are the cause of illness. This imbalance can be restored by the use of herbal potions, ointments, and other preparations.

Vedarala Sinhala term for a practitioner of Ayurvedic medicine.

References

Arseculeratne SN. (1999). *Our Orientations in Biomedical Ethics* (S R Kottegoda Memorial Oration). Colombo: Sri Lanka Association for the Advancement of Science. 5–24.

Arseculeratne SN, Simpson B, Premasiri PD, Kumarasiri PVR. (2008). Ethics, culture and relativism: some reflections on the teaching of medical ethics in contemporary Sri Lanka. *Biomedical Law and Ethics* 2(1), 131–160.

Babapulle CJ. (1992). Teaching of medical ethics in Sri Lanka. *Medical Education* 26:185–189.

Benatar SR, Singer PA. (2000). A new look at international research ethics. *British Medical Journal* 321:824–826.

Bhutta ZA. (2002). Ethics in international health research: a perspective from the developing world. *Bulletin of the World Health Organisation* 80(2):114–120.

De Castro L. (1999). Is there an Asian bioethics? *Bioethics* 13(3&4):227–235.

Dharmasiri G. (1997). *The Nature of Medicine: A Critique of the Myth of Medicine*. Colombo: Gunapala Dharmasiri.

Dissananayake VJ, Lanerolle RD, Mendis N. (2006). Research ethics and ethical review committees in Sri Lanka: a 25 year journey. *Ceylon Medical Journal* 51(3):110–113.

Garaffa V, do Prado M. (2002). Public health justice and market: a bioethical look on irreconcilable interests. *Perspectives in Health* 7(1):1. (Also see http://www.bioethciscongress.org.br/textos/hard.htm).

Gooneratna C. (2005). *A Doctor's Quest for Justice: Professor Priyani De Soysa versus Rienzie Arseculeratne*. Colombo: Vijitha Yapa Publications.

Hasbullah SH, Morrison BN. (2004). *Sri Lankan Society in an Era of Globalisation: Struggling to Create a New Social Order*. London: Sage Publications.

Jayasinghe S. (2002). Context of the health system. In *Health Sector in Sri Lanka: Current Status and Challenges* (pp. 1–11). Colombo: Health Development and Research Programme.

Kirthisinghe BP. (1984). *Buddhism and Science*. Delhi: Motilal Banarsidas.

Langlois A. (2008). The UNESCO Universal Declaration on Bioethics and Human Rights: Perspectives from Kenya and South Africa. *Health Care Analysis* 16(1):39–51.

NASTEC. (2003). *New Genetics and Assisted Reproductive Technologies in Sri Lanka: A Draft National Policy on Biomedical Ethics*. Colombo: National Science and Technology Commission.

Nichter M, Nordstrom C. (1989). A Question of medicine answering: health commodification and the social relations of healing in Sri Lanka. *Culture Medicine and Psychiatry* 13:367–390.

Nuffield Council on Bioethics. (2002). *The Ethics of Research Related to Health Care in Developing Countries*. London: Nuffield Council on Bioethics.

Pellagrino ED. (1992). Intersections of western biomedical ethics and world culture. In Pellagrino ED, Mazarella P, Corsi P (eds.). *Transcultural Dimensions in Medical Ethics* (pp. 13–19). Maryland: University Publishing Group Inc.

Pieris K. (2001). *The Medical Profession in Sri Lanka 1843–1980*. Colombo: Visidunu Prakashakayo.

Premasiri P. (1996). Indian Religions–Theravada Buddhism. Panel Discussion on Religion and Morality. Regional Training Workshop on Medical Ethics. University of Peradeniya, Sri Lanka.

Qiu RZ (ed). (2004). *Bioethics: Asian Perspectives. A Quest for Moral Diversity*. New York: Springer.

Simpson B. (2001). Ethical Regulation and the new reproductive technologies in Sri Lanka: perspectives of ethics committee members. *Ceylon Medical Journal* 46(2):54–57.

Simpson B. (2003). Localising a brave new world: new reproductive technologies and the politics of fertility in contemporary Sri Lanka. In Unnithan-Kumar M (ed.). *Reproductive Agency, Medicine and the State* (pp. 43–58). Oxford: Berghahn.

Simpson B. (2005a). Acting ethically, responding culturally: framing the new reproductive and genetic technologies in Sri Lanka. *Asia Pacific Journal of Anthropology* 5(3):227–243.

Simpson B. (2005b). Impossible Gifts: Bodies, Buddhism and Bioethics. *Journal of the Royal Anthropological Insititute* 10(4): 839–859.

Simpson B. (2007). Negotiating the therapeutic gap: prenatal diagnostics and termination in Sri Lanka. *Journal of Bioethical Enquiry* 4(3):207–215.

Simpson B. (2009). We have always been modern: Buddhism, Science and the New Genetic and Reproductive Technologies in Sri Lanka. *Culture and Religion 10* (2):137–158.

Simpson B, Dissanayake VHW, Wickremasinghe D, Jayasekera RW. (2003). Prenatal testing and pregnancy termination in Sri Lanka: The views of doctors and medical students. *Ceylon Medical Journal* 48(*4*):129–132.

Simpson B, Dissanayake VHW, Jayasekera RW. (2005). Contemplating choice: attitudes towards intervening in reproduction in Sri Lanka. *New Genetics and Society* 24(*1*):99–118.

Singer PA, Benatar SR. (2001). Beyond Helsinki: A vision for global health ethics. *British Medical Journal* 322:747–748.

Sumathipala A, Siribaddana S. (2003). *Research Ethics of From a Developing World Perspective*. Colombo: Vijitha Yapa Publications.

Ten Have T. (2006). The activities of UNESCO in the area of ethics. *Kennedy Institute of Ethics Journal* 16(4):333–351.

Uragoda CG. (1987). *A History of Medicine in Sri Lanka*. Colombo: Sri Lanka Medical Association.

Verhoeven MJ. (2001). Buddhism and science: probing the boundaries of faith and reason. *Religion East and West* 1:77–97.

Watson R, Crawford M, Farley S. (2003). *Strategic Approaches to Science and Technology in Development*. Number 3026, Policy Research Working Paper Series, The World Bank. http://econpapers.repec.org/paper/wbkwbrwps/3026.htm (accessed December 9, 2010).

Wickremasinghe N. (2001). *Civil Society in Sri Lanka: New Circles of Power*. New Delhi: Sage Publications.

Winslow D, Woost MD. (2004). *Economy, Culture and Civil War in Sri Lanka*. Bloomington: Indiana University Press.

World Health Organization. (2000). *Operational Guidelines for Ethics Committees that Review Biomedical Research*. Geneva: WHO.

II

A ROBUST RANGE OF SOCIOCULTURAL INTERESTS AND FORCES SHAPING BIOETHICS AROUND THE GLOBE

4 FRENCH BIOETHICS

THE RHETORIC OF UNIVERSALITY AND THE ETHICS OF MEDICAL RESPONSIBILITY

Kristina Orfali

Introduction

Despite sharing an intellectual history with the United States, France has followed its own path in relation to bioethics. France was the first country in the world to create a "consultative national council of ethics" in 1983; the Bioethics Laws, currently under revision, were passed in 1994. French bioethics, however, have largely prioritized biomedical issues of general scope, such as the impact of science, research, and technology on the human being. The early and very strong institutionalization of bioethics has had less impact on bedside ethics and medical practice than could be expected; and, despite legal changes, standard issues in clinical ethics, such as life and death decisions, still remain in the hands of the medical profession.

The dissonance between highly visible institutionalized and formal bioethics, linked to the state and to a still-powerful medical profession, on the one hand, and the late and limited impact of this institutionalization upon everyday care, on the other hand, is specific to the French context. Patients' voices and, in general, a public debate around ethical issues have had a hard time emerging as a driving force for change within the healthcare context. Mostly, these changes have been either politically initiated or intraprofessionally regulated, with little input from the lay world.

Another specific feature of French bioethics is—in the spirit of the Enlightenment—its strong claim to a universalistic mission in bioethics and to an "alternative path" of its own, often presented as a counter-model to American bioethics. France has positioned itself against the professionalization of bioethics, advocating an ethics of medical responsibility, and strongly emphasizing the concept of dignity (and solidarity), against the notion of autonomy paramount in the United States.

Bioethics and Clinical Ethics: An "Institutional" Dissonance

The U.S. bioethics movement emerged in the late 1960s as a response to questionable practices in human experimentation (Rothman, 1991), introducing a revolution in the patient's world of rights, promoting autonomy and informed consent. Few similar changes could, however, be observed elsewhere, particularly in France. In fact, "la bioéthique à la française," as referred to by a French minister (Lenoir, 1991), focused mainly and from the very beginning on modes of accountability to mankind and future generations, and very little on bedside ethics and accountability to patients. The main institutional changes concerned the creation of review boards (CCPPRB)[1] similar to IRBs, set up by the *Loi Huriet* as late as in 1988,[2] and the introduction of mandatory informed consent for patients enrolled in clinical trials.

The creation in 1983 of the CCNE, the first national consultative council on ethics, illustrates the specific path chosen by French bioethics. Its mission was defined as follows: "to give advice on the moral problems which are raised by research in biology, medicine, and in the field of health; problems that concern mankind, social groups, and society as a whole." This institution, despite its advisory role, has been very active in defining norms and producing expertise through numerous reports, becoming the most quoted source in Assembly debates on any related bioethical topic from assisted reproduction to (more recently) end of life. In fact, the CCNE can be viewed as a norm-producing institution, defining what should be considered as an ethical question. The prominence of issues related to the beginning of life in the French bioethics can be viewed less as the result of a Catholic heritage (Fox, 2008) than as part of the prevailing rhetoric about the future of humanity, and the responsibility toward society as a whole. CCNE members are mostly physicians or research scientists selected by the government,[3] although a few are philosophers or law professors from the academic world. Most, if not all, members of the CCNE are public servants; the private sector and the lay world are practically not represented. There are no members from the community. Of the thirty-nine members, five are personalities belonging to "the principal philosophical and spiritual movements."[4] Most of the Council's internal debates take place behind closed doors—further evidence of the weakness of any lay intrusion into French

1. CCPPRB: *comites consultatifs de protection des personnes dans la recherche biomédicale.*

2. Implemented, in fact, as late as 1990.

3. 64 per cent of the committee in the years from 1983 to 1993.

4. Quoted from the official site of the CCNE defining its mission. (. . .) "philosophical movements and Catholic, Protestant, Jewish, and Muslim religions."

bioethics (Orfali, 2002). While there were discussions in 1994 about extending the CCNE's role into clinical practice, the idea was never adopted, on the grounds that this function was already part of the jurisdiction of the *Ordre des Médecins.* Despite its powerful role (Memmi, 1996; 2003), the CCNE refuses to take an authoritarian jurisdiction over ethical matters. In fact the CCNE, while having no power to enforce any laws, and relying heavily on a nonauthoritarian rhetoric, remains the key player in the French bioethical framework. As expressed by one of its members, Professor Jean Bernard: "The power of the CCNE is not legal but moral. That is what gives its recommendations their value."[5]

The Bioethics Laws of 1994 created the *Agence de la biomedicine,* a public organization that has an oversight role regarding "good clinical practice" in the domains of transplantation, reproduction, embryology, and human genetics. This agency reports directly to the parliament, the government, and to the CCNE. Bioethics laws deal with the status of the human body (which cannot be "commodified"[6]), and with cloning and eugenism (which are considered as "crimes against humanity"). These laws are under revision today. Within the current working group for the revision of these laws—mostly high-ranking public experts from medicine, law or public administration—the focus remains again on regulating matters at the beginning of life, such as prenatal testing, research on embryos, assisted reproduction, and surrogate motherhood,[7] which seem to remain continuing, controversial topics among French experts.

Despite this strong institutionalization of bioethics, has the accountability to society through the CCNE, and to the human research subject with the *Loi Huriet,* extended to the patient who is not involved in any experimental protocols? Actually, changes regarding patients enrolled in clinical trials have been more or less enforced from outside, as the major Anglo-Saxon medical journals have imposed new ethical norms for any medical research to be published. The main debate in France regarding bedside ethics focused first on the right to information and the free access to one's own medical records, which were granted in 1995 with the revision of the *Code de Déontologie Médicale.* The publication of a "Hospital Patient's Chart," and a judgment by the highest appeals court, the *Cour de Cassation* in 1997, requiring physicians to prove they had given patients all the information they needed to consent to a procedure, subsequently

5. J.Bernard. «Le comité consultatif national d'éthique.» Rencontre avec le professeur Jean Bernard, *Catéchèse*, n98, janvier 1985, p. 71.

6. These laws are currently under revision.

7. Personal communication with Law Professor B. Feuillet, member of the working group for the Revision of the Bioethics Laws (July, 2008).

brought about changes to the Civil Code (Article 16-3) and a law on patients' rights, as late as in 2002. Yet, there are still many restrictions to patients' full autonomy as it is understood in American bioethics. A patient can still be not fully informed of a lethal diagnosis if her doctor considers that such information could be harmful for her. Interestingly, the *Code de Santé Publique,* in its new version of March 2002, while stating that each person has the right to information, mentions[8] that "each person makes, *with* the healthcare professional and according to the information and recommendations given, decisions regarding her health."[9] Despite increasing patient access to information, the physician still controls what kind of information is to be given, and the law does emphasize a participatory model more than a clear patient-autonomy norm. As S. Rameix (1996) remarks: "We are getting out of the paternalistic model; we are drawn to the autonomy model, such as it is in Northern Europe or in the U.S., but such an autonomy model is not compatible with the French moral and political representations."[10] In fact, several studies point to a discrepancy between the law and the reality within the clinical setting (Broclain, 2001; Fainzang, 2006).

While attention to bedside ethics has increased within the hospitals, with the creation of ethics committees, informal groups and, in 1995, the more formal *Espace Ethique,* by the largest French public hospital network (APHP), there has been hardly any widespread development of clinical ethics (Mino; 2002), as in the United States. There are no "ethicists" in France (DeVries et al., 2009) and the idea is even ridiculed (Hervé et al., 2004). The very first, and still single, clinical ethics center in France opened as late as 2002,[11] following the MacLean model at the University of Chicago (Orfali, 2003). Matters related to clinical ethics remain strongly in the hands of the medical profession, while matters related to bioethics are under the oversight of high-ranking public experts; both groups operate within a national healthcare system largely governed by civil servant experts, who are mostly linked to the medical profession. In contrast with the American legal context, in which the jurisprudence stemming from case-by-case court actions plays an active role, changes around bioethical questions are made

8. Article L.1111-4, *Code de la Sante Publique,* March 4, 2002. « *Toute personne prend,* avec *le professionnel de la santé et compte tenu des informations et des préconisations qu'il lui fournit, les décisions concernant sa santé.* »

9. The patient is supposed, as implied here, to decide with her doctor and, in a way, to comply.

10. Translated by author. S.Rameix, "Quelles sont les dimensions éthiques de l'expression et du respect du consentement aux actes médicaux,"in *Gazette du Palais,* du 1er au 5 janvier 1999.

11. The author, at the time Assistant Director at the MacLean Center for Clinical Ethics at the University of Chicago, introduced, for the first time, clinical ethics at a conference of the *Etats Géneraux de la Santé* on May 19, 1999, and worked closely with the French Ministry of Health to set up a center in Paris and train its current director in clinical ethics.

in France by laws enacted through the French parliament. Until very recently, few laws regulated clinical practice, leading to a professional self-regulation by hospital physicians facing new ethical dilemmas within a legal framework that was often obsolete, given the technological changes in medicine. French clinical practice has been under very limited outside scrutiny or accountability. As mentioned by J.F Mattei,[12] a Minister of Health and a physician himself: "The evaluation of (clinical) practice cannot be done by those who pay, or even by the state: it should be done by the professionals themselves."

The institutional dissonance between an elaborated, formal, and highly visible bioethical framework—dealing with such grandiose questions as the impact of science, research, technology, and medicine on the human being and the future of mankind—and a quieter, medically self-regulated world of clinical ethics, is largely due to the absence of lay voices[13] in the world of French medical ethics, and in hospitals in general (Orfali, forthcoming), despite a strong institutional rhetoric of healthcare democracy and patients' participation. After all, patients' associations (*Associations d'usagers*) took decades to be accepted within French hospitals. The more visible the institutional framework of bioethics is in France at the political and social (and even international) level and the less debated in the public opinion is the mundane world of bedside ethics—even though, from time to time, according to specific circumstances, the euthanasia debate rekindles within the media.

The Ethics of Medical Responsibility

In France, clinical ethics remain largely under medical authority, despite recent legal changes affecting patients' rights. The norm of informed consent, which today is a legal requirement for any medical intervention on a patient, is valid only if the patient is fully competent. Families and more generally lay surrogate decision making remain elusive in the clinic. Several studies (Ferrand et al., 2001; Pochard et al., 2001) have shown a better sharing of information with families in intensive care units, yet little role of families in decision making. In fact, French physicians, caught between a legal vacuum (or, more accurately, an obsolete legal framework outpaced by medical/technological changes) and new norms promoted by the bioethical rhetoric of the CCNE, have attempted to discuss ethical standards regarding their practice and, more specifically, to negotiate

12. Translated by author. *«L'évaluation des pratiques ne peut pas être faite par l'Etat ou le payeur : elle doit relever des professionnels eux-mêmes.»* *Le Figaro*, August 31, 2002.

13. Except for AIDS patients, strongly supported by several AIDS associations and support groups.

around the informed consent process before any specific law was enacted. In assisted reproduction, neonatal care, and end-of-life care, for example, professional self-regulation around a rhetoric of "ethical medical responsibility" has been set up to respond to the challenging issues of ethical dilemmas, and life and death decisions. In doing so, the medical profession has demonstrated both its autonomy and its "ethical concern," anticipating the law and endorsing a duty of ethical medical responsibility on behalf of society.

In assisted reproduction techniques (ART), a well-studied field in France in ethics (Novaes, 1992; 1994; Mehl, 1999; 2008 Feuillet-Liger et al., 2011), despite many calls for a more open debate, even from the CCNE, the whole selection system, remains entirely public and completely controlled by physicians within the framework set up by the 1994 Bioethics Law (Kunstmann, 2011). ART doctors[14] decide who should and should not benefit from ART. Responding to increased criticism of this overwhelming medical power, and what some critics view as somewhat a eugenist approach (Testart, 1989; 1990), ART physicians tend to put forward their medical responsibility (Novaes, 1992) more in moral terms than in legal ones. As the traditional public health approach in France is based on asking experts in a given field for normative guidance, ethical authority ends up being based on technical expertise (DeVries et al., 2009; Orfali, 2004). As a result, there is little ethical debate outside the professional world of experts and, again, little input from the lay world regarding clinical ethics.

However medicalized this ethical approach may seem, favoring the medical establishment and their authority, it has in fact brought about more changes within the medical profession itself than expected. Novaes (1992) showed, for example, how the ART experts[15]—dealing with decisions to allow or not to allow infertile couples[16] with a known genetic anomaly to get a child through ART—discussed at length the pros and cons, emphasizing strongly the moral nature of their medical responsibility. Never did these experts envision that the infertile couple should have the ultimate say in such a complex decision. Taking the risk of giving birth to a severely handicapped child is perceived as medically and ethically unprofessional—first toward the child herself, secondly toward her parents—notwithstanding the social and medical cost for society. The notion of medical responsibility is not directed solely toward the couple, but toward the outcome as a whole, involving society. Medical responsibility, perceived not as a legal obligation but as a moral contract, binding not only the infertile couple

---

14. From the CECOS, which is a network of around 20 gametes banks in France.

15. Commission de Génétique des CECOS.

16. Even if the couple is willing to take such a risk.

and the ART physician, but also the unborn child, and even society as a whole, becomes a guiding ethical principle within French health care. Individual rights and clinical decisions tend to be absorbed into the rhetoric of a larger bioethical framework of societal choices related to problems of normality, parentage, unknown consequences, and duties toward the unborn and society.

Another striking area for the study of challenging ethical dilemmas, and life and death decision making, is neonatal care. Empirical studies in pediatric and neonatal care are still scarce in France (Paillet, 1999; 2007; Orfali, 2004; Orfali et al., 2004) but they all point to professional self-regulation of neonatologists in dealing with difficult ethical issues. Despite the legal norm of parental authority over their minor children, most French parents, particularly in neonatology, do not decide their child's fate. Ethical decisions are viewed as medical decisions, relying on experts (Orfali, 2004). The current justification for such parental exclusion (Dehan, 1986), despite repeated calls by the CCNE and others for increased parental and lay intervention in medical care, is again that the moral duty of neonatologists is to "undo what they have done": by resuscitating babies at the threshold of viability, they have created the potentially extreme situation (and burden) of severely damaged premature infants. French neonatologists, therefore, consider it a matter of ethical responsibility toward the damaged child, the parents, and society to take care themselves of the dramatic decision to withdraw and withhold care. They even view it as cruel and unethical to explicitly ask the parents for consent in such dramatic situations (Orfali et al. 2004), especially as they consider the "making of such a situation" as their own burden. There is almost a professional consensus in France around this specific norm within neonatal care, with no public debate or many questions arising in the media about such issues.

Cases involving the ethics of end-of-life (EOL) decisions have, however, raised more controversy in public opinion. Some recent and dramatic examples (*Affaire Humbert* in 2003[17] and *Affaire Chantal Sébire* in 2008[18]) have triggered a debate on euthanasia. In France, as in most Western countries, more than 50%

17. In 2004, the Humbert case involved the mother and the physician of a young boy, severely handicapped after a car accident, who had repeatedly asked to die. The patient had tried to draw the attention of the media and the politicians by writing an open letter to the French president. With help of his mother, Marie Humbert, and the hospital physician, he finally died. The uproar around the Humbert case triggered the creation of the EOL law in 2005.

18. The recent case of Chantal Sébire (2008) involved a severely defigurated woman with a rare lethal condition, who demanded to be allowed to be euthanized. As she was not yet considered to be terminally ill, she therefore could not, under the current EOL law, be helped in any way. She ended up killing herself.

of deaths are linked to a decision to end life.[19] Still, until very recently, the obsolete legal framework gave hospital physicians a discretionary power to deal with these matters, with little external oversight. While there were considerable variations in EOL practice between units (although euthanasia was illegal, and still is), there has been considerable intra professional discussion at local and national levels (through professional associations in intensive care, etc.) to set up ethical norms regarding end-of-life practice (for instance, requiring that doctors make EOL decisions collegially instead of individually). For years, numerous commissions, meetings,[20] and reports by the CCNE (all involving little or no lay input) have worked on EOL matters. The Leonetti Commission, whose report was the basis for the highly expected EOL law in 2004, was again composed of experts. Not even Marie Humbert—who played a leading role in making the EOL debate an "open agenda," and who was widely praised in parliament—was interviewed by the commission. The weakness of the role of civil society, and of any lay intrusion into ethical matters in medicine, translates into clinical ethics remaining under public medical expertise and oversight. In the EOL Law of 2005, while a competent patient can refuse any further medical intervention, his family or his durable power of attorney have no decision-making power should he become incapacitated; they must be "consulted," but the EOL decision remains a medical collegial decision. Interestingly, the EOL law states that the opinion of the incapacitated patient's healthcare proxy prevails "*upon all non-medical opinions*"[21] (clearly implying that it cannot prevail upon *medical* opinions). Even advance directives, revised by the competent patient every three years, are simply "taken into account" by the attending physician. The wording of the French EOL law carefully avoids the language of patient autonomy and decision-making power. The law mandates in several sections, the physician's responsibility to "*protect the dying patient's dignity*."

By demonstrating that they act both responsibly and virtuously, the physicians, allied to institutional experts[22] through professional self-regulation, manage to respond to the new challenges regarding ethical dilemmas and ethical requirements, produced by the CCNE and others, by turning ethical decisions into

---

19. Memmi, p. 17, quoting *Le Monde,* November 12, 2001, p. 10.

20. The author was part of a specific meeting in 2001 on the subject of EOL (*Fin de Vie*) called by B. Kouchner with among others, Paul Ricoeur, Luc Ferry, A. Fageot-Largault, L.Badinter, representatives from the main religions in France, etc. The proceedings were published in *Fin de Vie, Ministère de l'Emploi et de la Solidarité,* May 31, 2001.

21. Although not on the patient's own advance directives.

22. These experts are often physicians named by the government as advisers in different political or scientific commissions, and institutions (CCNE, *Agence de la biomedicine,* etc.).

medical ones and by producing a consensual discourse on the ethics of medical responsibility. By negotiating carefully around the legal requirements of informed consent, and by avoiding any surrogate decision making, they tend to preserve their important discretionary role on matters of clinical ethics, such as life and death decisions, treatment decisions, and others. In the end, physicians act as if they were mandated both by the state and by society to be the "ethical gatekeepers" of the health care system. As mentioned by the novelist and physician M. Winckler,[23] the medical profession tends to keep EOL matters in their own hands, even stating (despite the 2004 law) that in such dramatic situations, "no law is possible."[24] By seeking to compromise with the concerns expressed by the CCNE (considered to be the speaker for "society's concerns"), by reshaping the norms of "good" clinical practice, by turning ethical issues into medical ones, and by being the consulted experts for the making of laws, French physicians have emphasized the moral obligations of their profession in new terms. Given the still-high trust in the medical profession within the French society,[25] and the overall satisfaction of the public with the nationalized healthcare system, the strategy of shifting medical accountability to society as a whole, instead of to the individual patient, has not been met by much resistance in France. The following recommendations by the CCNE, regarding end-of-life issues in the NICU as requiring a different approach than EOL in general, illustrate the specificity of the French approach:

> "(...) regarding the newborn, for whom can her life seem unbearable? Isn't it less the infant's suffering that is here the main concern, and more the fact that this vegetative life is being prolonged and becomes unbearable for her family, who alone will have to take care of her; for her healthcare team, who have failed her; for society, who will have to bear the costs of a life that will never ever develop and flourish ..." [26]

---

23. «Le paternalisme médical français interdit tout débat sur l'euthanasie», March 13, 2007.

24. Christophe Rufin, *Nouvel Observateur*, March 8, 2007.

25. Despite many scandals, such as the contaminated blood or the growth hormone affair (Orfali, 2001).

26. *« S'agissant du nouveau-né, pour qui sa vie apparaît-elle insupportable? N'est-ce pas moins la souffrance de l'enfant qui est en cause, que le fait que cette vie végétative se prolonge et en devient "insupportable" pour la famille qui en assumera seule la charge réelle, pour l'équipe soignante dont elle marque l'échec, ou pour la société qui doit engager des frais importants pour une vie qui ne se développera et s'épanouira jamais ?»* Translated by author. CCNE, Report no. 65: *"réflexions éthiques autour de la réanimation néonatale."*

After all, this approach might be consistent with a nationalized healthcare system and with institutions that all are public, and defend the same notion of "public good." In the Jacobin tradition, the public institutions, and the public leadership in general, are viewed as defenders of this general interest, defined as "universal," over particular interests (Schmidt, 1999; Prasad, 2005). The success of this French model lies in making the "public good" and the "patient's individual best interest" coincide as much as possible—which seems the case, at least at the rhetorical level of bioethical discourse.

A Counter-Model to American Bioethics?

As a nation with a self-appointed universal mission, France has developed an "alternative path," often presented as a counter-model to the American bioethics. Thus, the French bioethical enterprise has produced a unique rhetoric of universality, avoiding words such as "autonomy" or "decision making" and emphasizing the terminology of "dignity," "solidarity" and "ethical medical responsibility," while rejecting strongly any professionalization of ethics (Hervé et al., 2004: DeVries et al., 2009).[27] At the same time, while aspiring to a universal rhetoric, France[28] tends to constantly advocate (in bioethics, as in other fields) the notion of an *exception culturelle francaise.*[29] The French bioethical framework thus embodies the double reference of "universality and contextuality" (Callahan, 2003) without apparent dichotomy.

Most published papers dealing with bioethics and clinical ethical practices tend to systematically compare the medical practices in France with the prevailing American autonomy norm, viewed as a key reference. Generally speaking, most surveys and studies conclude that French physicians and French medical practice rarely follow the American path in matters of clinical ethics. Bioethical or medical works published in French tend to clearly position themselves "against" the American bioethical model, dismissing that model as irrelevant to the particular cultural context of French values, and contrasting the Anglo-Saxon bioethics with their own, solidarity-based bioethical framework. As Paillet (1999) shows in her study of pediatric intensive care units, there is a recurrent "rhetoric of nationalization" that is put forward as a model with equal, if not higher, ethical validity and claim to universality than the U.S. model. The American bioethics

27. There are no ethicists in France, and the word doesn't even exist. (The French Canadian uses the term "éthicien".)

28. This paradox is probably linked to the Enlightment model, considered, in a way, as both historically French and universal.

29. French cultural exception, translated by author.

model is to be dismissed and even rejected, as leading to the lack of trust and overwhelming litigation that characterize U.S. health care. In fact, the American autonomy norm is viewed less as a bioethical model than as a constraint externally imposed by the legal system on behalf of private health insurance companies. Parents are viewed as the "victims of this system," with a terrible burden imposed upon them, as mentioned in the neonatal ethical literature.[30] The high rate of litigation in the United States is, in fact, seen as the result of the American bioethical model gone awry.

Highly critical of the American autonomy paradigm, France has attempted to create a model that can be viewed as a compromise between the language of individual rights and the language of public good, more suitable for the context of socialized health care. The legacy of *human* rights, so specific to France and its inception in the bioethics rhetoric and project, has to be distinguished from *individual* rights, which has had little impact in the French public health model until very recently.[31] In reality, the French healthcare system's tardiness in addressing the needs and the role of its patients[32] undoubtedly reflects the separation between the medical and the social spheres, between the world of public experts and the lay world, so characteristic of the French system. Moreover, the French state is "strong institutionally: centralized (. . .) and politically guided by a corps of officials impervious (ideally, if not in fact) to outside pressure" (Nathansson, 2007); it remains a "deciding power" of public health. Thus, there are but few legitimate alternatives to action by the state. "Non-state groups that seek to advance their own ideas of the collective good are perceived as representing *intérêts particuliers* (private interests) and may be regarded not only as self-serving but as an impediment to action by the state." As a result, and compared to many other countries, the collective action (except for the AIDS movement) on behalf of public health goals by civil society remains weak in France. Thus, bioethics at the level of the CCNE, or clinical ethics in France, remain matters of medical and political experts, emerging less from any grassroots action or lay debate than from political will.

---

30. "The role given to parents, or actually imposed upon them, is due, in part at least, to the legal system, which itself is dependent on the insurance system, particularly in the United States." Translated by author. « *le rôle ainsi dévolu, pour ne pas dire imposé, aux parents, s'explique en partie au moins par le poids de la justice lui-même tributaire des assurances, aux Etats-Unis en particulier* » [Beaufils, Denizart, Meric, 1992).

31. The new-found importance of individual over collective interests represents a true but still limited break with the traditional model of public health policies (Orfali, 1997) and is, in France, very much linked to the AIDS patient and the policy surrounding the AIDS epidemic.

32. For example, the various hospital boards of directors were only opened up to patient advocates in 1996.

The notion of "participatory democracy"—born, in fact, from political will—is viewed as a recent alternative path, which has promoted the idea of an active patient, and a call for a fully informed patient (Caniard, 2001). In 1998, the so-called *Etats Géneraux de la Santé* attempted, through a system of surveys, to promote the idea of a "healthcare democracy"(*démocratie sanitaire*) (Orfali, 2001). The discrepancy between the reality of clinical practices, in which patient's autonomy and decision-making power isn't fully acquired, and the strong public and political rhetoric of participation, is one of the major characteristics of today's French ethics. The strong emphasis on patients' movements,[33] often born out of yesterday's mobilizations around AIDS (Barbot, 2002), and now around many other diseases (cancer, muscular dystrophy, etc.), is hardly representative of the ordinary hospital patient (Orfali, 1997; Fainzang, 2006) whose voice, in the current healthcare system, remains weak.

The overall weakness of any ethical debate in France within the public opinion, despite some more polemical cases around euthanasia (a topic with no closure yet) seems to suggest the existence of an implicit social consensus on such matters. While some authors mention the complex and contradictory relationship of French citizens to the state, made of reliance and trust and at the same time intense suspicion (Nathansson, 2007), in reality most ethical dilemmas, and most life and death decisions, are still today—despite legal changes—managed by physicians with little visible resistance from the lay world. The CCNE at one point recognized (2000) that active euthanasia could be allowed under exceptional circumstances as a "transgression," and the notion of *arrêt de vie*[34] still exists, for example, in neonatal care and even in published literature. ART, EOL, neonatal resuscitation, to mention but a few of the most challenging ethical issues, remain heavily under physicians' scrutiny and under medical intervention. Families remain under their physician's oversight regarding such choices. The medical establishment—particularly those who operate in public hospitals—have a crucial role as the ethical gatekeepers of "good clinical practice" within the healthcare system.[35] They tend to operate today less in a blunt, authoritarian way, avoiding the language of control, triage, and surveillance, and adopting a more libertarian paternalism (Sunstein et al., 2003), a pervasive and convincing rhetoric of ethical responsibility.

---

33. As mentioned by several sociological studies: (Dodier 2002, Aiach et al., 1994).

34. *"Arret de vie"* is the term used by French neonatologists to describe active termination of life despite the fact that intentional termination of life is considered illegal.

35. Among health professionals of all sorts, physicians today still hold a central position. In fact, the power held by hospital physician unions is all the more remarkable, given that it is in no way founded in law (Stasse, 1999).

Despite a public opinion already sensitized to serious institutional deficiencies by the recent scandals regarding blood contamination or growth hormone, there still seems to be surprisingly high trust in medicine (Hassentefeul, 1997)[36] and less litigation, compared to the United States. The medical standpoint has always held priority in France, in the chain of any health policy decision making and in the bioethical framework, possibly even at the expense of other social factors. Through the rhetoric of ethical medical responsibility and "healthcare democracy," the medical establishment, allied with institutional players, has been able to reshape the traditional power structure and create new modes of legitimization, focusing the ethical debate around issues related to information given to the patient, and retaining, in reality, decision-making authority under medical oversight. In that sense, patient autonomy has never gained any recognition in France as a rational, right-oriented notion empowering a fully informed decision-maker, as in American bioethics. Not only are there several limits to the information included, even in the French law, but the physicians are endowed with an ethical responsibility toward the patient, who is viewed as a "vulnerable" person. Thus the notion of "vulnerability" is strongly emphasized in French bioethics, and considered as a central concept in many medical ethics and philosophical writings (Levinas, 1961; Jonas 1991).

Conclusion

France has positioned itself against the professionalization of bioethics, defending an ethics of medical responsibility toward a "vulnerable" patient and emphasizing strongly the concept of *dignity* over autonomy (Orfali & Feuillet,working paper), and the notion of solidarity over individualism. While in the United States, the contested concept of dignity is debated at length,[37] often as "useless" (Macklin, 2003), "hopelessly vague," or too religious, it remains one of the core values of French bioethics. In French jurist Noelle Lenoir's view, it is the very task of human rights law to protect intrinsic *human dignity* in technological development, and to promote, through such goals, humanistic ideals. While self-determination is viewed as resting solely on an agent's capacity to exercise autonomous choices, dignity alludes to the notion of membership in the human species. Offending or betraying this membership, which is viewed as a

36. Several polls in France (Enquete SOFRES) and outside France (Harris Interactive, 2008, and OCDE) report that the French people's satisfaction with their health care and their physicians is higher than in any other country.

37. The President's Council on Bioethics, established in 2001 by President Bush, issued a contested report on Human Dignity and Bioethics.

"universal" world heritage, should justify state interference[38] as well as international oversight. In that sense, France, with its strong legacy of human rights, carries a powerful claim to a universalistic mission in international bioethics.

This French path has been quite successful among countries more concerned with principles of civic solidarity, and characterized by relationships between private and public, individual and collective, different from the United States—as shown in multiple texts of international organizations such as UNESCO and others. Today, following the French model of CCNE, more than 40 countries have implemented National Bioethics Commissions. The French rhetoric promoting dignity over autonomy seems to gain increased attention not only in the European context, but even in South and Central America, as observed recently at a UNESCO regional bioethical conference (2007).[39]

Finally, it is important to realize that the increased institutionalization of bioethics, observed not only in France but everywhere, at a national or even international level, does not necessarily generate transformation at the hospital bedside level, and does not systematically translate into more rights and empowerment of patients in everyday care. The 1994 Declaration on the Promotion of Patients' Rights in Europe, for example, allows the physician in exceptional cases to retain any information she deems harmful for her patient, showing the same limits to full disclosure as the French law, in the name of "therapeutic justification,"[40] and the same reluctance to embrace the autonomy paradigm so prevalent in the U.S. bioethics. While national ethics committees, hospital committees, and even laws appear almost everywhere around the globe, in fact they regulate research more often than care, and their weak impact upon bedside ethics and medical practice (as observed through still too-limited, empirical cross-cultural ethnographic work) should raise concern. Civil society, patients, families, or caregivers are less concerned with the future of humanity, or the moral issues involved in cloning, than they are with care or end-of-life decisions. Their highest concern is to have a say in matters of health. Has bioethics promoted such things, or has it remained more just a rhetoric of empowerment? As suggested by the French path and many of its followers, there might be more than a cultural dissonance between autonomy and dignity, between private and public—suggesting an incompatibility of models and systems between those who defend a public service, and those who believe first and above all in the individual's rights.

---

38. When the French Parliament in 2004 qualified cloning as "a crime against the human species," it explicitly referred to the impermissible violation of the very dignity of human nature.

39. Convencion Subregional de Bioetica. UNESCO, Santo Domingo, Dominican Republic, March 28–30, 2007.

40. Article 35 of the *Code de Déontologie*.

Glossary

Agence de la Biomedicine is a public institution created by the Bioethics Laws of 1994. It has an oversight and expertise role regarding "good clinical practice" in the domains of transplantation, reproduction, embryology, and human genetics.

APHP (*Assistance Publique des Hopitaux de Paris*) is a network of public hospitals, one of the largest in Europe. Providing health care, teaching, research, prevention, education, and emergency medical service in 52 branches of medicine, it employs more than 90,000 people in 44 hospitals.

CCNE, *Conseil Consultatif National d'Ethique pour les Sciences de la Vie et de la Santé* [National Consultative Ethics Committee on Life Sciences and Health] was created on February 23, 1983, by a decree of the President of the Republic, F. Mitterand.

Code de Déontologie Médicale established for the first time in 1947 by the *Ordre des Médecins,* regulates the professional duties of the physician. The Code is regularly updated.

Code de la Santé Publique created in 1953 and updated several times, is the legal code regulating matters related to health.

Loi Huriet named after then French Minister of Health, is the law of December 20, 1988, concerning the protection of the human subjects of biomedical research. This law (implemented in 1990) brought into existence the CCPRB.

CCPPRB *Comités consultatifs de protection des personnes dans la recherche biomédicale* are consultative committees for the protection of persons who undergo biomedical research. They are very similar to the IRB committees in the United States.

Espace Ethique was created within APHP in 1995 to discuss ethical matters among health caregivers.

Etats Généraux de la Santé Organized by the government, the *Etats Generaux de la Sante* was a vast survey of the healthcare system (and cancer patients) throughout the country, intended to find out the needs of the general population and foster a so-called "healthcare democracy" ("*Democratie Sanitaire*").

Lenoir, Noelle French stateswoman, was the leader of the report on bioethics to the French Prime Minister: *"Aux Frontières de la vie," Collection des rapports officiels, La Documentation Française,* Paris, 1991. She was the chair of the International Bioethics Committee of UNESCO, responsible for the Universal Declaration on the Human Genome and Human Rights, approved by the United Nations General Assembly in 1998. She has been the chairman of the European Group on Ethics with the European Commission.

Leonetti Commission named after Jean Leonetti, a deputy in the National Assembly who chaired the parliamentary mission on end of life. The end-of-life law was passed in 2004 following the recommendations of the Leonetti Commission.

Mattei, Jean-Francois pediatrician and geneticist, was a member of the CCNE until 1997 and has been one of the key persons involved in the preparation of the

1994 Bioethics Laws. He was the Minister of Health between 2002 and 2003, and is currently the President of the Red Cross in France. He is the author of numerous publications in the field of ethics and bioethics.

Ordre des Médecins In France, all physicians are required to register with the *Ordre des Médecins,* an institution created (under the Vichy government) to monitor access to the profession and maintain a professional deontology. The *Ordre des Medecins* is an oversight body that sanctions any physician who violates the *Code de Deontologie* (Deontology Code).

Wincler, Martin is a physician and well-known French novelist. One of his best-known novels, *The Case of Dr Sachs,* 1998, translated in several languages, was made into a film.

References

Aiach et al. (1994). « Crise, pouvoir et légitimité » in *Les métiers de la santé. Enjeux de pouvoir et quête de légitimité*, Paris, Anthropos-Economica.

Beaufils F, Denizart V, Meric M. (1992). La décision d'arrêt thérapeutique en réanimation néonatale. Rôle des familles et de l'équipe soignante. *Annales médicales de Nancy et de l'Est,* numéro spécial sur Les décisions d'arrêt thérapeutique en réanimation (adultes et nouveaux nés). *Journées d'éthique médicale*, Abbaye des Prémontrés, Pont à Mousson 21–22 (juin); 31: 355–357.

Barbot J. (2002). *Les malades en mouvements. La médecine en mouvements. La médecine et la science à l'épreuve du sida*. Paris : Balland.

Botti S, Orfali K, Iengar S. (2009). Tragic choices: autonomy and emotional responses in medical decision contexts. Leading Article in *Journal of Consumer Research*. 39(3): 337–352.

Broclain D. (2001). *La place de la personne hospitalisée dans la décision en cardiologie.* Paris : *Rapport pour la Fondation de l'avenir.*

Callahan D. (2003). Individual good and common good: A communitarian approach to bioethics. *Perspectives in Biology and Medicine* 46(4): 496–507.

Dehan M. (1986). Introduction in *Archives Françaises de Pédiatrie*, *43*, supplément spécial, Ethique et réanimation du nouveau-né et de l'enfant, pp. 543–544.

Dehan M. (1997). L'éthique et sa Pratique en Néonatologie. In Folscheid D., Feuillet-Le Mintier B., Mattei J.F. *Philosophie, éthique et droit de la médecine*, Paris, Presses Universitaires de France.

DeVries R., Dingwall R, Orfali K. (2009). The moral organization of the professions: Bioethics in France and in the United States. *Current Sociology* 57: 555–579.

Dodier N. (2002). Recomposition de la médecine dans ses rapports avec la science. Les leçons du sida. *Santé publique et sciences socials*, 8–9: 37–52.

Fainzang S. (2006). *La relation médecins-malades: information et mensonge*. Paris: Presses Universitaires de France.

Feuillet-Liger B. Orfali K., Callus T. (ed.) (2011). *Who is my Genetic Parent ? Donor Anonymity and Assisted Reproduction : a Cross-Cultural Perspective.*, Bruylant, Bruxelles.

Ferrand E, Bachoud-Levi AC, Rodrigues M, Maggiore S, Brun-Buisson C, Lemaire F. (2001). Decision making capacity and surrogate designation in French ICU patients. *Intensive Care Medicine* 27: 1360–1364.

"*Fin de Vie*" (2001). published in May by the Ministère de l'Emploi et de la Solidarité, Ministère délegué de la Santé. Paris, France.

Fox CR, Swazey JP. (2008), *Observing Bioethics*. New York: Oxford University Press.

Garel M et al. (2000). Attitudes et Pratiques des soignants confrontés à des problèmes éthiques en néonatologie, *Médecine thérapeutique/Pédiatrie*. 3(6): 443–449.

Hassentefeul P. (1997). *Les Médecins face à l'Etat, une comparaison européenne*. Paris: Presses de la FNSP.

Hervé C, Hirsch E. (2004). *Le Manifeste*, « Résister à l'idéologisation de l'éthique des professions de santé » May 7th, 2004, http : www.espace-ethique.org/fr/manifeste.php. (Resisting the ideologization of ethics in the health professions): a manifesto against the notion of « ethicist » as a profession.

Kunstmann J.M. (2011). « Medically assisted reproduction with a third party donor: rethinking anonymity in France. An insider's view. » in Chapt.1, in Feuillet-Liger B. Orfali K., Callus T., *Who is my Genetic Parent? Donor Anonymity and Assisted Reproduction : a Cross-Cultural Perspective.* Bruylant, Bruxelles

Jonas H. (1991). *Le principe de responsabilité. Une éthique pour la civilisation technologique*. Paris : Cerf.

Lenoir N. (1991). *Aux frontières de la vie*. Tome 1 : Une éthique biomédicale à la française, Tome 2 : Paroles d'éthique. Paris: La Documentation française.

Levinas E.(1961). *Totalité et infini: essai sur l'extériorité*. Paris: Livre de poche.

LOI (*Loi Huriet*) n88–1138 du 20 decembre 1988 relative à la protection des personnes qui se prêtent à des recherches biomédicales

LOIS (Lois dites de la bioéthique) de 1994 (Under the so called Bioethics Laws of 1994) :

Loi n94–548 du 1er Juillet 1994 relative au traitement de données nominatives ayant pour fin la recherche dans le domaine de la santé et modifiant la loi n° 78-17 du 6 janvier 1978 relative à l'informatique, aux fichiers et aux libertés.

Loi 94–654 du 19 Juillet 1994 relative au don et à l'utilisation des éléments et produits du corps humain, à l'assistance médicale à la procréation et au diagnostic prénatal *bioéthique*.

Loi 94–653 du 29 Juillet 1994. relative au respect du corps humain

LOI n°2002–2003 du 3 Mars 2002 sur les Droits des Patients et la Qualité du système de santé.

LOI n° 2004-800 du 6 août 2004 relative à la bioéthique (under revision 2008).

LOI n 2005–370 du 22 Avril 2005 relative aux droits des malades et à la fin de vie.

Macklin R. (2003). *Dignity is a useless concept.* Editorial. *British Medical Journal* 20(327): December: 1419–1420.

Mehl D. (1999). *Naitre? La controverse éthique.* Paris: Bayard.

Mehl D. (2008). *Enfants Du Don - Procréation Médicalement Assistée: Parents Et Enfants Témoignent.* Paris:R.Laffont.

Memmi D. (1996). *Les gardiens du corps.* Paris: EHESS.

Memmi D. (2003). *Faire vivre et laisser mourir et laisser mourir. Le gouvernement contemporain de la naissance et de la mort.* Paris: La Découverte.

Mino JC. (2002). Lorsque l'autonomie du médecin est remise en cause par l'autonomie du patient: le champ hospitalier de l'éthique clinique aux Etats-Unis et en France. In « Ethique médicale, biomédicale. Débats, enjeux, pratiques » *al La Revue Française des Affaires Sociales*, juillet- septembre n3. Paris, La Documentation française.

Nathanson, C.A. (2007). Chapter 7: Engines of policy and civil society. In *Disease Prevention as Social Change: The State, Society, and Public Health in the United States, France, Great Britain, and Canada.* New York: The Russell Sage Foundation.

Novaes (Bateman) S. (1992). Ethique et débat public, *Raisons Pratiques* 3: 155–176.

Novaes (Bateman) S. (1994). *Les Passeurs de gametes.* Nancy, Presses Universitaires de Nancy.

Orfali K. (2001). Chapter 17: The French Paradoxes. In W. Cockerham, ed. *The Blackwell Companion to Medical Sociology.* Oxford, U.K.: Blackwell publishers.

Orfali K. (2002). "Lingérence profane dans la décision médicale: le malade, la famille et l'éthique clinique [The lay intrusion in medical decision making: the patient, the family and clinical ethics]. In Ethique médicale et biomédicale. Débats, enjeux, pratiques", *La Revue Française des Affaires Sociales*, juillet- septembre n3., Paris, La Documentation française.

Orfali K. (2003). L'émergence de l'éthique clinique: politique du sujet ou nouvelle catégorie de la clinique? [Clinical Ethics : a patient-centered approach or a clinical category?] *Sciences Sociales et Santé* 21(2), 31–70.

Orfali K. (2004). Parental role and medical decision making: fact or fiction? A comparative study of French and American practices in neonatal intensive care units. *Social Science and Medicine* 58: 2009–2022.

Orfali K, Gordon EJ. (2004). Autonomy gone awry: A cross-cultural study on parents' experiences in neonatal intensive care units. *Theoretical Medicine and Bioethics* 25: 329–365.

Orfali K, Feuillet B. (2011). Dignity versus autonomy in bioethics. Work in progress.

Paillet A. (1999). Les pédiatres français sur la brèche de l'éthique : analyse de leurs publications depuis 30 ans. *Rapport MIRE,* (Mission Recherche) de la DREES, (Direction de la Recherche, de l'Evaluation, des Etudes et des Statistiques du Ministère de la Santé et des Sports) France.

Paillet A. (2007). *Sauver la vie, donner la mort. Une sociologie de l'éthique en réanimation néonatale,* La Dispute, coll. « Corps, santé, société », Paris.

Pochard F et al. (2001). *French intensivists* do not apply American recommendations regarding decisions to forgo life-sustaining therapy. *Critical Care Medicine* 29(10): 1887–1892.

Prasad M. (2005). Why is France so French? Culture, institutions and neoliberalism. *American Journal of Sociology* 111(2): 357–407.

Rameix S. (1996). *Fondements philosophiques de l'éthique médicale.* Ellipses: Paris.

Rothman D. (1991). *Strangers at the bedside.* New York: Basic Books.

International Bioethics Seminar "Towards a Subregional Convention on Bioethics". (2007). Proceedings published as a book" *Hacia una convencion subregional de bioetica.*" UNESCO, March 28–30, Santo Domingo, Republica Dominicana.

Schmidt V. (1999). The changing dynamics of state-society relations in the fifth republic. *West European Politics* 22(4): 141–165.

Stasse F. (1999). *Les acteurs de la politique de santé,* in Le Pouvoir Medical. *Revue Pouvoirs 89*: publisher, Seuil.

Sunstein C, Thaler R. (2003). Libertarian paternalism is not an oxymoron. *University of Chicago Law Review* vol. 70, Fall, number 4, pp. 1159–1202.

Testart J. (1989). *La responsabilité du Chercheur. L'Evènement Européen 5*: 19–27.

Testart J. (1990). *Sperme en banque, bébés en carte. Libération, 16*: 5.

5 THE SOCIAL FORMS AND FUNCTIONS OF BIOETHICS IN THE UNITED KINGDOM

Richard E. Ashcroft and Mary Dixon-Woods

Bioethics is a complex social and intellectual phenomenon, and a comparative sociology of bioethics has yet to be seriously attempted. There is a plurality of institutional and professional forms, discourses, and practices, as well as a range of individuals who claim to speak authoritatively and advise legitimately on bioethical matters of clinical or policy concern. In this chapter, we trace a variety of contexts in England (and, where appropriate, the broader United Kingdom) in which bioethics exists, or its discourses are mobilized, codified, and used. In so doing, we identify a range of social functions fulfilled by bioethics.

Our account here is largely descriptive, aiming to provide an outline of the emergence and current character of bioethics in the U.K. In part, this descriptive emphasis is because a social science of bioethics in the U.K. is only just beginning to emerge, in contrast with a more long-standing tradition in the United States.[1] We believe that understanding a complex, newly emerging social phenomenon requires close attention to where it emerges, the forms it takes, and the purposes it serves—either by being made to serve these purposes, or as aspirations. Moreover, treating the version of bioethics now characteristic of U.S. academic, clinical, and policy settings as normative for a definition of bioethics itself, and thus for assessing the degree and quality of "development of bioethics" in other countries, neglects the social, historical, legal, and cultural contingency of many features of the U.S. version.

---

1. For the most recent and most thorough contribution to the sociology of bioethics in the United States, see Fox RC, Swazey JP. *Observing Bioethics*. New York: Oxford University Press, 2008. The literature from the U.K. on the relationship between sociology and bioethics as competing discourses on the "social life of biomedicine" is somewhat more extensive; some recent contributions can be found in De Vries R, Turner L, Orfali K, and Bosk CL (eds.) *The View from Here: Bioethics and the Social Sciences*. Oxford: Blackwell, 2007. This volume collates work from several countries, and therefore provides some useful comparative data.

Bioethics as an Academic Field

U.K. bioethics is reasonably well established as an academic field, though its practitioners derive from an eclectic range of disciplines, including law, philosophy, theology, and social science, and are located in a range of departmental homes in U.K. universities. There are a number of Master's programs in medical law, medical ethics, bioethics, and related fields, such as applied philosophy, but as yet few formal PhD programs in bioethics.[2] Clearly, this makes bioethics difficult to characterize as a single discipline, but it is fair to say that it is generally committed to the use of methods of analytical philosophy and empirical social science, and, in the main, to liberalism in political philosophy. Bioethics with a particular theological affiliation is an exception to this general rule, though this has tended to be relatively self-contained as a field, with reasonably strong activist tendencies, to which we shall return later.

The academic field has been invigorated by a number of distinct developments. One was a requirement from 1993 onward that medical ethics be taught as part of the undergraduate medical curriculum, which created many new academic posts located mainly in medical schools. Another has been the growing attention given to ethical issues in the conduct of biomedical research. This has led both to a need for advice on these topics, and to the funding of research into ethical aspects of biomedical research. The latter has been stimulated by research funding, largely from the Wellcome Trust and the European Commission.

Though it has become increasingly well established academically, bioethics has been less successful in being seen as a resource called upon routinely to solve "real-life" problems. As we shall show in the discussion that follows, issues that are clearly "ethical" in character can become framed as another type of problem capable of resolution through various rules, contracts, consultation, or technical fixes. Conversely, even when something is defined as an "ethical" issue, the means used to adjudicate upon it may engage little in the way of formal bioethical reasoning.

From Professional Ethics to Governability

A recent focus of much debate has been on the professional ethics of the medical profession. Historical analyses[3] point to the critical importance of claims of ethics in the professionalization of medicine. Claims of trustworthiness, a service

---

2. Although there is a steady growth in PhD student numbers, we are only now seeing the beginnings of programmatic PhD training as distinct from individually tailored supervision on the traditional British model in the humanities.

3. See, for example, Starr P. *The Social Transformation of American Medicine*. New York: Basic Books, 1982.

orientation, and a fiduciary relationship with clients are evidently claims to the ethical character both of the corporate body of medicine and of its individual members. An influential body of work in sociology has traditionally been highly skeptical of these claims of ethical credentials, seeing their use as a strategic maneuver aimed at securing state protection for exclusive rights to particular titles and practices, and as part of a more general effort at gaining market monopolization, occupational enhancement, distinctiveness, autonomy, and status.[4] Critics within this tradition might point to the particular (even peculiar) values that such ethics expressed until relatively recently: one where the emphasis was on the maintenance of standards of collegiality and "gentlemanly" conduct, and where incompetence was rarely seen as justifying disqualification from practice.[5]

Also notable were the ways in which this form of ethics was codified and communicated: Medical ethics was not, until the last decade of the twentieth century, formally part of the curriculum of medical schools, and the specification of ethics by the regulator (the General Medical Council, or GMC) was at the level of broad principle. Until 1995, the GMC's guidance to the profession on ethical standards was contained in its "Blue Book," the major part of which was *Professional Conduct and Discipline: Fitness to Practice*. This document, which never extended to more than about 40 printed pages, gave guidance on the minimum standards expected of medical professionals, and related largely to traditional concerns of professional good practice (advertising, passing comment on fellow professionals, confidentiality and its breach, relationships with the pharmaceutical industry, and so on). Ethics was seen as something practitioners would naturally absorb through their socialization into the profession, and would be motivated to maintain through largely informal social sanctions and the need to perform a professional identity, with the regulatory code operating mostly as a background threat. Within this professional environment, it was argued that "detailed control over the professional judgment of the doctor, once admitted to the collegial community, was inappropriate. The fundamental purpose of regulation was to regulate the relationships between members of the collegial community and to preserve its solidarity."[6]

Consistent with this approach was a practice of handling ethical challenges in practice through informal discussions in private, rather than formal ethical consultation. At the institutional level, the relative lack of codification may be due to a suspicion inherited from the English common law culture of codification

---

4. Freidson E. *Profession of Medicine: A study of the sociology of applied knowledge*. New York: Dodd, Mead & Co. 1970.

5. Moran M, Wood B. *States, Regulation and the Medical Profession*. Buckingham: Open University Press, 1993.

6. Moran M. *The British Regulatory State*. Oxford: Oxford University Press. 2002: 50.

of the law, in the interests of flexibility and administrative or judicial discretion. This preference runs very deep. In part, it may explain some of the divergence between U.S. and English bioethics, in that U.S. legal and political culture is, to a far greater extent, constructed around common adherence to formally articulated constitutional principles with a moral or quasi-moral character. Ethical norms can perhaps fit into such a deliberative tradition more naturally than into English common law professional culture.

The formalization of medical ethics began, however, to change markedly during the 1980s, when the GMC expressed interest in the teaching of medical ethics in U.K. medical schools. A working party convened by the Institute of Medical Ethics, under the chairmanship of Sir Desmond Pond, reported in 1987. This was the beginning of a fresh flow of ethicists into academic medicine. From the late 1980s, medical schools began to appoint staff in medical ethics and law, though often part-time and teaching only. In 1993, the GMC published a wide-ranging policy document on the reform of medical education.[7] Among the changes required to be implemented by medical schools was the introduction of formal teaching and assessment of medical law and ethics as part of the undergraduate curriculum.[8] From then onward, medical schools appointed lecturers (i.e., full-status academic staff) more systematically in this area. The GMC did not itself produce a detailed curriculum specification of what might count as an adequate education in medical ethics and law, although a group of teachers in these areas at London medical schools and elsewhere in the U.K. produced a model core curriculum in 1997.[9]

At around the same time, the GMC radically revised its approach to issuing ethics guidance for practicing doctors, issuing a new publication, *Good Medical Practice*, and subsequently a series of specific booklets on particular topics,

7. General Medical Council. *Tomorrow's Doctors.* London: GMC, 1993. Downloadable from: http://www.gmc-uk.org/education/documents/Tomorrows_Doctors_1993.pdf (accessed July 1, 2008).

8. An influential approach to medical ethics education was developed by the Oxford Centre for Ethics and Communication in Healthcare (ETHOX Centre), as the Oxford Practice Skills Project. This combined ethics and communication skills, positioning ethics not simply as a body of formal rules or knowledge, but rather as a set of analytical skills to be used in practice, analogous to diagnostic or communication skills. See Hope T, Fulford KWM. "Medical Education: Patient Principles and Practice Skills" in Gillon R and Lloyd A (eds.) *Principles of Health Care Ethics* Chichester: John Wiley, 1994, ch. 59 pp. 697–709.

9. Ashcroft RE et al. Teaching medical ethics and law within medical education: A model for the UK core curriculum *J Med Ethics* 1998; 24: 188–192. (The authors of this paper were listed alphabetically; in practice, the lead authors were Prof. Raanan Gillon, Rev. Peter Haughton, and Prof. Len Doyal). A review of the implementation of medical ethics education and its assessment was published by Karen Mattick and John Bligh, based on a survey commissioned by the Institute of Medical Ethics in 2006. "Teaching and Assessing Medical Ethics: Where are We Now?" *J Med Ethics* 2006; 32: 181–185.

such as confidentiality. These were issued to all doctors, and to all medical students, and updated regularly. Their format was identical to other publications of the GMC in its role as guardian of professional education in medical schools and the early (nonspecialist) years post-qualification.[10] This positioned medical ethics as part of professional development, and not merely as standards against which doctors were to be measured. The documents were presented using "plain English" and were made available immediately on publication, on the GMC's public website. It was clear that the GMC wished its ethical standards to be widely available to patients and the public, as much as to doctors and students. The political governance of the NHS was increasingly emphasizing what patients could expect, and developing new ways to consult patients and to allow complaints to be handled (e.g., *The Patient's Charter*, 1991). At the same time, the GMC was also beginning, partly in response to external pressures, to move in a more democratic and consultative direction, rather than operating as regulator of the profession as a discrete "social system" with its own autonomous norms.[11]

Notwithstanding these changes in the specification of ethics and its teaching by the GMC, a number of weaknesses and dangers built into the self-regulatory model of the medical profession began to reveal themselves in dramatic fashion in the U.K. during the 1990s.

As far back as 1970, in a U.S. context, the sociologist Eliot Freidson had noted that self-regulation has a tendency to develop and maintain "a self-deceiving vision of the objectivity and reliability of its knowledge and the virtues of its members," arguing that medicine's "very autonomy has led to insularity and a mistaken arrogance about its mission in the world."[12] A series of medical scandals occurred over a period of about a decade, beginning in the early 1990s, that appeared to suggest that Freidson's analysis had some of the qualities of a prediction. One these scandals—which involved excessive death rates in children undergoing cardiac surgery at Bristol Royal Infirmary—well illustrates the way in which the autonomy of the medical profession came to be destabilized, and its claims of professional ethics, in particular, to be undermined. A public inquiry into Bristol, chaired by the academic medical lawyer Ian Kennedy, reported in 2001. Although Bristol was cast as an ethical scandal, the language of the report avoided the standard

10. Specialist medical training is regulated by the medical Royal Colleges (of Physicians, Surgeons, General Practitioners, and so on).

11. On this, see Hogg C. *Patients, Power and Politics: From Patients to Citizens* London: SAGE, 1999.

12. Friedson E. *Professional Dominance: The social structure of medical care.* Chicago: Aldine, 1970: 370.

tropes of medical ethics, instead focusing on the "club culture" of senior medical professionals, and the systems failure in management within the Infirmary. Rather than focusing on professionalism or education as the policy tools of choice, the Inquiry cast them as part of the problem: "systems" and management techniques were instead considered the appropriate tools for remedying the problems. The focus on failures of systems further marginalized a role for ethics, to the extent that ethics tends to be concerned with individual conduct.[13] The Inquiry recommended that systems for patient complaints about treatment and care, the law of torts relating to medical negligence, and professional self-regulation, all needed root and branch reform. Much subsequent government policy on the regulation of health care, from then on, can be considered the working out of a response to this.[14] A second scandal relating to organ retention following autopsies further added to the impetus to "do something" about the medical profession. The inquiry into the removal, retention, and disposal of human organs at the Royal Liverpool Children's Hospital (Alder Hey), which also reported in 2001, represented the conduct of the Professor of Pediatric Pathology as callous, immoral, and unconcerned with patient and parent well-being, and, further, that his professional colleagues did little to stop him.[15]

These and other scandals presented a challenge of disaster management for government. Though the particular subjects of the medical scandals were distinct, taken together they appeared to confirm that regulation of medical practice and conduct could not be safely left in the hands of doctors themselves. Further, they seemed to suggest that the ethics of the profession, far from protecting patients, in fact served the interests of the profession itself. The politically embarrassing nature of these scandals, and the ways in which they exposed the government to suggestions that it was not in control of the services it provided, made reform an imperative. In understanding the political imperatives operating in the United Kingdom, it is impossible to underestimate the importance of the National Health Service (NHS) as a public service, administered by central government and accountable to parliament and the electorate, as well as the courts, professional bodies, and patients. Thus, problems that in the U.S. system and elsewhere may be handled as

13. Of course, bioethics can contribute to the normative analysis of systems. But within the U.K. policy culture, systems tend to be evaluated against norms of efficiency and effectiveness, against a sort of informal utilitarian framework, rather than formally evaluated against principles of justice. Administrative law, for example, is much more concerned with legality and reasonableness, than with abstract principles of justice.

14. For a clear discussion, see Brazier M, Cave E. *Medicine, Patients and the Law.* London: Penguin, 2007 (4th ed.) chapter 1, pp. 3–25.

15. Royal Liverpool Children's Inquiry Report. Stationery Office, 2001. Available at http://www.rlcinquiry.org.uk/.

local issues of quality, performance, or ethics arising in a network of private actors (HMOs, hospitals, state medical boards, individual doctors), can, in the U.K., become political problems very quickly, and very potently.

The response to medical scandals in the U.K. was an attempt to make the medical profession more governable, though it also included widespread institutional reform. This included a move away from relying on the traditional agent-based model of professional practice, where professional ethics was part of the biography of the practitioner, to a more highly contractualized regulatory model, where powers of setting standards, monitoring of practice, and management of defaults from standards were largely relocated from inside to outside the profession. A new emphasis on seeing quality of clinical care and aspects of professional conduct as requiring external regulation was, for example, clearly evident.[16] By 1998, clinical governance (legal responsibility for the quality of clinical care) was imposed throughout the NHS, making it for the first time something for which managers, rather than clinicians alone, were accountable.

An important feature of these reforms also included the attempt to convert what had previously been ethical aspirations—for example, for fully informed consent to treatment—into forms of accountability that could be externally controlled. The Bristol Inquiry, for example, urged improved communication and information as part of the consent process, while consent was also institutionalized as a solution to the organ retention scandal through the Human Tissue Act 2004.[17] This recasting of consent represents both a "legalization" of bioethics and medical practice, and a particular social model of governance.[18]

Several critiques, both of the more general reforms of the medical profession and its relationship with the health service, and of the special role given to particular ethical principles such as consent, have been organized. One of these has come from a perhaps surprising quarter—the sociologists who previously had been so critical of professional ethics as simply tactics aimed at occupational closure and advancement. A new perspective has begun to distinguish more carefully between the way ethical credentials were mobilized by the corporate body of medicine, and the ways in which individual practitioners behave and understand to be their motivations for so behaving. In a U.S. context, Freidson has sought to rehabilitate professionalism as the "third logic," a form of practical and institutional ethics that could

16. Donaldson L. Clinical governance: a statutory duty for quality improvement. *Journal of Epidemiology and Community Health* 1998: 52: 73–74.

17. The Human Tissue Act (2004).

18. For authors otherwise quite alien in their theoretical approaches, who come to similar conclusions, see O'Neill loc. cit. n.15 and Rose N. *Powers of Freedom* Cambridge: Cambridge University Press, 1999.

defend against the excesses of market and bureaucratic/managerial forces.[19] Arguments that the new contractual forms of governing health professionals do damage to trust, and fail to serve the interests of patients, are now regularly heard in the U.K. also, prompting calls for a return to trust-based systems.[20]

Practices relating to consent have drawn criticism in this context. Consent is now central to medical practice. But other moral principles (in particular, principles related to justice and social participation) may take a back seat. Moreover, some commentators fear that this privileging of consent, in fact represents a transfer of risk to the patient, and also begins to support an argument to the effect that if the patient has consented, that in itself is sufficient moral justification for allowing it. Quite clearly, this argument would fail in many areas of law and public policy, most notably in the case of euthanasia: Consent of the deceased is not considered a defense to a homicide charge. But it may be powerful in other areas, such as participation in research.[21] Finally, the inevitable tendency for demands for accountability to be converted into procedural form means that consent may, in practice, be enacted as a ritual that frustrates the ethical purposes for which it was intended.[22]

From Medical Ethics to Clinical Ethics

There is a distinction between professional (medical) ethics—consisting of the norms of professional conduct, and the discourse supporting interpretation and practice of these norms in professional life—and the organization and deliberative means for resolving particular *cases* in clinical care. Frequently these overlap,

---

19. Freidson E. *Professionalism: The Third Logic.* Chicago: University of Chicago Press, 2001.

20. Checkland K, Marshall M, Harrison S. Rethinking accountability: trust versus confidence in medical practice. *Quality and Safety in Health Care* 2004; 13: 130–135.

21. The most sophisticated and intelligent analysis of the role of consent in law and ethics is now Beyleveld D, Brownsword R. *Consent in the Law.* Oxford: Hart Publishing, 2007. The research example has been quite important recently in a recent disaster involving a Phase I clinical trial at Northwick Park Hospital. What was striking about this disaster was that at no stage did the official inquiries challenge the ethical standing of the trial, the quality of the ethical review of the trial, or the quality of the informed consent process. Although 6 men were seriously injured in this trial, it appears that they have no legal remedy outside payments under an insurance scheme for "non-negligent harm." In this context it might be reasonable to say that the informed consent transferred the risk from sponsor to participant. See Medicines and Healthcare products Regulatory Agency (MHRA) Investigations into adverse incidents during clinical trials of TGN1412. Available at: http://www.mhra.gov.uk/home/idcplg?IdcService=GET_FILE&dDocName=CON2023821&RevisionSelectionMethod=LatestReleased (May 2006, accessed September 25, 2008).

22. Dixon-Woods M, Williams SJ, Jackson CJ, Akkad A, Kenyon S, Habiba M. Why do women consent to surgery, even when they do not want to? An interactionist and Bourdieusian analysis. *Social Science and Medicine* 2006; 62: 2742–2753.

naturally, but the growth of clinical ethics in the United States and elsewhere represents a shift both in ownership of the problem (from "what do I, the doctor, do?," to "what do we, the clinical team, the patient, and the family, do?"), and in preferred strategies for handling problems (from professional culture and informal discussion, to external consultation and deliberation by formal seeking of advice, framing of policy, or committee deliberation).

Ethical challenges in clinical practice have grown increasingly prominent for several reasons. One is the rapid pace of change in medical innovation and technology, particularly from the 1950s onward, but others include changes over time in the nature of doctor–patient relationships, and the declining authority of the medical profession itself as the sole arbiter of important decisions relating to people's health. An early example of how clinical ethics began to emerge as a distinct category of problem in practice can be seen in the emergence of the network of "medical groups" established in several U.K. medical schools from 1963 onward.[23] These groups were medical student societies, supported by like-minded clinical teachers in teaching hospitals and medical schools, established for the discussion of problems in medical practice. Their initial impetus came from the evangelical Christian organization, the Student Christian Movement (SCM), though they were formally ecumenical. By 1974, the groups had become sufficiently established that a society was formed to continue their work into post-graduate (that is, post-qualification and registration) medical training, the Society for the Study of Medical Ethics. This became the Institute of Medical Ethics, which still exists today.[24] In 1975, the Institute founded the *Journal of Medical Ethics*, which is now one of the leading journals devoted to medical ethics and bioethics. By 1987, 17 medical schools hosted a medical group. Since then, the GMC's educational reforms have led to formal teaching and the employment of academic staff, and the decline of the medical groups. The religious dimension of the Institute's orientation has almost completely vanished, although a minority of the board members are ordained ministers or priests. Inasmuch as it retains a religious orientation to medical ethics, it is in the form of seeing medical ethics education as a kind of ecumenical and nondoctrinal pastoral care, exemplified by the work of Prof. Alastair Campbell, an early member of the Institute and now a Vice President, and first editor of the *Journal of Medical Ethics.*

---

23. The factual information on the history of the medical groups and the Institute of Medical Ethics is derived from M. Whong-Barr, "Clinical Ethics Teaching in Britain: a History of the London Medical Group," *New Review of Bioethics* 2003; 1(1): 73–84.

24. One of the authors, REA, is a member of its Governing Body, ex officio as Deputy Editor of the *Journal of Medical Ethics*.

This strand of the development of bioethics in the U.K. is quite instructive. It suggests that one form of bioethics—that of clinical ethics—developed as part of the informal curriculum controlled by medical students, medical professionals, and medical educators, as an internal discourse on the problems of practice. This development can be interpreted to some extent as a response to the over-scientization of medical education, but also to the difficulties of making the transition from student to practitioner.[25] Other forces, such as the increasing pressure of demand for patients' rights, and patient-centeredness in teaching and practice, were no doubt also important.

Clinical ethics, conceived as the systematic application of principles of philosophical and ethical reasoning to resolve ethical dilemmas in clinical practice, remains, however, far from institutionalized in the U.K. Some hospitals do have clinical ethics committees, but these have grown only slowly in number over the last 10 years, and their workloads, legitimacy, and authority with either staff or patients vary considerably. Some research on clinical ethics provision has been conducted, mainly by the ETHOX Centre in Oxford, and training and support for clinical ethics committees is now provided with Department of Health support. Yet, the Department corporately has, by and large, avoided supporting the development of clinical ethics. Instead, there is a variety of alternate arrangements, largely managerial or professional in character.

In undergraduate education, establishing ethical deliberation as a core clinical skill is taking much longer than might have been expected 20 years ago, notwithstanding the GMC's original belief that training medical students in law and ethics would improve their patient-centeredness and the quality of their care and decision-making. In some ways, indeed, ethics has been taken up as a sort of scientific element of preclinical education. Formal examinations in ethics tend to split into examinations of knowledge (often by cognitive assessments such as multiple-choice questions) and of practice (in the form of tests of communication skills, rather than deliberative skills or attitudes).

The medical Royal Colleges have similarly played an often modest role in promoting clinical ethics. Some have shown a greater interest than others. The Royal College of General Practitioners established an ethical committee relatively early, and has issued documents on ethics and general practice, but is unusual in this regard. Its motivations may perhaps derive from a perception that general practice is the specialism concerned with the "whole patient" and the doctor–patient relationship as clinical phenomenon.[26] The Royal College of Physicians

---

25. See Whong-Barr op. cit. n. 4, at p. 75.

26. An idea which goes back to Michael Balint, *The Doctor, His Patient, and the Illness* (Various editions, first published 1959).

does have an ethical committee, and has published a number of influential reports, but has recently been focused on medical professionalism and medical humanities, perhaps at the expense of academic medical ethics.[27] This illustrates that bioethics is far from having achieved hegemony within the medical profession as the right set of institutions, individuals, and language for promoting and controlling ethical norms and values in the profession, but it may also reflect a degree of dissatisfaction with the way bioethics has become seen as a set of techniques for handling problems in public, rather than a vehicle for inward reflection by the professionals.[28]

Arguably more active in issues concerning clinical ethics are those bodies concerned with representing the interests of individual doctors in situations of conflict—the British Medical Association (BMA, the doctors' trade union) and the medical defense organizations (including the Medical Protection Society and the Medical Defence Union). The latter have almost no public role, but—partly to attract medical students into membership on qualification, and partly as a risk management strategy—play a small role in medical education about ethics and law, and, like the BMA, offer telephone advice. Their focus, naturally enough, is on the legal aspects of medical practice, counseling doctors about what might amount to a criminal offense, or give rise to claims in negligence. The BMA, on the other hand, has two important roles. First, it offers a telephone advice service for its members on medical law and ethics, and issues policy briefs, summaries of recent developments in medical law and ethics, and educational materials, including the BMA *Handbook of Medical Ethics* (which now runs to more than 800 pages).

---

27. Royal College of Physicians. *Doctors in Society: Medical Professionalism in a Changing World* (2 vols.) London: Royal College of Physicians, 2005. Kirklin D, Richardson R. (Eds.) *Medical Humanities: A Practical Introduction*. London: Royal College of Physicians, 2001. It should also be noted that the College produced an influential report on Clinical Ethics Committees: Royal College of Physicians. *Ethics in Practice: Background and Recommendations for Enhanced Support* London: Royal College of Physicians, 2005. Our point is that "clinical ethics" is not considered an "obligatory passage point" for advancing and defending the profession, or clinical quality, by the College.

28. For one such critique, by a former chair of the Royal College of Physicians ethics committee, professor of geriatric medicine, and well-regarded philosopher Raymond Tallis, see his *Hippocratic Oaths: Medicine and its Discontents*. London: Atlantic Books, 2005. More generally, see the critiques of the bureaucratic Research Ethics Committees, which appear very regularly in the medical press–although some of these critiques are targeted on the failure of RECs to be bureaucratic enough, in the sense of being fast, efficient, and predictable. Interestingly, there is a parallel critique of (philosophical) bioethics from within philosophy, led by Onora O'Neill, who argues that the technicization of bioethics, in the form of a rather mechanical approach to informed consent, both misrepresents the nature of moral problems in medicine, and undermines the social basis of its practice in trust, professionalism, and the moral responsibility of both doctors and patients. See O'Neill O. *Autonomy and Trust in Bioethics* Cambridge: Cambridge University Press, 2002.

The BMA's Ethics Committee prepares reports and position papers for consideration by the BMA executives and membership. The other chief function of the BMA in the field of clinical ethics takes place at its annual representative meeting, where its debates on issues such as voluntary euthanasia or physician-assisted suicide are routinely reported in the press as matters of great significance, and who take these motions as straws in the wind regarding doctors' attitudes.

"Patient" Pressure

The medical profession, its associated institutions, and the state are far from being the only players in the field of bioethics in the U.K. From the early days of the NHS onward, patients' groups have been more or less active in challenging medical, managerial, or policy agendas in healthcare and biomedicine. The Patients' Association, for example, was formed as a direct response to Maurice Pappworth's revelations in 1967 about ethical standards in clinical research.[29] Other civil society associations (such as patient groups), the official Community Health Councils (now defunct), and medical charities, all have had a significant role here. However, though their activism clearly concerns issues of bioethics, these agencies have generally not seen ethics as a suitable language or vehicle for their concerns, preferring the more natural activists' language of legal and civil rights. For the most part, these organizations find it more natural to construct issues as noncontroversial in principle, and focus on failures to deliver on promises or obligations, rather than identifying practices as unethical.

But this is by no means the only approach used by "lay" people. For example, conservative Christian groups campaigning against abortion, assisted reproduction, and embryo research have been highly effective both in getting press coverage of their positions, and using the courts (where they rarely win on points of law, but gain influential publicity). They have also become quite sophisticated about challenging "liberal elite" accounts of bioethics. Some of these groups seek to discredit bioethics as such; others seek to reclaim and reposition bioethics in a more conservative form. Much religiously led public activism around such issues has avoided engagement with academic bioethics, or even medical teaching, and is probably best understood as a form of social movement. Although religion is important in British society in many ways, public policy and professional bodies have tended in recent years to construct religious belief as a private matter, to which policy should be neutral (though respectful), and to consider certain

29. Hazelgrove J. The old faith and the new science: the Nuremberg Code and human experimental ethics in Britain, 1946–1973. *The Society for the Social History of Medicine*. 2002;15: 109–135.

arguments (for example, arguments referring to the sanctity of life) as inherently religious. Why this should be is a profoundly difficult question, which deserves serious historical investigation.

Adjudications of Contested Ethical Issues

Contestation about "ethical" issues, in part prompted by campaigning groups, but also a symptom of a more general move to an "ethics society," has led to increasingly visible processes of adjudicating upon highly contested areas of public policy. These range from the use of personal medical data for epidemiological research to organ recovery for transplantation. Precisely how (formal) bioethics gets mobilized, however, has varied considerably from one context to another. It might be expected that the courts would provide one context where bioethics might be expected to be influential. But in common law tradition, academic extralegal authority is no authority at all in legal reasoning; and, in the United Kingdom's constitution, appeal to abstract principle as distinct from formal legal rules is rarely, if ever, successful. Moreover, the structure of the NHS as a public service, forming part of the state apparatus, means that key roles are played by political argument on the one hand, and legal oversight on the other, so that ethics *qua* ethics can easily be marginalized or excluded.

One strategy for dealing with contested issues is simply to convert them into technical problems. Thus, problems of resource allocation within the NHS, which often erupt into the media when patients are denied treatments to which they feel entitled, are resolved not through ethical argumentation but, instead, through administrative arrangements in the form of the National Institute for Health and Clinical Excellence (NICE). Using technical assessments of cost-effectiveness, and consultation with interested stakeholders, NICE rules upon whether particular treatments should be made available to NHS patients.

Clearly, the remit of NICE is limited to a very particular domain, and some commentators have argued that there should be a national state bioethics commission to oversee policy on morally controversial matters in government biomedicine, and healthcare policy and regulation. None exists. Instead, the Nuffield Council on Bioethics was established in 1991, funded by the (state) Medical Research Council and the private charities, the Wellcome Trust and the Nuffield Foundation, to consult and produce reports on issues in bioethics, from pharmacogenetics to care of very premature newborn babies. The Council has no formal advisory role to government or Parliament. Its reports, while detailed and carefully written, rarely get into philosophical details of argument, and though they often make detailed recommendations, these are as much based on consultation evidence as on bioethical argument.

Thus, rather than a single voice on matters of bioethics in the public domain, a plurality of institutional arrangements, regulators, and processes can be seen. One important example is the regulation of human fertility. In 1991, the Human Fertilisation and Embryology Act was brought into force (though it is soon to be succeeded by a new Act). The Human Fertilisation and Embryology Authority established under the Act has been widely admired as an ingenious solution to the political challenges presented by assisted conception, around the regulation of morally and socially controversial issues such as embryo research, donor insemination, and preimplantation genetic diagnosis. Many commentators have argued that the Authority, by being independent of government but with strong licensing and regulatory powers, has preserved and promoted public confidence in assisted reproduction and embryology. However, as a statutory regulator it has also attracted controversy because of its decisions about matters of ethical policy, both as to the content of those decisions and as to its making ethical decisions at all. Critics have complained that the Authority has made decisions that ought properly be reserved to Parliament. On the other hand, its decisions have never been successfully challenged in public law on the basis of being made *ultra vires*, or of being irrational or unreasonable. In this regard, many would consider the HFEA as an exemplary public bioethics institution, having both a deliberative and regulatory function, and securing both high standards of practice, and high public confidence in it as regulator, and in the practices it regulates. However, following the 2010 General Election, the HFEA is to be closed and its functions merged with those of other regulators.

What is perhaps surprising, then, is that the HFEA model has not been more widely used in other areas of bioethical interest. Other attempts to deal with contested areas of public policy have instead used widely varying modalities of regulation and governance. For example, the Human Tissue Authority, established under the Human Tissue Act, has an almost exclusively regulatory role, and restricts itself to issuing codes of practice and policing the collection and use of tissues, organs, and bodies in teaching, audit, research, and museum collections. It avoids engagement with making ethical policy. On the other hand, the Genetics and Insurance Committee (GAIC), set up to license the use of genetic predictive tests by the insurance industry in the U.K., on the basis of an accord between the insurance industry and the government, does have some powers to regulate. But it has had very little work to do over its lifetime, has no statutory basis, and minimal public presence. The much better known Human Genetics Commission (HGC), explicitly concerned with bioethics in the field of genetics, both in the clinic and in society at large, has no powers, being purely advisory to ministers. Established in 1999, it produces reports and submits evidence to government consultations on topics within its remit, and conducts public engagement activities and public consultations of its own accord. The influence of the HGC is arguably quite limited, although it is well regarded by government and the academic community. Again, the reports it produces rarely lay out detailed ethical argumentation as a philosopher would recognize it, notwithstanding the membership of the committee including at least two philosophers or bioethicists at any given time. Instead, they concentrate on producing clear, plain-English discussions of the issues, often informed by social science or opinion poll data.

Indeed, whatever the regulatory modality adopted, a striking feature of many of the adjudicatory processes, where issues of ethical character are contested in England, is a concern with public consultation and public engagement, rather than ethical argumentation. The views of "the public" (itself a construct[30]) are frequently sought as part of the process of deliberation. Partly, this can be explained by the "consultation culture" of the British state, but the importance of consultation as a tactic aimed at securing legitimacy (or avoiding threats to legitimacy) should not be underplayed. The interest in conferring legitimacy on rulings (in whatever form) on ethical issues may go some way toward explaining why bioethics (as a formal, institutionalized field) itself may often tend to play a rather marginal role. It is notable, for example, that there are few "celebrity" bioethicists. Penetration of bioethics into popular culture is limited: Newspaper op-ed pieces by "bioethicists" are rare, and television appearances by bioethicists are relatively unusual. When an issue becomes ethically contested, the people called upon to speak in the media are usually clinical or scientific in background, and are arguably no better qualified to comment on ethical issues than anyone else not formally trained in the area. The ability of formal bioethical analyses to arrive at conclusions that are counterintuitive, or unlikely to command legitimacy (such as the argument that doping in sport is acceptable), may also be part of this story.

There is a deep sociological question here about why public opinion (however constructed, represented, and managed) should be a source of *legitimation,* where bioethics is not. We do not have an answer to this question, although a suggestion is that having dispensed with professional authority, replacing it with another source of expert authority (bioethics) is unlikely to succeed in a context where the credibility of the expertise was dubious (expertise *in ethics*, as distinct from expertise in *ethical argument,* which might be a technical matter), and where what may be under threat was social authority itself, rather than the authority of one specific group in society.

---

30. Dixon-Woods M, Wilson D, Jackson C, Cavers D, Pritchard-Jones K. Human tissue and "the public": the case of childhood cancer tumour banking. *Biosocieties* 2008; 3: 57–80.

Research Ethics

Research ethics is by far the most established form of "bioethical work" in England, and since the Medicines for Human Use (Clinical Trials) Regulations (2004), Research Ethics Committees (RECs) have had a formal legal existence. We have shown elsewhere that the development of RECs and associated processes of research governance can be understood as part of a history of scandal and disaster management,[31] the need for researchers to demonstrate their ethical credentials in the face of public skepticism, and the efforts of the pharmaceutical companies seeking harmonization of clinical trial processes (which found its expression, for example, in the European Clinical Trials Directive).[32] In England, NHS RECs are coordinated through the National Research Ethics Service. REC members serve on a voluntary basis, and may be either "lay" (independent of the NHS) or "expert" (having relevant methodological, clinical, or ethical expertise). Analysis of decision letters issued by these RECs shows that, once again, formal ethical reasoning is rarely an explicit feature; instead, the REC functions socially to produce a decision that fixes "what is ethical" through its location in the institutional structure.[33] In many ways, the functions of RECs can thus be understood as oriented, on the one hand, toward protection of research participants and their interests, but on the other, toward securing the social license for medical research and ensuring its continued legitimacy as an area of activity (though researchers may seldom recognize this benefit).

Conclusions

Bioethics constitutes an institutional field, in the sense of a recognized area of expertise or activity.[34] Our brief sketch of the emergence and characteristics of bioethics in England identifies it as a highly diverse field, containing a multiplicity of actors, interests, and organizational forms, and overlapping or interacting significantly with other institutional fields. The picture we have sketched here is partial and incomplete. We have said nothing about agricultural, environmental, and animal bioethics, though these are clearly important foci. But what we have

31. Dixon-Woods M, Ashcroft RE. Regulation and the social licence for medical research. *Medicine, Healthcare and Philosophy* 2008; 11:381–391.

32. We are grateful to Adam Hedgecoe for reminding us of the relevance of this.

33. Dixon-Woods M, Angell E, Ashcroft RE, Bryman A. Written work: the social functions of Research Ethics Committee letters. *Social Science and Medicine* 2007; 65: 792–802.

34. DiMaggio PJ Powell WW. 1983. The iron cage revisited: Institutional isomorphism and collective rationality in organizational fields. *American Sociological Review*, 48: 147–160.

perhaps made clear is that "bioethics as clerisy" has not become established in England.[35] Bioethics as an academic discipline, though thriving in its university settings, thus remains relatively marginal to the British polity, even while "bioethical issues" (such as abortion, euthanasia and assisted dying, genetic and embryo research) are widely discussed by the public, in the media, and in Parliament. Actors other than bioethics or bioethicists control and shape debates that have substantial ethical content.

Acknowledgments

Mary Dixon-Woods' work on the medical profession is funded through an ESRC Public Services Programme fellowship (Grant RES-153–27–0009). Both authors' work on research ethics is supported by ESRC grant RES-000–22–1908.

35. The allusion here is to Coleridge's early nineteenth-century concept of a semi-secular clergy who are a cultural and spiritual vanguard of the nation, in ST Coleridge, *On the Constitution of Church and State*, 1830 (various editions). Though it might be argued that, in contrast to the United States, bioethicists are the "missing intellectuals" in British public life, this is an argument that applies to several other disciplines (including sociology). See the work of Stefan Collini, in particular his *Absent Minds: Intellectuals in Britain* Oxford: Oxford University Press, 2006.

6 BIOETHICS BETWEEN TWO WORLDS

THE POLITICS OF ETHICS IN CENTRAL EUROPE

Bruce Jennings

Philosophy, Marx said, only interprets the world, but the point is to change it. Bioethics does both. Bioethics is a form of discourse that is shaped by particular social and cultural conditions, and that has a particular normative function in relation to these conditions. It operates on a theoretical level and on a political-cultural level. It must engage with moral philosophy and cognate disciplines (political philosophy, jurisprudence, theological ethics) to provide a basic normative conceptual framework. And bioethics must engage with the actually existing values, norms, and cultural belief systems that form the context for human behavior. Bioethics must meet actors and institutions where they are, but it cannot leave them there, because change in assumptions, commitments, understanding, and action is the entire point of the enterprise. If it is not critical, bioethics can become apologetic and ideological.

The "discourse" of bioethics is a sensitive barometer of the social context within which it germinates, because the basic subject matter of this discourse—the human experience and meaning of health and illness—moves so fluidly from the most intimate, personal needs and experiences, to the broadest social, systemic, and policy questions. Pain makes policy vivid and compelling; suffering makes systems come alive as tangible social agents, rather than as intellectual constructs or abstractions. Moreover, health-related conditions and services form a grid or microcosm for the most fundamental questions that a society must ask itself. These are questions concerning its deepest normative rules and beliefs, and concerning the legitimacy of its basic institutions, distributional structures, and communicative practices.

Every society needs to have a discourse with which to affirm and to contest power, equality, individual and group identity, knowledge, duty, and trust. Actually, it needs not one such discourse, but several layered and overlapping discourses. Repressive and stagnant societies tend to flatten and winnow this discursive landscape; more dynamic and open societies tend toward more diversity and argumentative conflict.

The bioethics that emerged in Central and Eastern Europe, after roughly 1989, provides a complex instance of this sociology of discourse.

In reflecting on the emergence of bioethics behind what was once the Iron Curtain, the preoccupations under discussion at that time, and the developments in the region during the intervening years, I find three salient, interrelated themes, which I propose to focus on in this chapter. These themes are: (1) factors impeding the development of bioethics during the Soviet period, and the blossoming of ethics with the discrediting of communism; (2) the ambivalence of Central European bioethics in the face of neoliberal values (e.g., individualism, competitiveness, and structured social conflict based on self-interest) and the implications of a market society; and (3) bioethics as an emblem of, and a discursive space for, a "Third Way" approach to social ethics between capitalism and communism—communitarian and solidaristic rather than individualist; pluralistic rather than collectivist.

Bioethics and Cultural Contradictions

Bioethics is a body of knowledge and a mode of analysis designed to address broad, but nonetheless bounded, questions, such as: how to promote health, how to respond well to human disease, disability, and death, and how to govern the practice of medicine and the social uses of biomedical technology. It was born in the West at a time when the range of social action and individual choice seemed on the verge of an era of tremendous expansion. And it was reborn again—partly from within and partly from outside—in the East when a similar opening of social horizons occurred, quite rapidly and to some, unexpectedly, there.

In the Western countries, for example, bioethics was given impetus by the notion that there was a cultural lag between normative and scientific knowledge, especially in the life sciences and the so-called "biological revolution."[1] What the new biology and the new medicine empowered us to do was changing faster than the ability of our repositories of normative knowledge and guidance—ethics, cultural mores, religion, the law—to guide and govern our use of that power. Consequently, a new form of power threatened to break loose from its moral moorings and its legal bridle. Individuals were confronted with unprecedented choices in reproduction, in plumbing the body's genetic secrets, in postponing or avoiding death. Physicians were becoming facilitators of this new power and range of choice. Investors sought to profit from them, governments sought to regulate them. But all were acting without a legal roadmap or an ethical compass. A new discourse, later dubbed *bioethics*, was needed to alleviate the danger inherent

1. Callahan, 1999.

in this cultural and normative lag. Those skilled in normative discernment and calibration should anticipate and adopt bodies of cases, rules, and regulations proactively. They should not merely react to scientific fait accompli, either with reactive negativity or with thoughtless affirmation and permissiveness.

If bioethics was needed for these reasons in North America and Western Europe in the late 1960s, it was needed for similar reasons in Central and Eastern Europe in the late 1980s and early 1990s.[2] However, the divergent conditions are as important as the parallels. In the West, bioethics was born amid economic affluence into a culture already thoroughly accustomed to the individualistic values that it promoted. In the East a generation later, bioethics emerged amid considerable economic scarcity and uncertainty into a culture that was both enamored and wary of market values and liberal individualism.

The reception of bioethics into the medical and philosophical circles of that region at that time was therefore complicated, and highly charged for the individuals and institutions involved, if not for the societies at large. The way bioethics was "exported" from the West and "reinvented" at home; how it intervened in the professional and political struggles that the fall and breakup of the Soviet Union brought about—these and other aspects form a story that has not yet been adequately researched or fully told.

It would require a wide linguistic competence, archival research, and the collection of oral histories to even begin such a study, and that is well beyond my intent and my capabilities in this chapter. Instead, what I propose is a reflection on some of my own experiences with colleagues, from Russia, and from Central and Eastern European countries. While on the staff of The Hastings Center, I had an opportunity to work with and learn from well over 100 colleagues from several countries in this region, in the immediate aftermath of the events of 1989 (e.g., the fall of the communist government in Moscow and the eventual disintegration of the USSR; the fall of Soviet satellite governments in Central and Eastern Europe; the reunification of Berlin, and then of Germany as a whole; and the intellectual and ideological discrediting of state socialism as an economic/political system and as a social ideal).

---

2. The political geography of Europe is nuanced and complex, and so is the terminology and self-identity of its various regions. I was introduced by visiting colleagues to the importance they attached to the distinction between "Central" and "Eastern" Europe. I am not certain I understand it exactly, but for the purposes of this paper I will mainly use the term "Central Europe," even though the American convention is to call the entire Soviet Bloc area "Eastern Europe." I do this because the core of the analysis in this paper actually comes from Hungry and Czechoslovakia (now the Czech Republic and Slovakia), which I gather are the countries that feel most strongly about the designation Central Europe. For an extended discussion, see Judt, 1996.

Some of these colleagues—from Russia, Hungary, Poland, the Czech Republic, Slovakia, and Lithuania—spent prolonged periods of time as visiting scholars at The Hastings Center from roughly 1988 to 1995, where I had an opportunity to converse with them at length. Many more attended three large conferences sponsored by the Center in these years. These were called East-West Bioethics Conferences, and were held in Dubrovnik, Pecs (Hungary), and Prague.[3] These conferences took place before the creation of the International Association of Bioethics, and were therefore among the first prolonged conferences bringing together bioethicists from what used to be called the "First World" with bioethicists from the Soviet Bloc countries (which used to be called the "Second World"), who aspired to make the field a niche in their own universities and professional structures.

When my colleagues and I organized these conferences and planned the agendas, we were concerned to avoid having Western speakers predominate, or to give any suggestion of one-way communication. On the contrary, the conferences were replete with presentations from Central European speakers, most often addressing both the history and current situation of their own countries and the important role that ethics education, consultation, and related activities and organizations could play in the new societies that they were trying to build. The conferences resulted in remarkably enduring personal friendships and intellectual networks, and opportunities for travel abroad, and assistance with curriculum development and library materials, grew out of them.[4]

Of course, since The Hastings Center did its pioneering work in the early and mid 1990s, many other, more extensive exchanges and collaborative work has been done. In particular, the European Union has been a significant force for such integration and collaboration. The EU funds bioethics research, bringing together scholars from both its "old" and "new" member states. The European Association of Centers of Medical Ethics (EACME) also devoted central attention to Central and Eastern European bioethics at its 2008 annual conference in Prague.

---

3. Donnelley, 1991. Among those with whom I was privileged to be associated, and from whom I learned a great deal, were: B. Blasszauer, J. Glasa, J. Payne, P. Tichtchenko, B. Yudin, and Z. Szawarski.

4. On a more somber note, a magnificent building where the Dubrovnik conference was held was destroyed a few years later in the civil war that accompanied the break up of Yugoslavia. On the other hand, one of our (then) East German colleagues presented The Hastings Center with a gift consisting of a chunk of masonry retrieved from the demolition of the Berlin Wall.

Bioethics under Communism

Prior to 1989 in the countries of the Soviet Bloc, there was very little in the way of what was called bioethics in the West.[5] Three forces converged to produce a political climate and a cultural soil uncongenial to a diverse, analytic, and relatively apolitical and ahistorical approach to ethical and value questions. The first was communist ideology itself. The second was the role of traditional professional physician ethics in Russia and, by extension of influence, in most of the other Central European countries as well. The third was the continuing role of religion, particularly Roman Catholicism in Central Europe.

Ideology. Communism, both in its Marxist origins and then much more strongly as it hardened into a dogmatic ideology under Stalin, was highly materialistic, positivistic, and utilitarian in its conception of ethics and morality.[6] All religious perspectives on ethics were dismissed, of course, but no secular versions of virtue ethics or deontological ethics (considered by some to be "bourgeois moralities") were encouraged, either. Human interests were taken to be straightforwardly material, tangible, and objective. Spirituality and aesthetic values were held to be decadent and corrupt, or a throwback to the false consciousness generated by a class society.

The contrast between the path taken by bioethics in the West, and the conventional understanding of "ethics" in the political culture of the East, could scarcely have been more sharp. Philosophically, this difference involved the distinctions between utilitarianism and rights-based theories, such as contractarianism. Socially, it was a version of the clash between collectivism and individualism. And, economically and politically, it mirrored the gap between centrally planned and market-driven economic systems.

From the perspective of communist theory, ethics can be looked at as a discourse that finally becomes authentic in a communist society, or as a discourse that is superfluous there. It becomes authentic because the real-world conditions necessary for the realization of ethical ideals have finally come into being. Or, it becomes superfluous because, since the social conditions of ethics have been met, the critical discourse of ethics goading the real toward the ideal is no longer necessary. In either case, the communist perspective on ethics generally is that it pertains to the good of the whole society (ethics is universal) and calls for a subordination of individual

5. Baker, 1992; Glasa, 2000; Luther, 1989; Prodanov, 2001; Tsaregorodtsev & Ivanyushkin, 1989.

6. For a general history and detailed discussion of Marxism, see Kolakowski, 1978.

liberty to communal equality and progressive solidarity ("from each according to his abilities, to each according to his needs").[7]

As a theory, utilitarianism is open to either a collectivist or an individualistic interpretation, and Marxism (and later the international communist movement) tended to incorporate utilitarianism in its former guise. It was attractive as well for its materialism, its sensationalist or associative psychology, and its penchant for quantification, making it a "scientific" approach to morality.[8] As for liberalism, social contract theory, or Kantian deontological ethics, these facets of Enlightenment and nineteenth-century thought were rejected by the Marxian left, little by little, in the years following Marx's death.[9] The final repudiation of a leftist version of deontological and rights theories was made complete in the ideological victory of Lenin's revolutionary thought over various rivals on the radical left, notably the "evolutionary socialism" of Edward Bernstein, which drew heavily from Kantian influences.[10]

Hence, in the 1960s and 1970s (despite de-Stalinization and Khrushchev's reforms), ethics remained rigid in the East, while in the West (particularly in the United States and the United Kingdom) bioethics was being born out of a variety of rights-oriented reconstructions of both philosophical and social ethics. For example, there was the postwar emphasis on universal human rights, and the spur of the Nuremberg war crimes and doctor's trials; the revival of contractarianism and neo-Kantianism in ethics in the work of Rawls and others, which has tended to translate in bioethics as an emphasis on autonomy; and the grassroots patients' rights and women's health movements, which were aimed at medical authoritarianism and paternalism.

The soil of the communist (or state socialist) version of utilitarian ethics was not hospitable to such developments in either theory or popular practice, and the virtual absence of such consumer or grassroots movements in these authoritarian systems also tended to repress the emergence of new thinking that would tap the same ideas and inspirations that bioethics was beginning to draw upon in the Western liberal democratic market societies. Yet, as events surrounding 1989

---

7. On the other hand, if we do not assume that ideal conditions have yet been realized in history and society, then ethics may retain its critical function even in a post-revolutionary (post-capitalist) era. This would be the case, for example, if the Communist Party, instead of truly representing the common good of the entire society, tends to promote instead the particular and separate interests of Party officials and bureaucratic elites.

8. Halévy, 1966.

9. Zalewski, 2000.

10. Kolakowski, 1978, 2: 98–114; 240–304; 381–528.

showed, the potential for these ideas was present in a subterranean sense; the new bioethics was as yet unimagined, but not unimaginable.

Medical professionalism. The medical philosophy and morality that did fit well with the ethical climate under communism was an exceedingly hierarchical and paternalistic culture and professional organization of physicians in Russia, and its example influenced the medical establishment in all the countries of the Soviet Bloc.[11] It is interesting that under communism the goal of creating a universal healthcare system of providing (at least *de jure*, if not *de facto*) equality of access could be achieved without direct recourse to a discourse or political argument about individual or patients' rights. In Western bioethics, it has been largely taken for granted that the recognition of an individual right or moral entitlement to equitable healthcare access is the *sine qua non* of just health reform.

Religion. Finally, throughout the communist period, religion—particularly orthodox Catholicism in Russia and Roman Catholicism in the Eastern European states, such as Poland—and religious ethics functioned as the counterculture to communism and collectivistic utilitarianism. This form of ethical discourse could draw upon traditional Catholic medical ethics, and it clashed with communist ethics on many medical matters, such as abortion. However, if the theology and traditions of the Church enabled it to be a source of counter-ethical discourse in relation to the official positions of atheism and materialism, this religious value system and worldview did not by themselves offer an opening for a secular and philosophical bioethics as an individualistic, rights-based orientation.

The papacy of John Paul II provides a prolonged and dramatic illustration of these tensions. He brought his long, oppositional struggle against the communist regime in Poland to Rome with him, but those same values—conservative respect for Church tradition and authority, deep commitment to human dignity, and the preservation of core human experiences such as marriage, family, labor; and an equally deep suspicion of technology that feeds consumerism and hedonism—could be, and were, turned with a sharp edge toward the culture and values of the secular capitalist West.

Finally, within the sphere of medical culture and the structure of medical professionalism in the Central and Eastern European countries, religious discourse or theological ethics did little to pave the way for a bioethics that would call into question well-established customs of paternalism and authoritarianism in the medical culture and everyday practice in these countries.

---

11. Lichterman, 2005; Tichtchenko, 2003; Doroszewski, 1988; Saunders, 1993; Tsaregorodtsev & Ivanyushkin, 1989.

Between Communism and Capitalism

It may take some effort now to recall how sweeping and rapid intellectual developments were in Central and Eastern Europe, just before and after 1989.[12] It is not an exaggeration to say that long-pent-up energies were explosively released. Seemingly irresistible bureaucracies and secret police organizations—the whole apparatus of long-standing repressive regimes—virtually crumbled almost overnight, not toppled by superior force of arms from outside, but undermined from within by corruption and incompetence. In this swirling, joyous, and often bewildering atmosphere, two large bodies of ideas emerged, one far more public and predominant, the other quiet and largely unobtrusive, except within philosophical and medical circles. The predominant one was neoliberalism and the reformist doctrines of economic competition, privatization, and efficiency. The quiet one was bioethics. Both were sought out and imported from the West.[13]

As it did in the United States in the 1960s, bioethics in Central Europe after 1989 developed slowly, out of the work of a few well-placed teachers, academics, and public intellectuals. Articles began to be written in journals and in languages that lacked a bioethics literature. Conferences and exchanges were held. Teaching positions were created. I met several individuals from Poland, Hungary, Czechoslovakia, and Romania, who had suffered dead-ends, blacklists, and other obstacles to their careers, and who were suddenly thrust into positions of authority in the major medical universities of their countries, where they could engage in and promote the teaching of bioethics. Younger colleagues began to see bioethics as a legitimate field of research and as a viable career path. With some funds and freedom of international travel, they sought advanced degree and training programs in bioethics abroad.

Looking back at this period (roughly 1989–1995) and these developments, I believe that bioethics in Central and Eastern Europe should be interpreted as striving to achieve a type of "Third Way" intellectual formation, at once rejecting the past ethic of communistic utilitarianism and resisting the most extreme forms of the emerging ethic of neoliberal capitalism.[14] There are two specific manifestations of this that warrant further study beyond the confines of this chapter, but I want to note them briefly here.

The first is discussions of the physician–patient relationship within medical practice in the East. Unlike their American counterparts, such discussions do not focus primarily on paternalism, informed consent, and the like. Instead, they focus

12. Judt, 2005: 585–749.

13. Blasszauer, 1986.

14. Haderka, 1992. On the notion of Third Way social theory generally, see Giddens, 1998.

on financial conflicts of interest and micro-access to care. In formally universal systems, where resources were limited and physicians as a group were not highly paid, inequalities of access emerged in the form of queues and the practice of "tipping" or buying one's way to the front of the line for consultation, elective surgery, or other services, through private payments to physicians.[15] This was a form of market medicine, *avant la lettre*, but its implications were clearly troubling, both from a communist point of view and also from the perspective of the rights-based bioethics that was now available to Central European ethicists to use in their critiques.

This prefigured a larger and more ethically troubling discussion. State socialism and central economic planning were discredited, and indeed had not performed well in the 1970s. Yet, to many intellectuals at least, Western market practices looked more attractive from across the Iron Curtain than they were beginning to look once the curtain had lifted and these practices came flooding in. Indeed, the collapse of communism created several layers of quandary for emerging bioethicists in Eastern Europe.

For example, in Czechoslovakia the memory of Prague Spring in 1968 was a factor that intertwined with the stance of the new bioethics among many scholars I talked with. Reformist thinking at that time, critical of party hierarchy and privilege and critical of human rights abuses, had risen to the surface.[16] This produced the possibility of a more progressive and humanistic ideological left, "socialism with a human face," as it was called.[17]

If this reform had been permitted to continue, I believe that something like bioethics would have emerged in Czechoslovakia, and perhaps some other Soviet Bloc countries, twenty years earlier. However that may be, the Soviets quickly repressed this movement by invading militarily and setting up a much more compliant and repressive regime. Remarkably, however, in the 1989 collapse of that regime, there was little bloodshed, recrimination, or revenge. The "velvet revolution" restored many exiled leaders, including President Václav Havel, who seemed set to pick up where the reformers of 1968 had left off, albeit in a much bolder fashion, both in the embrace of Western liberal democratic values and in the more wary embrace of market economic policies.

I believe that Czech bioethics reflected, and took some direct part in, precisely this ideologically complex situation. Neither a full embrace of liberalism nor a full repudiation of socialism seemed desirable for society as a whole, and in particular,

15. Adam, 1989; Kovacs, 1991.

16. Payne, 1993.

17. Kolakowski, 1978, 3: 450–493.

it was not desirable in health care. Those policymakers who advocated a rapid transition of the healthcare system to privatization, and market competition among providers and insurers, experienced opposition not only from President Havel and his supporters, but also from many in the emerging bioethics community, who were concerned about the loss of solidarity that an overly individualistic orientation in healthcare delivery would cause. They were mindful of the social and civic effects that Thatcherism was having in the U.K. and that Reaganism was having in the U.S. In general, I would say, they were much more comfortable with the example provided by the healthcare systems of most other Western European countries, but continued to be nervous that those systems too would eventually succumb to a fiscal crisis, or fall under the neoliberal spell of the United States and the United Kingdom.

Communist utilitarianism is not the only perspective that permits one to value such social solidarity, and to support the preservation of a universal healthcare system. Yet, the stigma of the failure and even the moral brutality of that ethical orientation—and many of the emerging bioethics scholars had experienced that brutality first hand—made it difficult to argue for any kind of egalitarian progressivism or communitarianism.[18]

It would also have been possible for Central European bioethics to turn to progressive, social justice traditions within the Roman Catholic tradition to reinforce ethical arguments against the privatization and dismantling of the socialized medical system. But many factors concerning the social position of the Church in Central European society and history tended to bring its authoritarian face to the fore, and that quarter did not seem promising for the development of an egalitarian but secular version of bioethics, either.[19]

Conclusion

Neoliberalism and its free market ideology proved to be a much more powerful force than bioethics in the post-communist transition of Central and Eastern Europe. The possibility of a velvet revolution in values, as well as political action, which would have perhaps led to a transition that preserved (and made more genuine, less cynical) the ideals of the socialist worldview, has not been realized for the most part. Bioethics continues to grow and expand as a discipline in the

---

18. I discovered this complexity and nuance myself on an occasion in Prague, when I was lecturing on health policy reform discussions in the U.S., and took what was then being called in the U.S. a "communitarian" position. After the lecture, several Czech colleagues pointed out to me that my argument would not be publicly acceptable in their country at that time, because it was far too reminiscent of the spirit of Prague Spring.

19. Zalewski, 1997.

medical profession and healthcare systems of Central Europe, but it is my impression that in the past decade or so it has not developed a distinctive perspective, but has tended instead to follow Western philosophical and theoretical leads, applying them to a local or regional context.[20]

Much of this can be explained by the very difficult economic circumstances this entire region faced. Without the Soviet sphere to bolster and provide markets for the Central European economies, they were forced to fend for themselves in a global context. They continue to struggle with this today; membership in the European Union or other Western-oriented alliances has not been a panacea.

Socially, as well, Central Europe has had to endure hard times and a difficult transition. In the last decade, the advantages promised by neoliberalism (such as greater personal liberty, political and civil liberties, and a rising standard of living) have only partially been delivered, or have proven somehow less satisfying than they seemed to many in the immediate aftermath of 1989. Meanwhile, the dangers of neoliberalism (such as greater inequality, personal anxiety, and loss of communal solidarity) are manifesting themselves in many disturbing social and public health indicators. The precipitous decline in population health status in Russia since the breakup of the USSR is one marked example, and less dramatic but similar trends also exist in Central and Eastern Europe.[21]

On the world stage, the field of bioethics seems to be turning away somewhat from the preoccupation with high technology, acute care medicine, and biotechnological applications of genomics, which had characterized work on bioethics in the United States, and toward questions of population health, the ethical issues related to the social determinants of health and health disparities, and questions of global equity. In this work, a secular ethic that has not lost touch with the vision of a socialism with a human face can make an important contribution. Central Europe can be a source of a third-way bioethics that draws on that memory and that legacy to good effect.

References

Adam, G. (1989). Gratuity for doctors and medical ethics. *Journal of Medicine and Philosophy* 14(3): 315–322.

Ashcroft, R.E. (2005). Ethics committees and countries in transition: a figleaf for structural violence? *BMJ* 331: 229–230.

20. Ashcroft, 2005; Bankauskaite & Jakusovaite, 2006; Borovecki et al., 2004; Borovecki et al., 2005; Borovecki et al., 2006; Glasa, 2000; Glasa et al., 1999; Glasa & Glasova, 2001; Marusic, 2005.

21. Garrett, 2000: 121–265.

Bankauskaite, V. & Jakusovaite, I (2006). Dealing with ethical problems in the healthcare system in Lithuania: achievements and challenges. *Journal of Medical Ethics* 32(10): 584–587.

Baker, R. (1992). Medical ethics in a time of de-Communization. *Kennedy Institute of Ethics Journal* 2(4): 363–370.

Blasszauer, B. (1986). In Hungary, the old medical ethics meets the new. *Hastings Center Report*, June 16(3): 25–27.

Borovecki, A., ten Have, H. & Oresković, S. (2004). Developments regarding ethical issues in medicine in the Republic of Croatia. *Cambridge Quarterly of Healthcare Ethics* 13(3): 254–262.

Borovecki, A., Oresković, S. & ten Have, H. (2005). Ethics and the structures of health care in the European countries in transition: hospital ethics committees in Croatia. *BMJ* 331: 227–229.

Borovecki, A., ten Have, H. & Oresković, S. (2006). Ethics and European countries in transition—the past and the future. *Bulletin of Medical Ethics* 214: 15–20.

Callahan, D. (1999). The Hastings Center and the early years of bioethics. *Kennedy Institute of Ethics Journal* 9 (1): 53–71.

Donnelley, S. (1991). Political sea changes and bioethics—Prague 1991. *Hastings Center Report* 21(6): 5–6.

Doroszewski, J. (1988). Medical ethics in Poland. *Theoretical Medicine* 9(3): 351–370.

Garrett, L. (2000). *Betrayal of trust*: The collapse of global public health New York: Hyperion.

Giddens, A. (1998). *The third way*: the renewal of social democracy Cambridge: Polity Press.

Glasa, J. (2000). Bioethics and the challenges of a society in transition: the birth and development of bioethics in post-totalitarian Slovakia. *Kennedy Institute of Ethics Journal* 10 (2), June: 165–170.

Glasa, J., Bielik, J., Dacok, J., Glasová, H., Mojzesová, M., & Porubský, J. (1999). Bioethics in the period of transition. *Med Ethika Bioetika* 6(1–2): 4–8.

Glasa, J. & Glasova, M. (2001). Ethics committees and consensus in the post-totalitarian society. *Medical Ethika Bioethika* 1–2: 5–9.

Haderka, J.F. (1992). Why is cooperation in medical ethics in Central European area advisable and how to achieve it? *Journal Internationale Bioethique* 3(4): 229–235.

Halévy, E. (1966). *The growth of philosophical radicalism*. Boston: Beacon.

Judt, T. (1996). *A grand illusion: An essay on Europe*. New York: Hill and Wang.

Judt, T. (2005). *Postwar: a history of Europe since 1945*. New York: Penguin Press.

Kolakowski, L. (1978). *Main currents of Marxism (3 Volumes)*. Oxford: Oxford University Press.

Kovacs, J. (1991). Bribery and medical ethics in Hungary. *Bulletins of Medical Ethics* 66: 13–18.

Lichterman, B.L. (2005). Soviet medical ethics (1917–1991). *Journal Internationale Bioethique* 16(3–4): 33–41;167–168.

Luther, E. (1989). Medical ethics in the German Democratic Republic. *Journal of Medicine and Philosophy* 14(3): 289–300.

Marusic, A. (2005). Ethics in health care and research in European transition countries: reality and future prospects. *BMJ* 331:230.

Payne, J. (1993). Ethics and healthcare in Czech Republic. *Bulletin of Medical Ethics* 85: 13–16.

Prodanov, V. (2001). Bioethics in Eastern Europe: a difficult birth. *Cambridge Quarterly of Healthcare Ethics* 10(1): 53–61.

Saunders, J. (1993). Polish medical ethics: an outsider's view. *Bulletin of Medical Ethics* 5 (Feb.): 20–22.

Tichtchenko, P. & Yudin, B.G. (1992). Toward a bioethics in post-communist Russia. *Cambridge Quarterly of Healthcare Ethics*, 1 (4): 295–303.

Tichtchenko, P. (2003). Changing roles in Russian healthcare. *Cambridge Quarterly of Healthcare Ethics* 12(3): 265–267.

Tsaregorodtsev, G.I. & Ivanyushkin, A. (1989). Trends in the development of medical ethics in the USSR. *Journal of Medicine and Philosophy* 14(3): 301–314.

Zalewski, Z. (2000). What philosophy should be taught to the future medical professionals? *Medicine and Health Care Philosophy* 3(2): 161–167.

Zalewski, Z. (1997). On medical ethics in Poland and its impact on public life. *Biomedical Ethics* 2(2): 50–53.

7 BIOETHICS IN CHILE AND THE NEED FOR LATIN AMERICAN BIOETHICS

Miguel Kottow and Moisés Russo

Introduction

Most Latin American countries, including Chile, share a common historical development and a comparable social and cultural heritage, which can be summarized under four aspects: (1) a strong colonial past, evolving into a still partially prevailing neocolonialism; (2) the sustained influence of the Catholic Church in social and political matters; (3) economic dependence on the exploitation and export of natural resources, subject to the vagaries of international markets; and (4) persistent socioeconomic inequities.

Severe socioeconomic differences in Chile have favored extreme, if temporary, political conditions, ranging from a socialist government (Allende, 1970–1973) to a prolonged conservative military dictatorship (Pinochet, 1973–1988), consequently perpetuating a widespread social divide that also affects bioethical issues, such as the inequities of a two-tiered medical system, and disparities in social security plans. These historical and contextual realities have led Chilean mainstream bioethics to emphasize the debate on social protection and the quest for justice, universal access to medical care, and the allocation of scarce resources. Furthermore, secular bioethics has been involved in controversial polemics with an outspoken and very influential brand of religious orthodoxy. The main concern of this chapter is to address issues arising from the fact that Chile is a representative but not participatory democracy, facing crucial issues in bioethics that need to be known and discussed by the civil society.

Latin America's Common Background

Latin American nations constitute a fairly uniform subcontinent with common features that distinguish them from other underdeveloped parts of the world. The region was conquered by Spanish and Portuguese explorers, not gaining its independence till the beginning of the nineteenth century.[1] Nevertheless, the effects of 250 years of colonialism were not easily shed, and for much of its republican history, the region was to live under neocolonial conditions that still persist in some enclaves.

When, in the fifteenth century, the Catholic monarchs obtained financial support from Pope Alexander VI, they had to commit their expeditions to seek not only gold and silver, but also to support a strong missionary activity. The Catholic Church took part in the conquest of America by actively converting Indian populations, as well as taking care of a number of civic tasks, predominantly in education and health care. The Church's presence in public service remains active up to the present, in form of excellent schools and universities, as well as high-quality hospitals, thus upholding a solid influence in social and political matters.

To a great extent, social stratifications remain fixed in classes that show only minimal mobility. Class distinctions are both socioeconomic and ethnic, with Indians occupying the lowest ranks and living in permanent, at times violent, tension between the quest for assimilation and the need to preserve their cultural identity. Less than 2% of the population is Indian (*mapuches*=people of the earth), and another 4% consider themselves to be of Indian origin.

As independence was proclaimed, the local oligarchy took over, but was unable and unwilling to completely sever ties with Spain and Portugal, thus prolonging colonial dependence in cultural, economic, and technical matters. Each country developed an economy based on some kind of monoculture (fruit, wheat, coffee) or monoproduction (tin, oil, Chilean nitrates in the past, replaced by copper in the twentieth century), and remained dependent on foreign capital, know-how and marketing, thus recreating the colonial situation of a periphery that produces for the benefit of a foreign economic power—a trend also followed nowadays by biomedical research programs.[2]

As a direct consequence, Latin American countries have fluctuating economies, with some submerged in chronic poverty, while others have enjoyed periods of bonanza, during which they have been unable to definitely solve their social problems (Brazil, Chile) or solidly defend their economies against relapses (Argentina, Venezuela). Economic growth has been irregular and at times elusive, suffering lost decades in which the region did not develop substantially in spite of harboring pockets of high industrialization, sophisticated exports, as well as focal areas of excellence in science, higher education, and the arts.

1. Bethell L. (ed.) *The Cambridge History of Latin America*. Cambridge, Cambridge University Press. 12 vols. 1984 onward.

2. Nundy S & Gulhati CM. A new colonialism? Conducting clinical trials in India. *N. Engl. J Med* 2005; 352:16–19.

The region has one of the largest inequities of income distribution in the world (average Gini index of 0.57, as compared to 0.30 for developed countries), extreme wealth coexisting with severe poverty.[3] Many indicators show the economy of Latin America, like that of all Third World regions, to be increasingly outdistanced by the rich nations. National inequities are also on the rise between the well-to-do and the destitute within the same society, with an extreme concentration of wealth at the top of the income pyramid.[4] Knowledge and academic output disparities are also increasing, to a good measure induced by the alarming "brain drain" of Latin American professionals.

A Touch of Statistics[5]

Chile has a population of nearly 17 million, 85% of whom are urban dwellers. Demographic growth has stabilized at 1.3% annually. The per capita income is around USD $10,000, inflation rate is currently under 10%, and unemployment ranges between 6% and 8%. Average life expectancy is 75.21, slightly higher for women. Fertility is down from 5.4 children per fertile woman in 1962, to 1.9 at present, with somewhat higher rates in the distant provinces. Infant mortality has reached a low of 10.3 per 1000 live births. The epidemiologic transition has brought cardiovascular diseases and cancer to the forefront of mortality causes, whereas infectious diseases have declined, following the trend of highly industrialized countries.

The country presents a number of striking contrasts, having some of the finest universities in the region with strong scientific commitment, as well as two Nobel laureates in literature, and at the same time harboring vast sectors of the population who can read and write but show deplorable comprehension skills. Santiago's skyline is filled with modern high-rise buildings, but shantytowns can still be found, where drug dealing and delinquency are rampant. The statistical analysis of poverty leads to widely differing results, ranging from 20% to 29% of the population considered to be living under the poverty line.

In spite of these social inequities, bioethics is rarely and very briefly touched upon by the mostly conservative media, usually in relation to some controversial

3. Almeida C. Health systems reform and equity in Latin America and the Caribbean: lessons from the 1980s and 1990s. *Cad. Saúde Pública* 2002; 18 : 905–92

4. De Ferranti D, Perry G, Ferreira FHG, Walton M. *Inequality in Latin America and the Caribbean: Breaking with History?* World Bank, Washington, DC. 2003.

5. This text was written in December 2008, when the economic crisis was little more than a threat. By 2010 it became clear that the Chilean economy had not suffered major ill-effects from the global financial crisis.

local or international case concerning permanent vegetative conditions, assisted suicide, or abortion of anencephalic fetuses. The media may interview an expert or two, but will not take pains to ensure pluralism, whereas academia almost never engages in opinion-forming debates, precluding bioethics from taking up advocacy for disempowered minorities or the defense of liberal stances.

Political and Social Scene in Chile

Throughout its history, Chile has only occasionally been plagued by social unrest, at times eliciting aggressive official responses.[6] A few exemplary social laws have been passed, including social security and medical benefits for the working class, but for a long time these legislative efforts had more the character of appeasement than of social conquest,[7] which explains, in part, why social mobility is so limited.

The country has enjoyed a stable representative democracy, only interrupted by a brief military coup in 1932, and the long de facto dictatorship of Pinochet (1973–1988) after Allende's democratically elected government was violently overthrown. The military regime was repressive and conservative, dismantling social securities, prohibiting all sorts of elections, and discouraging political or cultural criticism. Most efforts went into reactivating the economy under the guidance of neoliberal economists. International bank loans were negotiated, accepting the earmarked conditions that encouraged private investments in schools, universities, medical services, and social security schemes.[8]

Reinstated in 1988, democracy basked in superb macroeconomic conditions but was slow in taking up pending social issues like the reconstruction of public healthcare programs and facilities. At the end of almost two decades of solid economic expansion, there has been no major breakthrough in health, education, or social security, with painful deprivation still affecting one-fifth of the population. Many hospitals and schools are in a severely rundown condition, ill-equipped and understaffed, and yet fiscal policy holds tight to the surplus revenues obtained from copper exports, arguing that reserves have to be stockpiled for the uncertain future, and that too much social spending would unleash inflation.

As sophisticated private medical and teaching institutions proliferate, they compete successfully with the impoverished public hospitals and educational

---

6. Deves E. "Los que van a morir te saludan: historia de una masacre : Escuela Santa María, Iquique, 1907." Eds. Documentas, 1989.

7. Illanes MA. "En el nombre del pueblo, del Estado y de la ciencia, (...)" Santiago, Colectivo de Atención Primaria, 1993.

8. Labra ME. Neoliberal reinvention of inequity in Chile: the case of the health sector. (Spanish). *Cadernos de Saúde Pública* 2002; 18:1041–1052.

establishments, which have been forced to exact fees from their clients in order to remain viable. Private health care is available under different schemes for about one-fifth of the population, including fee-for-service, HMOs, and private insurance plans; the rest make use of public services, with co-payment being graded according to income. Medication is very rarely provided free of charge for either private or public prescriptions, thus constituting a major expense that severely cuts into the budgets of the less affluent, and those whose low pensions are often exhausted by their medical needs.

Bioethics in Chile

This article has definitely preferred the emic, or insider, approach that social sciences may employ, in spite of some peculiarities and shortcomings. Much of what is reported relies on impressions and empathic sensitivity, as well as on informal sources of information like the media, political opinions, anecdotal interviews, narratives, and experiences, as well as ephemeral written or published material.

The Actors

Bioethics in the mid-1980s was still under the strong influence of principlism. Scholars with theological background had authored groundbreaking publications in bioethics, just as men of the cloth were among the first to present bioethics to Chilean medical and academic audiences. At present, the strongest graduate and postgraduate bioethics programs show a fervent and highly vocal religious commitment.[9, 10] Professions like medicine have traditionally been conservative in their views and in their practice, as illustrated by a staunch and persistent paternalistic doctor–patient relationship, and by the fact that only one-third of physicians are willing to take poorly paid, part-time jobs in public hospitals. Consequently, the major trend in the country is a smooth mix of normative bioethics blending into a society steeped in tradition, and an academia committed to conservative and religious values.

Chile has almost no full-time bioethicists, with most university centers hiring health-care professionals and some social scientists, with part-time teaching assignments. Training in bioethics is haphazard, with a very small number of

---

9. Lavados MM & Serani AM. *Etica clínica.* Santiago, Ediciones Universidad Católica de Chile. 1993.

10. Lavados MM. *Problemas contemporáneos en bioética.* Santiago, Ediciones Universidad Católica de Chile. 1990.

people taking a degree abroad. In recent years, major local universities have begun to offer a master's degree in bioethics, but of those who graduate, only a handful devote themselves to bioethics because academic salaries are low compared to freelance work as a healthcare professional. Financial support has clearly favored private universities with ecclesiastic commitment, so that, at present, there is only one secular Unit for Bioethics in the country. The vast majority of those engaged in bioethics agree with the traditional principlism of Georgetown. European Catholic bioethicists—e.g., Gafo, Screggia, Scola—have been very influential and are carefully studied. Specific issues are discussed on a conservative and religious basis. For example, "respect for life" will triumph over "autonomy" when the patient rejects treatments that might jeopardize his life. The production of written material remains sparse. A minority of bioethicists publish in Latin American and English-language journals; some have gained regional reputations as teachers and lecturers, and are engaged in programs sponsored by international organizations like Pan American Health Organization (PAHO) and UNESCO. In 1995, PAHO created a Regional Program of Bioethics, with offices in Santiago and with the mandate to foster and support bioethical activities throughout the region, with a strong emphasis on Fogarty-sponsored research ethics training. In recent years, the program has been financially weakened, has become less connected with all local bioethics centers, and concentrates on non-participatory academic activities.

Ever since the so-called "double standard" research ethics was presented, Third World countries like Chile have been wary of getting a second-best, situational kind of bioethics[11]. Major scientific centers have research ethics committees that evaluate protocols dealing with humans or animals; increasingly, investigations are initiated by contract research organizations (CROs)—that is, foreign commercial research institutions, along with commercial site management organizations (SMOs). Following mostly pharmaceutical interests, and relying on external ethics committee evaluations, these protocols will not allow any modifications in their procedures, instead catering to local institutional and academic interests, in order to get approval of protocols even though they show ethical deficiencies.

The Strategies

It may be difficult for outsiders to understand the enormous influence of the Church on political matters. Countries with strong Catholic majorities have dictated laws and regulations that legalize and publicly finance abortion (Italy),

---

11. Macklin R. *Double standards in medical research in developing countries.* Cambridge UK, Cambridge University Press, 2004.

allow assisted reproduction for the unmarried (Spain), and the use of pre-embryos for research (France). These and other liberal bioethical stances have all been adamantly and publicly criticized by the Chilean Church, which, incidentally, did not allow divorce to become legal until 2004. Extrapolating from statistics in other Latin American countries, Chile can be estimated to have an observant population of about 15%–20%, and yet analysts conclude that "[T]he Church in Chile, in contrast to the rest of the Southern Cone, had a strong voice in public affairs."[12]

Needless to say, the civil society is therefore in urgent need of secular representation. "[T]he dilemmas of legitimacy and public morality in health policy allocation may find their only viable solution, not in ethical or economic theory, but in the public process and the political imagination embodied in a democratic consensus."[13] The prime model is, of course, the grassroots procedure of the Oregon model, which is exemplary in respecting priorities in medical care as expressed by the people, although the process has not been free of controversies and failures. A recent survey of healthcare priorities in developed countries concludes that engaging the public in decision-making processes is essential to "ensure fairness and legitimacy." These experiences have been closely followed by some Chilean bioethicists, and brought to the attention of authorities at the Ministry of Health and to parliamentary health committees. It has been an unfortunate experience that bioethicists, having been called in to present their views to authorities and lawmakers, find the final legal product to contain little of what they contributed. Public forums, discussions in the media, or public participation scenarios—a National Bioethics Committee—have not yet been implemented to allow the civil society to participate in debates on bioethical issues.[14]

With its history of strong political conservatism, religious intransigence, and both social and professional paternalism, Chile is in particular need of opening spaces for a kind of public deliberation that is sensitive to social needs, respectful of individual autonomy, and tolerant toward the diversity of multicultural societies. Following M. Weber's ideas, bioethics evolves from an ethics of convictions that internalizes norms and principles, to an ethics of responsibility that requires avoiding harm to others. Chilean tradition has yet to modify its unrelenting commitment to an ethics of convictions, for it is not rare to hear politicians, bioethicists and practitioners state that they will put their beliefs before any rational

12. Lynch J. La Iglesia católica en América Latina, 1830–1900. In Bethell L. (ed.): *Historia de América Latina 8*. Barcelona, Editorial Cítica1991: p. 100.

13. Jennings B. Health policy in a new key. In Bayer R, Gostin LO, Jennings B & Steinbock B. *Public health ethics.* New York, Oxford University Press. 2007: 231–245 (232).

14. Kottow M. *Bioética y acción social.* Santiago, Universidad Diego Portales. 2008.

argument or even voter's injunction. Conscientious objection, also derived from such conservative ethics, is often mentioned as a last resort whenever liberalization is discussed.

The Issues

Public Health

Chile's only public health school has graduate MPH and PhD programs, including an extensive bioethics course, from which one of the first textbooks in the Spanish language, *Bioethics in Public Health*, has emerged.[15] From this vantage point, bioethicists have engaged in debates on the public aspects of values, right to health care, reproductive issues, occupational medicine, patients' rights, death, dying, transplant medicine and, more recently, non medical issues like environmental ethics.

Both public health policies and medical care are major issues in less developed nations, persistently but with little effect, striving to find the consistent political will to assign the fiscal resources needed to implement nationwide preventive measures, and secure a minimum of medical care for the poor and the less affluent. The Chilean national budget assigns a meager 3% of its GNP to health, increasing to slightly over 6% if private expenditures are included. Public health care is needed for somewhat less than four-fifths of the population, the rest negotiating with health insurance companies for whatever partial or full coverage they can afford. The idea of state-run medical services was actively discouraged in Chile and other Latin American countries by the World Bank, when it provided badly needed fiscal loans in the 1980s.[16] These healthcare policies are inspired by economic considerations and political agendas, causing a number of conflicts to which bioethics is especially sensitive since, in the final analysis, individual health care and survival are at stake.

In countries with marked socioeconomic disparities, health issues become all the more dramatic when accompanied by unfortunate biological conditions like undernourishment, endemic diseases, or stunted development, exacerbating socioeconomic deprivation and lack of social empowerment. Latin American bioethics has repeatedly stressed its role in protecting human beings by demanding that the state recognize the priority of comprehensive public health and medical care programs. As political interests limit resources to less than what is needed, bioethics is forced to reflect on rationing procedures, allocation criteria

15. Kottow M. *Bioética en salud publica.* Santiago, Editorial Puerto de Palos 2005.

16. See Ref. 3.

for scarce resources, and the setting of priorities, although its true advocacy is to secure health care especially for the deprived population, rather than participating in, or justifying, the allocation of insufficient resources. These social aspects of bioethics can hardly be tackled from the perspective of academic theory, for it requires deliberations that include people's needs and desires, as well as the acknowledgment of common sense morality.

The country's sanitary policy was taken to task in recent years by a nationwide public healthcare plan, now renamed *Garantías Explícitas Sanitarias* (GES = explicit healthcare guarantees), committed to delivering timely, effective, and "cost-neutral" (i.e., subsidized) medical services for a list of 56 diseases, expected to be increased to 80 in the next two years. This healthcare plan has shown three major flaws: (1) Coverage is incomplete, either because of poor accessibility and unduly long waiting lists, or because treatment is restricted within certain age limits or disease severity—for example, cataract patients only qualify with visual acuity below 20/100. (2) Diseases included were selected in a top-down manner, with only sporadic consideration of focal group deliberation. (3) As additional diseases are included, bottlenecks become more frequent, affecting also the medical care for diseases not included in GES.[17,18]

The weaknesses of this major healthcare reform, strongly based on rationing, illustrate that bioethical considerations and the civil society should be called upon to participate in the deliberation on sensitive social issues. If high-income groups hold not only economic but also political power, and own the most influential media, social issues become skewed and decisions will, more often than not, favor liberal policies, and dump on a small and weak state the tasks and duties to take care of the insolvent, because they are of no financial interest to free enterprise. Chile, being a mid-level, robust economy, is not accordingly strong in its social development, since educational, medical, and environmental issues have received insufficient attention in relation to these needs.

Reproductive Policies

Bioethics concerning reproductive issues also present peculiar aspects in Chile, and in other nations with a similar cultural profile.[19] In liberal states, reproductive

17. Unger J-P, De Paepe P, Solimano GC, Arteaga OH. Chile's neoliberal health reform: An assessment and a critique. *PLoS Med* 2008: 5(4):e79. doi:10.1371/journal.pmed0050079. Accessed October 21, 2008.

18. Zuñiga FA. Sistemas sanitarios y reforma AUGE en Chile. *Acta Bioethica* 2007; 13:237–245.

19. Jiles Moreno X. *De la miel a los implantes.* Santiago, CORSAPS. 1992.

decisions are increasingly placed in the hands of individuals. Developed nations tend to respect reproductive autonomy that includes the possibility of seeking abortion and sterilization, the use of routine and emergency contraception, as well as access to artificial fertilization in any of its forms, including embryonic selection. Most of these interventions are anathema to the Roman Catholic Church, in whose view they thwart the lives of potential human beings and act against the laws of nature; consequently, under the influence of the Church, laws are passed that prohibit these interferences with human reproduction.

In a 1976 Gallup poll that has never been updated,[20] 74% of Chileans were in favor of legalizing or at least tolerating abortion, much before Pinochet, in 1989, at the behest of political leaders linked to the Catholic Church, and especially to its *Opus Dei* movement, tightened the existing law to an absolute proscription. Therapeutic abortion was abolished as the last remaining indication, resulting in a legal framework that punishes both the woman who has an abortion and the healthcare personnel who provides it. Public health authorities consistently estimate clandestine abortions at about 150,000 annually, or approximately one of every three pregnancies—a third of which suffer complications that require medical care. Unsafe abortion causes the death of 400 women each year.[21] Often-proclaimed reproductive rights (Beijing, 1995) are ignored, with the exception of voluntary sterilization, practiced in public hospitals since 1975. And yet, most initiatives to reinstate a discussion on abortion have been thwarted before reaching Congress, with the argument that the abortion issue is not fit to be presented even for preliminary political discussion.

Official pro-life policies have witnessed an enormous increase in adolescent pregnancies (which occur in 14.9% of all births), with all the problems they entail, not the least being loss of educational opportunities and increased socioeconomic inequity.[22] Related reproductive issues, such as the distribution of levonorgestrel—emergency contraception that might have benefited from a less turbulent discussion than the abortion issue—are also held hostage by a national climate that stifles debate and discussion around bioethical issues. Emergency contraception was, in fact, recently banned by the Constitutional High Court from being freely distributed by the public health system, even if requested by rape or incest victims. The argument brought forth was that scientific evidence has been unable to

---

20. Ibid. p. 317.

21. Casas BL & Dides CC. Objeción de conciencia y salud reproductiva en Chile: dos casos paradigmáticos. *Acta Bioethica* 2007; 13:199–206.

22. Molina C, Ramiro, Molina G, Temístocles y Gonzalez A, Electra. Madres niñas-adolescentes de 14 años y menos: Un grave problema de salud pública no resuelto en Chile. *Rev. Méd. Chile* 2007; 135(1):79–86.

convincingly rule out a potential abortive effect of levonorgestrel, even though overwhelming scientific data consider the pill to act by inhibiting ovulation before fertilization occurs.[23] As an additional argument, the Church, right-wing politicians, and conservative scholars agreed that easily available contraception would slacken sexual mores and gnaw at fundaments of the traditional family concept, a point of view that might be agreeable to some conservative moral views, but does not purchase sufficient general agreement to support public policy.

Assisted fertilization has been a major issue for the Church, and certainly of great concern to society. Only a few private fertility clinics cater to the wealthy who can afford expensive reproductive treatments. Legal regulations are lacking, and practices are carried out behind a gray veil of ignorance. In all these issues, the Church does not really enter the arena of bioethical deliberation; it rather acts as a gatekeeper rejecting any proposition that might endanger its immutable principles. By using such emblematic phrases as "respect for life," "sanctity of life," "dignified dying," "solidarity," "playing God," "natural law," discussion is stultified, and any reflection is finally a zero-sum exercise that makes changes improbable.

Restrictive policies on fertility and reproduction, and the public health problems involved—high illegal abortion rates, rising number of adolescent pregnancies, unwanted children, child abuse—are prime examples of what French sociologist A. Touraine described as the invasion of the private realm by the public sphere. All these issues have hardly been discussed beyond a few newspaper interviews and TV panels, and a serious academic deliberation is lacking. Bioethics theories and practices are developing in institutions that are still young and insufficiently empowered to influence the cultural meanings of these and other sensitive issues.

Other Issues

A miscellany of topics concerning medical and bioethical themes are equally subject to restrictive regulations. Healthcare committees will be required by a law, which has been under parliamentary discussion for 9 years, to oversee rights and duties of patients and healthcare personnel. The most contentious item of this law on patient's rights has been disagreement about whether the right to refuse treatment also applies to life-saving interventions, which detractors interpret

23. International Consortium for Emergency Contraception (ICEC) & International Federation of Gynecology & Obstetrics (FIGO). How do levonorgestrel-only emergency contraceptive pills (LNG ECPs) prevent pregnancy? Available at: http://www.figo.org. Accessed October 21, 2008.

as euthanasia. The law will, in fact, disallow patients from taking life-threatening decisions, thus not only limiting patient autonomy, but also disregarding court decisions that have upheld the right of Jehovah's Witnesses to reject blood transfusions even in emergency situations.

When the Ministry of Health initiated a campaign favoring condoms as a protection against HIV/AIDS, the Church countered by discouraging any form of extramarital sex, reasoning that abstention was the best preventive—which of course it is, but such a suggestion flies in the face of modern sexual mores.

Universities, research centers, and teaching hospitals have created research ethics committees tailored after the American IRBs, where all research done with human beings or animals is subject to ethical evaluation. A recent law mandates the Ministry of Health to regulate and oversee the work of such committees, a necessary but not easy task to accomplish, in view of an unknown but increasing number of imported research protocols sponsored by international pharmaceutical companies, often insensible to local ethical needs. Most research committees abide by the Declaration of Helsinki, but there are other influences, like that of the John E. Fogarty International Center of the National Institutes of Health, which has carried out its own training programs in this and in other Latin American countries, requiring the local investigators whom it finances to take its online ethics course.

Environmental issues are a slow-growing concern in Chile. In 1994, a National Commission for the Environment was created, and a few laws were passed concerning protection of whales, and the basics of preservation of the environment. Some actions have been taken to secure clean water and air, as well as taking care of industrial waste. The Commission will evaluate new projects as to their environmental impact, but there has been little interaction with bioethics.

Institutionalization

Socioeconomic inequities, and ensuing educational disparities, make it very difficult for the disempowered and underprivileged to voice their needs or unite in social actions. Our democracy is more elitist than representative, as Schumpeter would have it, and hardly at all participative.[24] Public deliberation in a truly participative democracy requires certain social conditions that are, as yet, absent in Chile, but much can be learned by observing participative democracy operating in other countries. What is needed is a deliberative body of people who have

24. Cohen JL & Arato A. *Civil society and political theory*. Cambridge, MIT Press. 1995.

the know-how, are responsive and responsible to the civil society, and remain immune to the influence of power.[25]

Most developed nations, and many in the Third World, have created permanent National Bioethics Commissions, and UNESCO is offering its ABC (Assisting Bioethics Committees) Program to help in planning and setting up such commissions, always keeping in view the efficiency and social impact of the French National Committee which, since 1983, ably gives bioethics a voice at the level of public policies.[26]

Chile has become aware that broad-based academic bioethics has not been able to influence political decisions to the satisfaction of a pluralistic and, to some extent, multicultural society. In 2006, Congress passed a law requiring the creation of a permanent National Bioethics Commission and, although implementation has unfortunately not yet begun, a few caveats are already necessary. First, the law dictates that the Commission will have 9 members, which is less than most commissions have, and can easily upset plural parity. Furthermore, such a reduced number of members can hardly tackle the variety of problems at hand, nor will they possess the agility to probe in depth and yet come up with timely proposals. Hopefully, the suggestion will be heeded to create sub-commissions that might function simultaneously.[27] Otherwise, we might be getting a National Bioethics Commission that contradicts its essential mandate by failing to be broad-based, pluralistic, and with members chosen for their knowledge and prudence, not for their commitments to interest groups. Furthermore, in order to avoid navigating in political waters, a National Bioethics Commission should not be under the administration of the legislative branch of government.

National Bioethics Commissions should not wield direct political power, their task being advisory, but in no way mandatory or decisional: "bioethics commissions should be assessed primarily as agenda-setting rather than as expert bodies, and be judged successful according to their capacity to facilitate a wider public dialogue over ethical questions in the medical domain, rather than by their ability to find the best possible answers to the questions."[28] One of their main tasks is to educate the public and consider its opinion in bioethical matters where

---

25. Annas GJ. Will the real bioethics (Commission) please stand up? *Hastings Center Report* 1994; 24:19–21.

26. Isambert F-A. Ethics committees in France. *Journal of Medicine and Philosophy* 1989; 14: 445–456.

27. Kottow M. El rol de una Comisión Nacional de Bioética. In León CFJ (Coord.): *Libro de Actas VIII Jornada Nacional de Bioética*. Santiago, Sociedad Chilena de Bioética 2008: 15–32.

28. Dzur AW & Levin D. The primacy of the public: in support of bioethics commissions as deliberative forums. *Kennedy Institute of Ethics Journal* 2007; 17:133–142 (134).

such essentials as human rights, individual autonomy, and harm avoidance are at stake. Such proposals hope to place bioethics commissions in the midst of civil society's concerns, provided three basic tenets are accepted: (a) commissions are not regulatory bodies; (b) bioethical questions transcend the medical domain and include public health issues, biomedical research policies, and environmental concerns; and (c) lest it become sterile, dialogue should be widely participative and go beyond unending deliberation in search for the ultimately best possible answers to bioethical questions. To qualify as the best, these answers ought to remain revisable, and the laws suggested should be of the crepuscular variety, that is, valid for a specific period of time.

Conclusion

The particular Chilean historical and cultural background, as well as its socioeconomic development, show this country to be an interesting scenario to study the social impact of bioethical issues. Conservative forces slow down any attempts to revise moral values, even when the status quo is damaging and unwanted. Urgent issues like right to health care, reproductive rights, status of the embryo, end-of-life decisions, and many more, require a new approach with strong civil participation, which will, hopefully, be guided by a competent National Bioethics Commission providing top-down flow of information to the public, as well as a bottom-up stream of suggestions for appropriate public policies.

Finally, another reason to press matters in this direction is the emergence of a strong current of community investigations, especially in the field of population genetics, and the need to develop ethical norms to protect and benefit the communities being studied. As in most other areas of biomedical research, communities are being primarily tapped in less developed countries and, for the most part, by industry-subsidized ventures, thus providing convincing reasons why ethical surveillance must be expertly and democratically carried out.

Bioethics in Chile should seek the active participation of civil society, so as to broaden participation, help educate the citizenry, and increase public awareness about the issues of bioethics, as these concerns reach the personal life of each individual and are, therefore, not be decided upon in the absence of those affected. In addition, the flux in public health policies, the proliferation of community investigations, and increasing interest in population genetics require the citizenry to reach an informed and active participation in these matters.

8 BIOETHICS IN COSTA RICA

ORIGINS AND CHALLENGES

Fred Gifford and Ana Rodriguez

This chapter examines some important strands of the origin of bioethics in Costa Rica, as it arose beginning in the 1990s, thus elucidating certain characteristics of, and challenges for, present-day Costa Rican bioethics, and also revealing political interests underlying these developments. The analysis reveals how bioethics in Costa Rica, both its content and its profession, is shaped by cultural background features, social and political agendas, and historical contingencies. It also indicates that counterforces of tradition and economic interests pose challenges for those hoping to introduce bioethics into the healthcare system in a way that can have a positive effect on individual thinking and public policies.

Costa Rica is an especially interesting country in which to examine bioethics. A small, developing Central American nation, with a population of about 4.3 million and a gross national income per capita of $9,220 (PPP international $) in 2006, its total expenditure on health per capita in 2005 was $684, or 7.1% of GDP. Yet, its health statistics are in line with those of the industrialized nations. For instance, life expectancy is at least as good as that in the United States. (In 2006, these figures were 80 and 76 for life expectancy at birth for females and males, respectively, compared to 80 and 75 for the United States.[1]) These impressive results have been achieved through a broadly universal government-run healthcare system—called "the Caja"[2]—and through emphasis on primary care, public health, and such social determinants of health as education, addressed by programs and policies of the Ministry of Health.[3] Yet, healthcare reforms introduced primarily in the 1990s, a result of both international pressures and

1. World Health Organization, 2008.

2. *Caja Costarricense de Seguro Social*, or Costa Rican Social Security Fund.

3. Ministerio de Salud, 2002; Ministerio de Salud, 1999.

local decisions, are transforming the system, and they threaten Costa Rica's successes by a covert privatization of the system.[4]

Recently, bioethics has begun to emerge in Costa Rica institutionally and professionally. National committees for the oversight of human subjects research arose in the mid-1990s. Academic activity in bioethics has begun, with a small number of courses and occasional conferences at universities.

Yet, one must not be too sanguine here. The start had by research ethics committees has been unsteady and controversial. Not only is the overall number of bioethics courses small, but very little bioethics is taught in the medical schools. There remain strong political interests relevant to health sector reform, as well as entrenched interests of the medical profession that will resist critique. Thus, there are serious uncertainties about what Costa Rican bioethics will become. The directions it takes, how it is perceived, and what success it comes to have, will all continue to be shaped by the social and political agendas it advances and contests, and this will affect what useful role it can play. Those attempting to advance bioethics in Costa Rica must bear this in mind.

Main Background Strands

In what follows, we focus on two important strands of the origins of bioethics in Costa Rica, broad bioethical topics brought to the fore by particular practices and events in recent Costa Rican history: justice and the structure of the healthcare system, and research involving human subjects.

Health Care System Reform and Justice. Costa Rica's government-run system of healthcare provision (the Caja) was put into place in 1943, based on the principles of universality, equality, and solidarity.[5] It has been widely praised for its fairness and effectiveness, and strongly valued by the Costa Rican people. But, along with rising health care costs, certain reforms put into place in the early 1990s have been argued to threaten the integrity of the system. These reforms have confronted Costa Ricans with a number of moral tensions, and they have caused some to see the need for bioethical debate and reflection.

Research Involving Human Subjects. Ethical concerns about clinical trials in the 1990s resulted in the attempt to set up regulations and regulatory bodies. This history has been filled with controversy. Government regulations, along

---

4. Homedes, Nuria. Privatizacion de los servicios de salud: las experiencias de Chile y Costa Rica, in *Gaceta Sanitaria*. Vol. 16, n. 1 (Barcelona), Feb. 2002, p. 1.

5. Miranda, Guido, 1995. "Development of the Social Security Institute," in Carlos Muñoz and Nevin S. Scrimshaw, eds., *The Nutrition and Health Transition of Democratic Costa Rica*. International Foundation for Developing Countries (INFDC). Boston, MA.

with a research ethics committee set up by the Caja, were subsequently terminated, leading to the later emergence of a private committee. There remain serious worries about whether the present system of oversight of human subjects research is adequate.

Before we examine these healthcare reform and human subjects research strands, it is worth mentioning some other background factors—in particular, religion, the power of the medical community, and a culture of secrecy and corruption.

The Roman Catholic Church is the official religion of Costa Rica, and has considerable influence over both policy and public opinion. The most obvious effects of this involve topics concerning reproduction (for instance, in 2000, the Constitutional Court of Costa Rica (the Sala IV) declared in vitro fertilization unconstitutional). But the implications are, in fact, more general.[6]

Another important social and cultural background factor is the power of the medical profession. Certain cultural factors make this an especially potent force in Costa Rica. Physicians are highly regarded; several of the country's presidents have been physicians. There is a strong tendency toward paternalism in the medical profession, and a strong tendency among patients to acquiesce in or contribute to this.

There is a culture of secrecy, in the medical profession and in the government. (The policy changes concerning healthcare reform and experimentation discussed below were made outside of the public eye.) Also worth mentioning as a background factor is the culture of corruption in Latin America; corruption is denounced, yet at a certain level it is seen as inevitable.

The resultant failure to question authority is exacerbated by a particular cultural feature of Costa Ricans—a strong desire to get along peaceably and not confront others about disagreements.[7] This makes it even harder to challenge the medical profession, as well as to have explicit and frank discussion of bioethical issues that are controversial, or challenging to some interest group.

We should also note the role of the legal system. Patients in Costa Rica don't have the prospect of bringing a malpractice suit (as they would in the United States), nor do they tend to view themselves as having rights to such. In part, this reflects the general unempowered position of the average Costa Rican; it may also be a function of their viewing themselves as receiving their health care for free.

---

6. Marlasca, Antonio. 2001. *Introducción a la bioética*. Heredia, Costa Rica: Facultad de Filosofía y Letras, Universidad Nacional.

7. Mavis Hiltunen Biesanz, et al., 1999.

These factors may affect how the challenges sometimes posed by bioethics are taken seriously or not, and how the medical profession is able to retain its hegemony on these issues more strongly than, say, in the United States.

We now address in more detail the strands of healthcare reform and human subjects research.

Healthcare Reform

From the 1960s to the 1980s, the government-run healthcare system in Costa Rica worked quite well. While the Caja's coverage of the population began small, with just 8% of workers at its inception in 1943, it has expanded consistently over time, reaching 88% in recent years.[8] The near-universality and fairness of the system elicited the commitment of both practitioners and patients. While there has long existed a private healthcare sector, there have not, until recently, been strong reasons for patients to move to the private sector in large numbers, nor a strong monetary incentive to offer private services. Medical expertise has been similar within the private and public systems. The commitment of the health care practitioners within the government-run system, along with the fact that the system covered almost everyone, encouraged a feeling of contentment, loyalty, and trust among the populace, one strengthened by an already-existing culture of trust in authority, especially medical authority.

In the late 1980s and early 1990s, some crucial reforms in the financing of health care were planned and put into place, and their consequences still reverberate today. Central to these reforms was the institution of *compromisos de gestion* ("management contracts"), whereby various administrative units (notably, "health areas" overseeing a certain geographical area) take a more active role in making decisions about how to utilize their budget to obtain results. Such "purchasers" would then make contracts with "providers" of particular services, with the aim that the resultant accountability and competition would advance the overall goal of efficiency. But there were a number of other effects of the range of reforms put into place at that time, including a set of incentives that have changed the culture of medicine for the worse. An important feature of the reform was that the Caja was allowed—indeed, encouraged—to buy services from the private-sector doctors, clinics, and hospitals. The way this has played out has benefited the private sector by substantially enhancing the amount of profit to be made there. At about the same time, the government was made able to divert funds from the Caja to other, non-health-related, projects that it wanted

8. James Cercone and Jose Pacheco Jimenez, 2008.

to fund. This exacerbated the financial problems of the Caja, which in turn were used to justify the claim that reform was needed.

According to the official story, as described in the documents setting out the plan for reform,[9] the purpose of this reform was to prevent economic collapse of the healthcare system in the face of the country's economic crisis, by increasing the efficiency of the system, thus allowing lower costs and increased quality of services. Such a story was necessary in order to justify any dismantling of an institution as popular as the Caja, but it provides a misleading picture of the reasons these changes in fact came about. First, it leaves out the role of international financial institutions, such as the World Bank. More importantly, because more hidden, it leaves out the interests and agendas of those in the Costa Rican government and the medical profession.

There was indeed a serious crisis of the Costa Rican economy beginning in the late 1970s. Along with the rising costs of medical technology and an aging population, this led to a crisis in the healthcare system, with long waiting lists and lack of resources. This generated both a need to look for ways to cut costs, and a need to rely on loans from the World Bank and the International Monetary Fund. But such international agencies, of course, had their own agenda, seeking to tie such loans to the privatization of various government agencies and the reduction of public spending, the so-called "structural adjustment programs."[10] The World Bank had developed its own model for healthcare system reform, one designed at the 1994 "Cumbre de Las Americas" in conjunction with the Pan American Health Organization (PAHO) and the World Health Organization (WHO), and which was to fit all of Latin America.[11] Costa Rica was able to resist employing all the suggestions made by the World Bank, but the main features of these were ultimately embraced.

But these changes were also made possible in part because they fit with the interests of Costa Rica's *Colegio de Medicos*, the professional group of physicians with influence over various medical policies. To them, it was a benefit to lessen the degree to which doctors would work for the government, and to provide them with opportunities for substantial profit. Indeed, it should be noted that the *Colegio de Medicos* had never been completely supportive of the Caja or its universalization in the first place.[12]

---

9. Caja Costarricense del Seguro Social, 1997. *Hacia un nuevo sistema de asignación de recursos. Proyecto de modernización*. San José, Costa Rica.

10. Garnier, L. et al., 1997.

11. Ministerio de sanidad y consumo, 1998.

12. Clark, Mary, 2001.

These reforms changed the practice of medicine in fundamental ways. They brought business decisions and a focus on efficiency into the way clinics and other healthcare settings were run, and the way in which doctors thought. They provided economic incentives for physicians to move to the private sector. Especially important has been the *interaction between* the public and private sectors. Many doctors now work in both the public and private systems, spending part of the day in each, and the public sector purchases health services from the private sector. This has resulted in the stimulation of the private sector, and in less work in the Caja (doctors often leave the public hospitals early, in order to begin working in their private clinic). Further, it has led to corruption of various sorts that, among other things, strain the resources of the Caja further. Such corruption includes what are termed *biombos*, where physicians, seeing patients within the public system, offer to see them in their private practice and, at the same time, enable them to move ahead in a (public system) queue for procedures for which there are waiting lists. At a deeper level, these reforms have brought about a profound cultural change in the healthcare system, including a change in its underlying values from solidarity to competition.

On the other hand, some doctors and other healthcare professionals saw these changes, the ethically dubious motivations and behavior of their colleagues, and the kind of mentality that was developing in primary care, as disturbing. They were concerned that a weakening of solidarity and a strengthening of competition would be bad for Costa Rican health care. Discussions among these doctors led to the idea that some instruction in bioethics would be useful for counteracting this new model, and for helping healthcare practitioners think more carefully about these emerging issues. Hence, these controversial reforms were also, in a sense, one of the sources of bioethics in Costa Rica.

It is noteworthy that many of these doctors were in primary care (rather than from the hospitals), and that many of them had worked within the Ministry of Health (rather than within the Caja). The Ministry of Health (established in 1927) has always had an importantly different perspective concerning the approach to addressing health and health care—one that takes public health, preventive care, and primary care more seriously. It was responsible for the rural health program, whose success in the 1970s had made such an impression on the discussions at the International Conference on Primary Health Care in Alma-Ata in 1978.[13] But the Ministry has had, in recent years, a sort of "outsider" status in the Costa Rican healthcare system. Reforms already being completed in the 1980s included the transfer of all responsibility for the actual provision of health care to the Caja from the Ministry of Health, and a drastic cut in the latter's

13. Organización Mundial de la Salud. Alma-Ata 1978.

resources. In the process, several people from the Ministry of Health (those who didn't accept early retirement) were transferred to the Caja, and this brought to the surface some conflicts between these worldviews. The deep, longstanding tension and power differential between the Caja and the Ministry is likely to have an influence on who does what in bioethics, and who takes what seriously. In addition, the Caja's predominant role in medical education will affect the task of trying to insert bioethics into medical school curricula.

Research Involving Human Subjects

In the early 1990s there was considerable human subjects research in Costa Rica, much of it sponsored by universities and companies from the United States and Europe. Reasons for this include the existence of an ample number of well-trained local medical scientists, a useful population (with a health profile similar to that of developed nations, due to the successes of the health care system over decades), and the lack of effective regulations.

Before 1996, ethical review of human subjects research in Costa Rica consisted simply in sending the protocol of the proposed research to the Minister of Health. The Ministry of Health had no precedent for how such review should take place; there were neither resources for careful review, nor an understanding of how such review should take place.

In this environment, certain private organizations such as ICIC (*Instituto Costarricense de Investigaciones Clinicas*) arose, which acted as facilitators of clinical trials. International sponsors of trials were attracted to such local entities that could serve them in this way. In 1996, conflicts between ICIC and the Ministry of Health, along with the increased volume of research proposals, led to the appointment, within the Caja, of the first national "research ethics committee," composed mostly of physicians, but including a philosopher. This group was very divided. Some, in effect, opposed all research on human subjects. Others were motivated primarily to enable research to go forward, and saw the concern with bioethics and regulation mostly as an improper imposition that would hinder research. This committee did, however, create Costa Rica's first regulations for research involving human subjects,[14] relying (in significant part) on the Declaration of Helsinki.

There was also division among administrators about this committee and whether to have such regulations, and in 1998, with a change of administration, the committee and the regulations were eliminated. Later, a private research committee arose at a private university called UCIMED (*Universidad de Ciencias Medicas*).

---

14. "Reglamento para la investigacion en los servicios asistenciales de la CCSS." March, 1998.

As a result, research in Costa Rica was submitted only to UCIMED and other private entities, no longer to the Caja, so all research oversight was now done "privately." Among other effects, this changed the experience and culture of clinicians in the Caja with respect to experimentation.

There are now in Costa Rica several "research ethics committees," or RECs (called "institutional review boards," or IRBs, in the United States). Seven are listed on the website for CONIS (Consejo Nacional de Investigaciónes en Salud, or National Council of Research in Health), an entity within the Ministry of Health.[15] But questions remain about the expertise, training, and functioning of these RECs, and thus their ability adequately to protect human subjects. This is especially of concern in a cultural climate where there remains resistance to oversight of research among some groups, and considerable variation concerning how seriously the regulation of trials is taken. CONIS issued a decree in 2003[16] that all RECs be certified as adhering to certain standards, but in fact only a few are officially certified, and the certification process is not very stringent. In principle, CONIS should have the power to enforce this, and shut down substandard RECs, but this does not happen. This may be due to fears that they would be sued, and the realistic worry that the Ministry of Health may not be able to back them up in the event of such a lawsuit.

As well as the whole range of ethical issues concerning human subjects research (informed consent, vulnerable populations, etc.), especially prominent in this environment are conflicts of interest. These come first from the fact that individual researchers can make money enrolling their patients in trials, but also from the fact that private RECs not only charge for their services, but do so in a manner that could be expected to bias their judgment. (For example, if they approve a protocol, they'll be able to charge for further services as time goes on.) Clearly, there are a number of important institutional weaknesses standing in the way of proper oversight.

And, note the following two cultural reasons for concern about how well these committees work: First, experience in the United States suggests that effective oversight by committees is not just a matter of regulation but requires, in addition, education and the development of a culture that takes seriously and understands how to have serious discussion and perform oversight. This cultural change is something that develops only over time. Second, the Costa Rican cultural tendency to avoid confrontation may act as a further impediment to adequate oversight, by dissuading some from pushing hard questions about a given protocol. Plausibly, non-doctors might act in this way in relation to

15. http://www.ministeriodesalud.go.cr/comconis.htm.

16. http://www.ministeriodesalud.go.cr/reglamentos/31078-s.pdf.

doctors, resulting in an especially potent challenge to the adequacy of community representation on committees. But between doctors, this tendency not to confront would dovetail with other pressures to go along with the protocols put forward by their colleagues.

Implications

Healthcare system reform and experimentation came to the fore just as bioethics in Costa Rica was generating its self-consciousness—so these topics will be seen as central, as part of the agenda of those studying bioethics. In both cases, it is clear that there have been, and continue to be, political and economic interests at play. In the case of research issues, the focus is on regulation, and there has been a battle concerning where the regulation will take place, what will be considered adequate regulation, and who will take part and be considered expert in this area. Some will come to see these issues as intrinsically important, including the importance of protecting human subjects; some will see this regulation (and bioethics) as an inappropriate imposition from the outside. Some will come to see bioethics expertise simply as instrumentally useful toward the goals of getting research done. And, some will see it as a source of status or (if there is money to made in trial oversight) financial gain.

It is also worth mentioning that the way in which these currents of healthcare reform and experimentation have arisen results in an especially high level of divisiveness (including between different physicians). The role of religion in bioethics in Costa Rica also contributes to a certain amount of divisiveness. Further, the issues surrounding healthcare reform, coming to the fore just as bioethics was beginning in Costa Rica, is likely to affect the orientation of bioethics in Costa Rica in a way that embraces questions of social and political philosophy—especially concerning the role of the state, rather than only ethics and ethical theory.

But the following, more specific, points should be noted by way of comparing the origins of bioethics in Costa Rica and the United States. Bioethics emerged in the United States at an earlier time, and in a different cultural context. Interestingly, the ethics of human experimentation was also an important force early on in bioethics in the United States—beginning with the revelation in 1972 of the Tuskegee syphilis study, and subsequent legislation in the 1970s. But Costa Rica has come to these issues at a different time and place, in a context where there is now a well-developed set of regulations in other countries, and where a central question is the regulation and evaluation of trials generated in other countries by pharmaceutical companies that propose to utilize Costa Ricans as research subjects.

Further, even more central to the development of bioethics discussion in the United States were cases concerning paternalism and autonomy in the doctor–patient relationship, especially cases concerning the right to die or to refuse life-saving medical treatment. (For a variety of reasons, this has *not* been such a central factor in the rise of Costa Rican bioethics. The strong paternalism of the medical profession, the blind trust in doctors and of the medical system, and the influence of the Catholic Church kept patients and their families from questioning these things.) Even though observers of the U.S. healthcare system in the 1960s and 1970s noticed issues of access to health care, and the growing tendencies toward medicine being a business, these issues were not front and center. They did not constitute the *crisis* that they do now; they were not perceived as the most important worries about medicine, especially compared with end-of-life decisions and other issues of paternalism, autonomy, and patient's rights. But to a larger extent in Costa Rica, at least some Costa Rican healthcare professionals saw these healthcare reform issues around them as the central concerns, and this is likely to affect the perspective of those studying bioethics in Costa Rica.

Who Does Bioethics, and What Bioethics is Taught?

Arising from the foregoing discussion, there are a number of other things to say about the nature of bioethics in Costa Rica. First, who does bioethics? Before 1990, doctors and priests wrote about bioethical issues, but the issues raised were limited mostly to those concerning experimentation and reproductive issues, and they did not focus on access to health care or the power of physicians. Philosophers entered the discussions in the mid-1990s for reasons described above. Today, there are also lawyers and journalists. The journalists, for instance, report various scandals, such as the practice of biombos (mentioned earlier), or members of the board of the Caja found to be taking bribes.

Concerning education in bioethics, there are a few university courses, and one in CENDEISSS (*Centro de Desarrollo Estratégico e Información en Salud y Seguridad Social*—Center for Strategic Development and Information on Health and Social Security), part of the Caja. There have been occasional conferences at the universities. But bioethics is still not a strong part of the curriculum in universities, even in most philosophy departments. Nor is it a part of the curriculum of medical schools. A couple of the private medical schools (UNIBE—*Universidad de Iberoamérica*—and UCIMED) have recently begun courses in bioethics. But these have not involved discussions of the philosophical analysis of ethical issues in either research or clinical practice. (Note that students in Costa Rica enter medical school directly from high school, not after an undergraduate degree, so such students will, of course, not have had any bioethics course prior to medical school, either.) In 2005, Universidad Nacional (jointly with Universidad de Costa Rica) began Costa Rica's first graduate (Master's) program to train specialists in bioethics, which arose with the support of Universidad Nacional's rector and the country's Minister of Health.

For bioethics to flourish and have a positive impact, there needs to be much more teaching and research in bioethics in Costa Rica. But, just as importantly, there needs to be a change in the culture of both medicine and academia, so that there is receptiveness to the importance of bioethics in medical education, and to the importance of bioethicists participating in discussions of ethics and oversight of medical research and practice.

Concluding Remarks

As in other countries, ethical issues concerning health care increasingly present themselves in Costa Rica. There is a need for honest reflection concerning how to confront and resolve these questions. Bioethics has the potential to be a real aid in this process. But the progress is slow, and there is uncertainty concerning the degree to which those practicing bioethics will have the right interests and expertise, and whether there will be an adequate system of oversight. The worry, in the case of RECs, is that this will become merely a rubber stamp for the research that medical researchers would like to get done. There is thus a danger that bioethics will not well serve its function of critical discussion.

Such cooptation of bioethics is, of course, not unique to Costa Rica or developing nations. In the United States there are interests of various sorts at play, and there is a danger that bioethics (or research ethics) can be "embraced" but used as a "cover" or "public relations." But in the United States, a number of factors have typically been sufficiently weighty so as eventually to make the bioethical reflection (and regulations) have real significance. For example, the power of consumer and patients' rights groups (and perhaps the power to bring legal action) have served as a countervailing force in this regard. Further, the culture of medicine in the United States, while conservative in important ways, has been such as to allow bioethics—and regulations concerning human subjects protection—to be taken seriously. One reason may be that despite being seen as a threat, bioethics has also been seen as a potential help with the unavoidable and vexing ethical dilemmas that physicians have faced, and which are uncomfortable to face on one's own.

There is, and will continue to be, debate and struggle at various levels concerning what bioethics will become—what its role will be, and who bioethicists will be: Will doctors (and other healthcare professionals) dominate the discussions, or will those outside the field (academics, patients) have a strong voice? Will philosophers play a central role? Will religious perspectives be dominant? Questions are raised here of both divisiveness and power. Groups who already hold power, whether the medical profession or the Catholic Church, want to keep that power, and so it is important to them that bioethics not become something that could challenge their authority. At the same time, as bioethics discussions emerge and seem compelling, and questions of regulation arise, bioethics is seen as a useful expertise to be able to claim. Doctors would like to say that they have things under control, and don't need to be regulated from without.

A different challenge for Costa Rican bioethics can be seen by noting the relation to bioethics in other countries. There is debate concerning what identity *Costa Rican* bioethics is to have. Will it be *sui generis* or (more) derived from the bioethical discourse of other nations? If the latter, will this be that of the United States, Spain, Chile, Brazil? (We can also ask more generally whether *Latin America* will have its own distinctive bioethics.) This may affect what topics are seen as central, and what sort of foundational discussions occur. This will also both be influenced by, and have an impact on, who in Costa Rica is to be taken seriously and have an effect on the terms of the debate.

One implication of all this is that the *foundation* of bioethics in Costa Rica is more contested and controversial than, say, in the United States. Perhaps this will mean that, to a larger extent than in the United States, much of what is written and said will be ignored (because not understood or recognized) by others with different points of view about foundations. This makes more difficult the creation of a single bioethics community that functions as a connected discipline. It will also mean that, to a larger extent than in the United States, much of what is written and said will be about the foundations rather than the more practical, substantive analyses of particular bioethical issues.

It can thus be seen that the various strands and forces at play in the origin and development of Costa Rican bioethics have a variety of important implications for understanding the field, and in particular, for those interested in advancing bioethics in Costa Rica to understand the challenges that exist.

Glossary

Caja Costarricense de Seguro Social (Costa Rican Social Security Fund): the government entity, begun in 1943, in charge of the provision of heath care in Costa Rica ("the Caja").

CENDEISSS (*Centro de Desarrollo Estratégico e Información en Salud y Seguridad Social,* Center for Strategic Development and Information on Health and Social Security): the branch of "the Caja" dealing with medical education.

CONIS (*Consejo Nacional de Investigación en Salud*, National Council for Health Investigation): A council within the Ministry of Health advising concerning research involving human subjects.

ICIC (*Instituto Costarricense de Investigaciones Clinicas*): a private medical research organization, founded in 1991, involved in the performance of clinical trials in Costa Rica and other Latin American countries.

International Conference on Primary Health Care at Alma-Ata 1978 conference central to the international recognition of the concept of primary health care.

Sala IV Costa Rica's constitutional court, established in 1989.

References

Biesanz, Mavis Hiltunen, Richard Biesanz, and Karen Zubris Biesanz, 1999. *The Ticos: Culture and Social Change in Costa Rica.* London: Lynne Rienner Publishers.

Caja Costarricense del Seguro Social, 1997. Hacia un nuevo sistema de asignación de recursos. Proyecto de modernización. San José, Costa Rica.

Cercone, James and Jose Pacheco Jimenez, 2008. Costa Rica: "Good Practice" in Expanding Health Care Coverage–Lessons from Reforms in Low- and Middle-Income Countries, in Gottret, Pablo, George J. Schieber, and Hugh R. Waters, eds., *Good Practices in Health Financing: Lessons from Reforms in Low- and Middle-Income Countries.* Washington, DC: The World Bank

Clark, Mary, 2001. *Gradual Economic Reform in Latin America: The Costa Rican Experience.* Albany: State University of New York Press.

Garnier, L. et al., 1997. Costa Rica: Social Development and Heterodox Adjustment, in Mehrotra and Jolly, eds., *Development with a Human Face: Experiences in Social Achievement and Economic Growth*, Oxforf: Oxford University Press.

Homedes, Nuria. Privatizacion de los servicios de salud: las experiencias de Chile y Costa Rica, in *Gaceta Sanitaria.* Vol. 16, n. 1 (Barcelona), Feb. 2002, 54–62.

Marlasca, Antonio. 2001. *Introducción a la bioética.* Heredia, Costa Rica: Facultad de Filosofía y Letras, Universidad Nacional.

Ministerio de Salud, 1999. *Memoria Anual.* San José, Costa Rica.

Ministerio de Salud, Caja Costarricense del Seguro Social, Instituto Costarricense de Acueductos y Alcantarillados, Organización Panamericana de la Salud, Organización Mundial de la Salud, 2002. "Indicadores de Salud Cantonales Costa Rica." San José, Costa Rica.

Ministerio de sanidad y consumo, 1998. "Salud: la llave del desarrollo," *Jornadas de cooperación sanitaria.* Madrid: Edita Ministerio de Sanidad y Consumo, pp. 307–323.

Miranda, Guido, 1995. "Development of the Social Security Institute," in Carlos Muñoz and Nevin S. Scrimshaw, eds., *The Nutrition and Health Transition of*

Democratic Costa Rica. International Foundation for Developing Countries (INFDC). Boston, MA.

Organización Mundial de la Salud. Alma-Ata, 1978: Atención primaria de la salud. Serie "Salud para todos, num 1." Ginebra: Organización Mundial de Salud.

World Health Organization, 2008. Available at: http://www.who.int/whosis/data/Search.jsp

9 THE SOCIAL FUNCTIONS OF BIOETHICS IN SOUTH AFRICA

Anton A. van Niekerk and Solomon R. Benatar

Introduction

For the purposes of this chapter, the term *bioethics* will not only refer to the outcome of systematic reflection (mainly occurring in an academic context) on moral problems raised by health care and the life sciences and informed by a range of multidisciplinary perspectives (e.g., philosophical, political, medical, anthropological, etc.), but also to institutional practices that provoke or are influenced by such reflection. In short, while bioethics will refer to what is done on the level of academic training and research in the discipline, it will also refer to practices and institutions that occur and operate on the basis of social endeavors that are fundamentally informed by moral ideas and concerns.

How did bioethics come to South Africa? This question has no simple answers. Bioethical reflection in the developed world was mainly stimulated by the unmasking of the serious violations of human rights in the medical context that occurred during the Holocaust, as well as the surge of unprecedented technical prowess in medicine, epitomized by the Scribner shunt and the progress in organ transplantation in the course of the 1960s. South Africa as a state in the 20th century was the product of (mainly British) colonialism, interspersed with nationalist movements (like that of the Boer republics in the nineteenth century, and African nationalism that developed since the creation of the African National Congress [originally the South African Native National Congress or SANNC] in 1912). As a former British colony, the country maintained strong links to the academic institutions of Britain and the European continent in the first half of the twentieth century. As such, bioethical interest gradually "spilled over" to South Africa.

We shall, in the rest of this chapter, explore the cultural meanings and social functions of bioethics, particularly since the developments of the 1960s. Because space is limited, we concentrate on the following broad themes: bioethics training, the Biko history, the situation with abortion and euthanasia in South Africa, patient rights, the AIDS debacle, clinical ethics, and capacity building in research ethics.

Social Impact through Training in Bioethics

The extent to which bioethics has attained distinct cultural meanings and social effects in South Africa depends, to a large extent, on the success with which bioethics as an academic discipline and a public discourse has become entrenched in this society, and also by whether the ideas associated with the field are compatible with, and are not rejected by, local cultural and social concepts.

While South Africa's population is predominantly black African, and there is a black African government, the economic infrastructure, educational, and health systems are entirely "Western" in their orientation—a consequence of the country's colonial past. Yet, traditional medicine is and continues to be widely practiced. Indeed many, if not most, Africans who consult Western physicians also consult traditional healers. If, as predicted from a long-term perspective, the role of Western medicine in Africa could be evanescent (Van Rensburg & Benatar, 2001; Benatar & Van Rensburg, 2001), then the future of bioethics would be even more so.

However, in the short term we should acknowledge that the battle to free South Africa from apartheid, and the resulting political transition have been driven not only by the liberation movement, but also by Western liberal ideology, language, and values that included the concepts of human rights. We should also acknowledge that Western medicine, as well as a Western style bioethics, will continue to be influential—at least among those privileged to have access to these. It is therefore not surprising that, in the initial phases of bioethical awareness in South Africa, the context was characterized by typical Western-inspired concerns, such as the moral uncertainty created by the application of new technologies. In this sense, one may argue that bioethics initially attained the meaning of a concern regarding adequate etiquette and sound professionalism in the practice of medicine. Its function was essentially to complete or "round off" the professional training of healthcare workers. It was only gradually, and parallel to the intensification of the liberation struggle in the country, that bioethics became linked to more indigenous concerns and started to function in a way that was more focused on local, social, political, and humanitarian concerns. This will become clearer in the next section.

So, since the 1980s the increasing inclusion of bioethics in the curricula of several philosophy departments and medical faculties in South Africa has been largely in synchrony with the Western tradition of medicine and the associated advances being made in bioethics thinking and education in the Western world. While some effort is being made to refract such ways of thinking through the lens of African culture, the anthropological skills and cultural knowledge required to do so are not a significant part of the armamentarium of bioethics educators. Godfrey Tangwa, an African philosopher/bioethicist, who teaches in South Africa (vide infra) within the International Research Ethics Network of South Africa (IRENSA) Diploma course, has made significant efforts over many years to bring into view African perspectives on bioethics (Tangwa, 2006). However, we do not have any empirical evidence of the compatibility or acceptance of bioethics within African cultures.

While it can be questioned whether an enhanced level of ethical practice in society is influenced by bioethics education, we view sensitization to ethical issues, and some understanding of the underpinnings of ethical arguments, as one of the most important contributions that bioethics education and training can bring about. While there is also no good empirical evidence that bioethics is significantly affecting medical practice, it seems that the effects of bioethics training are slowly filtering through to medical practice in South Africa. The Health Professions Council of South Africa has made continued professional development (CPD) compulsory for all healthcare professionals, and continued ethics training constitutes a necessary part of those training programs. This is in line with the international trend that increasingly regards ethics as an integral part of medical training and research. There is, in other words, also in South Africa a tendency to understand bioethics as the recognizable face of a more humane and holistic approach to medical education and practice. The hope is often expressed that it will thus function as a humanizing influence on a discipline that has, in the past, because of a reductionist, mechanistic view of the method of clinical practice, forfeited the holistic approach to patients that a sound medical methodology requires (Kriel, 2000).

The message is hopefully being brought across that ethics in medicine requires significantly more than a mechanistic compliance with enforceable rules, and that ethics is not limited merely to following codes required in order to avoid litigation and punishment. Indeed, the motive behind the current-day emphasis on ethics is the humanization of medicine, the protection of patients and research subjects, and the fostering of a rational and reflective society with sound moral values.[1]

1. We are not implying that the "humanization of medicine" can only be achieved through bioethics training. The introduction of the humanities in general into medical education, as well as the adoption of a philosophically sound anthropology (i.e., freed from Cartesian dualism; cf., Kriel, 2000), can also contribute significantly to this ideal.

The Death of Steve Biko and the Function of Bioethics in South Africa's Liberation Struggle

The events surrounding the death of Steve Biko in 1977 were instrumental in linking bioethics with significant trends in South Africa's struggle against apartheid and even, to a limited extent, to an aspect of the liberation struggle. In this sense, one can argue that the Biko history contributed to an indigenization of bioethics in South Africa in the sense that now, the formulation, interpretation, and application of bioethical concerns took their inspiration from an indigenous South African tragedy.

The Biko case history is well documented; we only provide the essential facts. While detained without trial in September 1977 by the security police in Port Elizabeth, Biko sustained serious head injuries (probably as a result of acts of torture) that were grossly misdiagnosed and treated by two white doctors who colluded with the police. The physician who initially examined Biko, Dr. Ivor Lang, at the time noted in writing on more than one occasion that he could find "no pathology" in the patient. Biko was consequently driven 750 miles from Port Elizabeth to Pretoria Central Prison, lying semicomatose, naked, and handcuffed on some cell mats at the back of a Land Rover. He was not accompanied by a doctor and no medical records were sent with him. After arriving at the prison in Pretoria, he was again inadequately examined by a doctor, who administered an intravenous drip and a vitamin injection. He died on the night of September 12, 1977, unattended on a mat on the floor in his cell (McLean & Jenkins, 2003, pp. 78–80; cf. also Damster, 1998).

When these facts became known, failure of the SAMDC (the South African Medical and Dental Council, established in 1928 with the responsibility for licensing medical professionals and overseeing their professional and moral conduct) to exercise its duty to protect the public by acknowledging the unethical behavior of state-employed medical practitioners toward Biko, and failing to take appropriate disciplinary action against them, met with resounding criticism nationally and internationally (Jenkins 1986; 1987; 1988; Nightingale et al., 1990; Benatar, 1990). This shameful medical response was aggravated by the heartless statement in parliament by the then South African Minister of Justice, Jimmy Kruger, that "Biko leaves me cold."

In a protracted process that lasted almost a decade and a half, the SAMDC initially declined to admonish and discipline the culprit physicians. A small group of members of the profession (Professors Frances Ames, Trefor Jenkins, and Phillip Tobias) nevertheless took legal action, which led to a Supreme Court injunction against the SAMDC, resulting in a reversal of its previous decisions and the imposition of disciplinary action against both doctors who acted negligently in the treatment of Biko (Jenkins, 1988; Benatar, 1990). The fact that they were a small group, who persisted in these efforts in spite of opposition from the authorities, shows how public and even professional debates on ethical issues in medicine were limited in a repressive, authoritarian society lacking a patients' rights movement and unaccustomed to public discourse on civil and political liberties (Benatar, 1988; 2004).

The Biko affair was one of the most high-profile and reprehensible moral aberrations of the apartheid era. Yet, it was, at the same time, an important stimulus to heightened moral awareness in the country in general, and in the medical profession in particular. The way in which a small number of medical professionals stood their ground against both a professional body (the SAMDC) and a professional society (The Medical Association of South Africa, or MASA) for whom protection of colleagues was more important than upholding moral standards in the profession, demonstrated a commitment to ethical awareness and moral conduct that was not widely accepted up to that time. The affair spilled over in significant reforms to both bodies, culminating in the establishment of the Health Professions Council of South Africa that replaced the SAMDC in the 1990s, and the South African Medical Association, which was the amalgamation of the old MASA with the National Medical and Dental Association (NAMDA), created in 1982 as a result of discontent in progressive medical circles with MASA's actions in the aftermath of the Biko affair. Bioethics, which essentially inspired the actions of Biko's defenders, thus came to be interpreted as not merely an academic enterprise but indeed a motive, not only for social action generally, but for the prudence and efficacy of resistance to tyranny.

In this sense, the Biko affair, and the way in which it highlighted the importance of a moral orientation in the practice of medicine, directly contributed to a reorganization of the institutionalized medical profession in South Africa. Greater attention to ethical responsibilities toward prisoners, detainees, and hunger strikers was another gratifying response to the Biko case (Jenkins, 1987; 1988; Benatar, 1988; 1990; Kalk & Veriava, 1991). The public confession of guilt by the district surgeon, who bore major responsibility for Biko's medical care, emphasized the need to maintain professional independence in the face of state security and other coercive pressures.

The Biko affair might not have sparked an immediate or widespread revolution against an inhumane social and political dispensation in the late 1970s or early 1980s. But, together with an event such as the Soweto uprising of June 1976, Biko's death made it clear that all rhetoric from government leaders about the intended justice of the homeland system, and other alleged feats of apartheid, was bogus, that the system was morally corrupt, and that its demise was merely a matter of time. At the same time, it highlighted the depths to which a society can sink when gross violations of human rights occur and are tolerated. It is no exaggeration to claim that the Biko affair, together with other factors, played an important role in sensitizing the country at large about the dire need of a culture of human rights in South Africa. The Bill of Rights that today introduces the South African Constitution (finalized in 1996) is, therefore, in a special way, a testimony to the important lessons learned in South Africa from the Biko affair, and from the canons of medical ethics. In this sense it can be argued that the Biko affair was also a very significant turning point in South African history, and an illustration of the social and political impact that a severe violation of medical morals had on South African society.[2]

Debates about Abortion and Euthanasia

The advent of the new South African democracy in 1994 generated a general climate in which people were intensely aware of the need for change on most fronts. This included views about and legal provisions for medical practices such as abortion and assisted death. It is not surprising that international debates on abortion and euthanasia, often regarded as pivotal markers for renewed bioethical debate,[3] should have impacted on the intellectual climate of a society in radical transition, such as the "new South Africa" in the 1990s. In addition, the growing women's movement in South Africa, with increasing influence following the advent of democracy in 1994,[4] had, through its advocacy of women's right to choose, a notable impact on the speedy reform of abortion legislation that occurred in the mid 1990s.

Such impact became most obvious in the sphere of abortion legislation. Under pre-democracy South Africa's draconian conservative legislation, an abortion was only permitted when continued pregnancy endangered the pregnant woman's life, when the pregnancy was the result of incest or rape, when the fetus would be born with severe congenital defects, or when continued pregnancy would cause severe mental disease. This overly conservative abortion act of the old South Africa was changed in a new abortion law, adopted in 1996 and entitled the Choice on Termination of Pregnancy Act (Act 92 of 1996),

2. Sadly, events at Guantanamo Bay and Abu Ghraib reveal that even those countries that have been most vociferous about human rights abuses may similarly default when faced with security threats.

3. See Singer, 1993 and 2002 (including the articles jointly authored by Singer and Kuhse in Singer, 2002, pp. 179–198, 233–245), as well as Tooley, 1983.

4. South Africa's ruling party (the African National Congress) has a target that 50% of its members of parliament should be women; currently, more than a third of members are indeed women—a situation very different from the parliament of apartheid South Africa.

which became one of the most liberal sets of abortion provisions currently available in the world.

It is clear that South Africa has moved from a disposition where abortions were mostly illegal, and generally only obtainable abroad or by backstreet practitioners, to a thoroughly liberalized situation where the principle of a woman's right to choose, in view of her autonomy over her own body, is accepted and protected.

While it is difficult to determine whether the changed abortion practice in South Africa is the direct or indirect outcome or social effect of the study of bioethics, we venture to propose that it is unlikely that the abortion situation in this country could have been so dramatically reversed without some role played by the study of, and reflection on, bioethics (Oosthuizen et al., 1974; Benatar et al., 1994a). While it can reasonably be claimed that the utilitarian, liberal strain in abortion bioethics played a significant role in creating South Africa's new abortion law, human rights considerations also had a marked effect. At the same time, a conservative orientation to issues pertaining to the status of prenatal life, as demonstrated by the concerted action of Doctors for Life in fighting the new law, is also apparent. It remains safe to argue that bioethics of a varied orientation did play, and continues to play, a significant role in the propagation and contestation of ideas and practices concerning abortion in South Africa.[5]

We therefore conclude that bioethics' libertarian discourse on an issue such as abortion provided an intellectual framework on the basis of which the liberation of women, as the latter is expressed through the right to choose, achieved a more vocal, articulate, and effective vehicle for promotion and elucidation.

Regarding euthanasia or assisted death, the story is much briefer (Oosthuizen et al., 1973). In South Africa, no form of "active euthanasia"[6] in the sense of active assistance in bringing about death is legal in the clinical situation. Withholding treatment in situations where the treatment is futile and death is inevitable has been defended in South Africa (Benatar et al., 1994b) and is legally permitted. The "new South Africa" has seen a seemingly provocative reinvestigation of this position on assisted death. At the time following the adoption of South Africa's new constitution (1996), the South African Law Commission launched a comprehensive research project on this issue and brought out a report.

While this report and recommendations of the Law Commission were tabled in parliament more than 10 years ago (1998), and its recommendations were

5. See on this issue also Hoffman et al., 2006.

6. Bearing in mind all the problems that can rightfully be identified with the alleged distinction between "active" and "passive" euthanasia or "killing" and "allowing to die." Cf., Brock, 1998, pp. 235–239.

widely reported and commented on in the press (for example, Soal, 1999), there has been no further effort by the government of the day to take these recommendations further in terms of legislation.

The earlier referred-to status quo, therefore, still prevails on this issue in South Africa. Whereas it is fair to surmise that bioethical teaching, reflection, and discussion might well have contributed significantly to the formulation of the Law Commission's report (many bioethicists, including the authors of this chapter, made inputs to the commission at the time), the absence of further action and legislation bears testimony to the limited impact of bioethics in South Africa as far as this issue is concerned.

Patient Rights in South African Healthcare Practice

A formal acknowledgment of the rights of patients in the healthcare setting is one of the significant outcomes of the transition to democracy in South Africa. The Department of Health (Department of Health, 1996) accepted and published a formal Patients' Rights Charter in 1996. This Charter was also included as Booklet 13 of the *Guidelines for Good Practice in Medicine, Dentistry and the Medical Sciences* of the Health Professions Council of South Africa (Health Professions Council of South Africa, 2002).

In addition to the formulation of patients' rights, patients' responsibilities have also been stipulated. It is praiseworthy that the culture of human rights reintroduced to South Africa via the constitution—a model of a well written and balanced liberal democratic document—has generated a Patients' Charter. Heightened awareness of bioethical discussions since the 1980s has probably contributed to the National Department of Health's emphasis on patients' rights.

It is, however, an entirely different question whether what is professed in theory is being translated into actual practice. The situation at several hospitals in the public sector in South Africa bears testimony to practices that are, in fact, the direct opposite of what is so loftily professed in the Charter. To substantiate, the examples are plentiful. We rest with the findings made in two research reports of the Ethics Institute of South Africa (EthicSA) about conditions and practices at two of South Africa's biggest and best known hospitals, viz. the Chris Hani Baragwanath Hospital in Johannesburg, and the Universitas Hospital in Bloemfontein (Landman, Mouton & Nevhutalu, 2001; 2002). These findings show that there is a significant gap between theory and practice in terms of the rights of patients espoused in the Charter. In this respect, bioethics has not yet made the desired impact on the practice of South African health services. Ethical conduct should not only be considered in the sphere of individual behavior in the clinical setting, but also from the perspective of what institutions provide to enhance the care provided by healthcare workers. The problem is thus not, fundamentally, only one of promoting ethical conduct by healthcare workers, but also of improving the ethics of how institutions operate.

The fact that a charter of patients' rights has been formulated shows how powerfully the idea of human rights and its concomitant ideology of liberal individualism currently pervades—at least on the rhetorical level—the discourse of medicine in South Africa. In this country, bioethics and human rights discourse have indeed become noteworthy partners in the rhetoric that has been and is being created to underpin the transformation of society. It is therefore not surprising that bioethics and human rights discourse are often simply associated or equated. As indicated in the previous paragraph, this, however, provides no guarantee that the actual lives of patients in practice are significantly improved.

Bioethics and AIDS

The HIV pandemic poses a major challenge to the new South Africa. The social, ethical, and economic implications of HIV/AIDS were foreseen many years ago, but are only now becoming widely appreciated. The intense suffering, loss of human labor power, and the increased work required to care for AIDS sufferers, will increasingly and profoundly affect the lives and well-being of all in South Africa. Adverse effects on the economy affect all aspects of development: income, access to food and basic living requirements, interpersonal, class, and gender relationships, government credibility in caring for their citizens and in upholding human rights. In brief, HIV/AIDS is resulting in medical and social disasters in Africa (Barnett & Blaikie, 1992; Van der Vliet, 1996; van Niekerk, 2002, Benatar 2001, 2004), and how to deal with these raises many complex ethical considerations.

It surprises many that, despite considerable attention to HIV/AIDS, so little has been achieved in slowing the pace of the pandemic (Whiteside, 2006). Clearly the denialism promoted and sustained by the Mbeki government must be considered to play a prominent role (Nattrass, 2004; Feinstein, 2007). However, it is also necessary to consider the nature of the disease, how it arose, the factors associated with its propagation, and the limited role of medicine in controlling a pandemic with such deep roots in social structures and human behavior.

Clearly, scientific progress and the delivery of modern medical care make major contributions to dealing with disease, as illustrated by the development of effective antiretroviral drugs for the treatment of AIDS, their impact in wealthy countries, and the successes achieved in lower income countries such as South Africa (Coetzee et al., 2004). However, the role of extreme poverty, subhuman living conditions, lack of access to basic education, poor sanitary and living conditions, dysfunctional families, lack of recreational facilities, sexual freedom, and high crime rates should not be underestimated. All are endemic to Africa and are fueled by the powerful forces that have been promoting global disparities for many generations (Benatar, 2001, 2002b). While acknowledging such considerations, it is also necessary to be critical of inadequate attention from governments to the pandemic, most especially in South Africa (van Niekerk, 2003a), and to be supportive of the courageous efforts of activists like the Treatment Action Campaign (TAC), an activist organization under the leadership of Zachi Achmat. Although the TAC does not present itself as an organization that explicitly promotes bioethics, it has been significantly successful—more successful than any other organization—in forcing the South African government through legal action and injunctions to act in a more focused and humane way to alleviate the plight of the needy living with AIDS.

Some blame can also be laid at the doorstep of major international institutions driven by the imperialist economic and ideological power of wealthy nations. For the past two decades, the World Bank and the IMF have held the balance of power in formulating global health policy. In so doing, they have imposed structural adjustment programs, encouraged liberalization of economies, cut subsidies from basic foods and shifted agricultural policy to promote export crops to the detriment of home-grown food production—all resulting in devastating malnutrition and starvation that have caused billions to suffer, especially in Africa. It is a sad reflection on organizations that promote public health that these adverse forces are not adequately acknowledged or discussed. HIV/AIDS cannot be dealt with unless these underlying conditions are gradually reversed (Logie and Benatar, 1997). Recognition of the adverse effects of overt racial apartheid in South Africa, while failing to recognize the adverse effects of covert economic apartheid at the global level, regrettably reflects a form of "*selective moral blindness*." It is becoming an increasingly important social function of bioethics in South Africa to unmask these forces and to insist on a broader contextualizing of bioethical discourse. As both of us have argued elsewhere, bioethics should become operational, not only on the micro level of interpersonal, clinical relationships between patients and healthcare workers, but also on the meso level of institutions, as well as on the macro level of relationships between states and the operations of multinational corporations (Benatar et al., 2003; van Niekerk, 2006).

Education about safe sex and about the use of condoms are important aspects of the thrust against HIV/AIDS, but these are not remotely sufficient to overcome the deeply entrenched suspicion of such advice that interferes with procreation, and that goes against centuries of socially accepted and psychologically driven sexual practices in African and many other cultures. Failure to recognize the pervasive social, economic, behavioral and political aspects of HIV/AIDS—both in terms of its origins and its control—is self-defeating. The complexity of the scientific endeavor required to understand the pathobiology of the disease, and to develop appropriate treatment, is more than matched by the complexity of understanding and dealing with the social underpinnings of HIV/AIDS and other plagues (van Niekerk, 2002), locally and globally (Benatar, 2002b).

The example of antismoking campaigns illustrates the difficulty in achieving behavioral change even for acquired habits with only mild addictive effects. The greater challenge of achieving change in relation to such basic drives and needs as sexual relations should not be underestimated—especially when interacting with people whose social and sexual mores differ, and who may be suspicious of the underlying motives of imperialistic "educators" (van Niekerk, 2002). Bioethics as a force for the motivation of a moral course of action in relation to AIDS is, in other words, in this regard up against the powerful, pervasive, and seemingly impregnable forces that govern human behavior.

Establishment, Training, and Effects of Research Ethics Committees for Medical Research

As in the rest of the world, clinical research has become a major enterprise (and an instance of big business) in South Africa and, increasingly, in other parts of Africa. In their chapter on health research in South Africa in the 1999 edition of the *South African Health Review*, Mbewu and Mngomezulu write that, for many years prior to democracy, South Africa had been regarded as a "researcher's 'paradise' . . . because of its first world technology alongside a third world captive population, largely unprotected by codes of conduct and with extremely poor human rights protection" (Mbewu & Mngomezulu, 1999, p. 370). Consequently, health research done in South Africa and other African countries was often not submitted to rigorous ethical scrutiny in a manner that would have been required in developed countries, and the benefits (if any) of that research were often not made available to the populations among whom the research was originally done. A lot of what is currently done in bioethics in South Africa deals with capacity building in research ethics—in particular, capacity to participate in the ethical review of research protocols. Research, including the research initiated and executed by multinational conglomerates in the developing world, has always, prima facie, been considered to have a beneficial intent. Yet, these multinational corporations at the same time have commercial, profit-seeking agendas that do not always operate with altruistic intent and to the demonstrable benefit of research subjects in these countries. Bioethics therefore faces a special responsibility not to be hijacked by those same agendas, and to exercise its morality-seeking responsibility with real integrity.

Nothing focused the attention more clearly on this problem than the debate about trials for shortened regimens of antiretroviral drugs for HIV/AIDS in Africa.[7] This debate illustrated the serious moral concerns that exist about issues such as equipoise in terms of research questions and minimum and/or normal standards of care. Such debates have made it clear that not only does ethical review of clinical trials in the developing world require special attention to special concerns, but that the review ought also to occur in the host countries themselves, in cooperation with the countries in which the research is initiated. That, in turn, raised the issue of adequate capacity for such ethical review in the developing world, and constitutes the context within which the training of research ethics committees has become an issue of pivotal importance, both in Africa at large, and in South Africa in particular. (National Bioethics Advisory Commission, 2001; Nuffield Council on Bioethics, 2002; Benatar, 2002, Benatar and Landman 2006, Cleaton-Jones and Wassenaar 2010.)

Growing interest in research in developing countries since the HIV/AIDS pandemic thus reflects renewed and encouraging interest in, and concern about, the nature of the relationship between researchers and their subjects. Appreciation of concerns regarding research in developing countries requires some knowledge of the growing global disparities in wealth and health, and of the lifestyle and worldview of potential research subjects. Against such a background, it is apparent that the ethical dilemmas faced in conducting collaborative international research can only be addressed satisfactorily if research ethics is seen as being intimately linked to health care, to human health globally, and to the promotion of social and economic processes that could begin reversing widening global disparities in health—an idea propagated by Africans (Benatar, 2001).

When those in privileged positions and in wealthier countries consider undertaking collaborative research with colleagues in developing countries, it is necessary for them to understand both their own framework of thinking, and the implications of very different mindsets and environments in which research projects may be carried out in developing countries. The mindset of researchers from industrialized countries, and in which the debates on research ethics are taking place, is characterized by a biomedical approach to disease, and a neoliberal approach to economics and trade (Lee & Zwi, 1996). These powerful forces shape the world through a dominant worldview. We have argued for greater sensitivity to the fact that not all, and especially not those who are disadvantaged or who have been exploited, see the world through the same prism (Benatar, 2002).

---

7. For this debate, which we cannot deal with now, given the scope of the chapter, see van Niekerk, 2003a; Lurie & Wolfe, 1997; Angell, 1997; Resnik, 1998; De Zulueta, 2001; Schuklenk, 1998; Benatar, 2008.

In "developing" countries, where cultural, linguistic, economic, and other barriers may prevail between researchers and subjects, it is especially important to ensure effective communication. Anthropologists and others have documented the many pitfalls and difficulties that need to be faced in obtaining meaningful informed consent under these circumstances (Marshall, 2001; Slack et al., 2000). However, despite many cross-cultural barriers, it should not be assumed that disadvantaged people cannot grasp the concepts involved in research. Most of the goals of ethical research can be achieved when dealing with impoverished and illiterate people if sufficient time, skill, interest, and resources are devoted to communication and consultation. Attention to many cross-cultural considerations in international collaborative clinical research has been a specific focus of our capacity-building program and from this experience, approaches have been developed toward resolving seemingly intractable dilemmas in research (Benatar, 2004b). Bioethics, in this regard, increasingly serves the function of a facilitator of effective communication in South Africa's multicultural and multilingual context.

It seems reasonable to expect that profits from well-conducted trials should also benefit the citizens of developing countries in which the research was undertaken (Benatar, 2002). While it may be difficult to undertake harm/benefit calculations in advance of knowing what research will reveal, and how valuable the information may be, the debate that is beginning on how safeguards can be built into the contract to promote justice in the distribution of benefits at a later time, is being encouraged in the quest to achieve greater fairness in the international research endeavor (Shapiro & Benatar, 2005).

Clinical Ethics

Because medical schools and hospitals have not actively embraced and supported bioethics, there are very few well-trained bioethicists in South Africa with the skills and credibility to provide effective and appreciated bioethics consultations in the clinical care setting. Much of the focus has been on research ethics education and practice, because these activities have been promoted, encouraged, and funded by organizations outside of South Africa—notably, the Fogarty International Center at the U.S. National Institutes of Health and the Wellcome Trust in the United Kingdom. Regrettably, clinical bioethics receives minimal financial support from South African universities or hospitals.

The University of Cape Town Bioethics Centre has, for more than two decades, offered and provided a clinical ethics consultation service at the UCT academic hospitals, as well as to practitioners in the private sector when invited to do so. A similar consultation service is now also provided in Tygerberg Hospital in Bellville, by the Tygerberg division of the Unit for Bioethics (part of the Centre for Applied Ethics) of Stellenbosch University.

The development of clinical bioethics, and of well-trained and effective clinical bioethics committees within our healthcare system, is one of the many challenges to be faced in the future. A significant part of this challenge is to understand how such African values as hierarchical decision-making processes, *ubuntu* (the concept of interdependence), and other cultural concepts can interface with ideas of individualism, autonomy, informed consent, and civil and political rights. Medicine in Africa is largely assumed to be beneficent, and physicians enjoy considerable trust. This is largely because Africans appreciate what Western medicine can offer them without rejecting the role of the traditional healer. This area is ripe for further study and research.

Conclusions

We conclude that bioethics has made significant contributions to medicine and health care in South Africa. We have illustrated how the Biko affair was, on the one hand, symbolic of the moral shortcomings in providing health care for the majority of South Africans under apartheid and, on the other hand, brought about a turn for the good in resensitizing South Africans about moral issues in medical practice. We have suggested that bioethics has contributed a small, but nevertheless relevant, role in the South African transition. This contribution assisted in transforming attitudes toward practices such as women's right to choose in the abortion debate, and the acceptance, at the level of official health policy, of the idea of patients' rights. Bioethics also played a central role in the creation of new institutions, and new educational programs in bioethics at a number of universities that significantly facilitated and continue to facilitate an enhanced moral awareness in health care, business, and other organizational practices.

However, in spite of these and other small islands of success, bioethics has, overall, had a limited effect on the moral fabric of South African society. In particular, we note that in areas such as the regulation of humane and morally defensible health-related practices such as assisted death, as well as in actual clinical and service-rendering practices that occur in large South African hospitals, there is a sad lack of both moral deliberation and expressed concern for the rights and dignity of patients, with attention to cross-cultural considerations.

The vast task of transforming South Africa beyond a fledgling democracy struggling to maintain this status, into a caring society that optimizes the opportunities and life quality of the majority of its citizens, is the major challenge that lies ahead. Hopefully, bioethics will have some positive impact on this process and Western bioethics will benefit from insights into the values of solidarity and interdependence that are characteristic of traditional African culture, and that have allowed many to live relatively good lives in the face of very limited resources.

References

Angell M. (1997). The ethics of clinical research in the third world. *New England Journal of Medicine, 337*,847–849.

Barnett T & Blaikie P. (1992). *AIDS in Africa: its present and future impact*. London: Belhaven Press.

Benatar SR. (1988). Ethical responsibilities of health professionals in caring for detainees and prisoners. *South African Medical Journal* 74: 453–456.

Benatar SR. (1990). The South African Medical and Dental Council: some proposals for change. *South African Medical Journal*; 78:179–180.

Benatar SR, Abels C, Abratt R, et al. (1994a). Abortion - some practical and ethical considerations. *S Afr Med J*. 84: 469–472.

Benatar SR, Abels C, Abratt R, et al. (1994b). Statement on withholding and withdrawing life-sustaining therapy. *S Afr Med J*. 84: 254–256.

Benatar SR. (2001). South Africa's transition in a globalizing world: HIV/AIDS as a window and a mirror. International Affairs, 77 (2) 347–375.

Benatar SR, Van Rensburg HCJ. (2001). Medicine in Africa: present and future. In: J Last & S Lock (Eds.). *The Oxford Illustrated Companion to Medicine*. 2001: 18–23.

Benatar SR. (2002). Reflections and recommendations on research ethics in developing countries. *Social Science and Medicine* 54: 1131–1141.

Benatar SR. (2002b). The HIV/AIDS pandemic: a sign of instability in a complex global system. *Journal of Medicine and Philosophy* 27: 163–177.

Benatar, SR, Daar, A, & Singer PA. (2003). Global health ethics: the rationale for mutual caring. *International Affairs* 79(1): 107–138.

Benatar SR. (2004). Health care reform and the crisis of HIV/AIDS in South Africa. *New England Journal of Medicine* 351: 81–92.

Benatar SR. (2004b). Towards progress in resolving dilemmas in international research ethics *Journal of Law, Medicine and Ethics*. 32: (4) 574–582.

Benatar SR, Landman WA. (2006) Bioethics in South Africa. Cambridge Quarterly of Healthcare Ethics. 15: 239–247.

Benatar SR. (2008). Global health, Global health ethics and cross-cultural considerations in bioethics. In: PA Singer & AM Viens (Eds.). *The Cambridge Textbook of Bioethics*. Cambridge: Cambridge University Press: 341–349.

Brock DW. (1998). Medical decisions at the end of life. In: P Singer & H Kuhse (Eds.). *A companion to bioethics*. Oxford: Blackwell: 231–241.

Cleaton-Jones P, Wassenaar D. (2010) Protection of human subjects in health research – a comparison of some US federal regulations and South African research ethics guidelines. *South African Medical Journal 100*: 710–716.

Coetzee D et al. (2004). Outcomes after two years of providing antiretroviral treatment in Khayelitsha, South Africa. *AIDS* 18 (6): 887–895.

Damster G. (1998). *MASA and justice: the role of the institutionally organised South African medical profession in response to human rights violations within the apartheid era, with special emphasis on Steve Biko*. Unpublished MPhil dissertation, University of Stellenbosch.

De Zulueta P. (2001). Randomised placebo-controlled trials and HIV-infected pregnant women in developing countries. Ethical imperialism or unethical exploitation? *Bioethics 15* (4): 289–311.

Feinstein A. (2007). After the party: a personal and political journey through the ANC. Jonathan Ball Publishers Jeppetown.

Health Professions Council of South Africa. (2002). *National Patients' Rights Charter*. Available at: http://www.doh.gov.za/docs/pamplets/patientsright/chartere.html Accessed 13th December 2010.

Hoffman M., et al. (2006). The status of legal termination of pregnancy in South Africa. *South African Medical Journal* 96 (10), October 2006: 1056.

Jenkins T. (1986). The organised medical profession on trial. *South African Journal of Human Rights* 2: 236–241.

Jenkins T. (1987). Ethical issues in the medical care of prisoners and detainees. *South African Journal of Continuing Medical Education* April 5, 1987: 40a–49.

Jenkins T. (1988). The health care of detainees–the law, professional ethics and reality. *South African Medical Journal* 74: 436–438.

Kalk WJ, Veriava Y. (1991). Hospital management of voluntary total fasting among political prisoners. *Lancet* 337: 660–662.

Kriel JR. (2000). *Matter, Mind and Medicine: transforming clinical method*. Amsterdam: Rodopi (Value Inquiry Book Series 93).

Landman WA, Mouton J, & Nevhutalu K. (2001). *Chris Hani Baragwanath Hospital Ethics Audit* (EthicSA Research Report No. 2). Pretoria: Unpublished.

Landman WA, Mouton J, & Nevhutalu K. (2002). *Universitas Hospital Ethics Audit* (EthicSA Research Report No. 4). Pretoria: Unpublished.

Lee K & Zwi AB. (1996). A global political economy approach to AIDS: ideology, interests, and implications. *New Political Economy* 1: 355–373.

Logie D E, Benatar S R (1997) Africa in the 21st Century: can despair be turned to hope? *British Medical Journal* 315: 437–441.

Lurie P & Wolfe S. (1997). Unethical trials of interventions to reproduce perinatal transmission of the Human Immunodeficiency Virus in developing countries. *New England Journal of Medicine* 337: 853–856.

Marshall PA. (2001). Findings and recommendations from the case study on informed consent for genetic epidemiological studies of hypertension, breast cancer, and diabetes mellitus in Nigeria. *Consultation Report for the President's National Bioethics Advisory Commission: The Relevance of Culture for Informed Consent in U.S. Funded International Health Research*. Bethesda, MD: National Bioethics Advisory Commission.

MBewu A & Mngomezulu K. (1999). Health research in South Africa. In *South African Health Review*. Durban: Health Systems Trust, pp. 369–384.

McClean GR & Jenkins T. (2003). The Steve Biko affair: a case study in medical ethics. *Developing World Bioethics 3* (1): 77–95.

National Bioethics Advisory Commission (2001). *Ethical and policy issues in international research: clinical trials in developing countries*. Bethesda MD: Author.

Nattrass N. (2004). *The Moral Economy of AIDS in South Africa*. Cambridge: Cambridge University Press.

Nightingale EO, Hannibal K, Geiger J, Hartman L, Lawrence R, & Spurlock J. (1990). Apartheid medicine: health & human rights in South Africa. *Journal of the American Medical Association* 264: 2097–2102.

Nuffield Council on Bioethics. (2002). *The ethics of research related to healthcare in developing countries*. London: Author.

Oosthuizen GC, Shapiro H, & Strauss S. (1973). *Euthanasia*. Cape Town: Oxford University Press.

Oosthuizen GC, Abbot G, & Notelowitz M. (1974). *Great Debate: Abortion in South Africa*. Cape Town: Howard Timmins.

Resnik D. (1998). The ethics of HIV research in developing nations. *Bioethics 12* (4): 286–306.

Shapiro K, Benatar SR. (2005). HIV prevention research and global inequality: towards improved standards of care. *Journal of Medical Ethics 31*: 39–47.

Soal J. (1999). "Mercy killing laws reviewed." *The Cape Times*, July 29, 1999: 1

South African Department of Health. (1996). *Charter of Patients' Rights*. http://www.doh.gov.za/docs/legislation/patientsright/chartere.html.

Singer P. (1993). *Practical Ethics* (2nd Edition). Cambridge: Cambridge University Press.

Singer P. (2002). *Unsanctifying human life* Helga Kuhse (ed.). Oxford: Blackwell.

Slack C., Lindegger G., Vardas G., Richter L., Strode A., & Wassenaar D. (2000). Ethical issues in HIV vaccine trials in South Africa. *South African Journal of Science* 96: 291–295.

Tangwa G. (2006). The HIV/AIDS pandemic: African traditional values and the search for a vaccine in Africa. In: van Niekerk & Kopelman, pp. 179–189.

Tooley M. (1983). *Abortion and Infanticide*. Oxford: Clarendon Press.

Van der Vliet V. (1996). *The Politics of AIDS*. London: Bowerdean Publishing Company.

Van Niekerk AA. (2002). Moral and social complexities of AIDS in Africa. *The Journal for Medicine and Philosophy 27*(2): 143–163.

Van Niekerk AA. (2003a). Mother-to-child transmission of HIV/AIDS in South Africa: moral issues. *Jahrbuch für Wissenschaft und Ethik 8*: 149–171.

Van Niekerk AA. (2006). Principles of global distributive justice and the HIV/AIDS pandemic: moving beyond Rawls and Buchanan. In: AA van Niekerk & LM Kopelman (eds.). *Ethics and AIDS in Africa* (pp. 84–110). Cape Town: David Philip.

Van Niekerk AA & Kopelman LM.(Eds.) (2006). *Ethics and AIDS in Africa*. Walnut Creek, CA: Left Coast Press.

Van Rensburg HCJ, Benatar SR. (2001). The history of Medicine in Africa. In: J Last & S Lock (eds.). *The Oxford Illustrated Companion to Medicine*. New York: Oxford University Press: 14–18

Webb D. (1992). *HIV and AIDS in South Africa*. London: Pluto Press.

Whiteside A. (2006). AIDS in Africa: facts, figures and the extent of the problem. In Van Niekerk & Kopelman (Eds.) (pp. 1–14).

10 TOWARD AN AFRICAN *UBUNTUOLOGY/ uMUNTHUOLOGY* BIOETHICS IN MALAWI IN THE CONTEXT OF GLOBALIZATION

Joseph Mfutso-Bengo and Francis Masiye

A Short History of Malawi and the Rise of Bioethics in Malawi

Bioethics in Malawi is as old as humanity itself. The first settlers in Malawi had creation myths that talked about ethics and morality. According to the myths, ethics arose as a result of conflicts among human beings. Ethics also manifested itself during colonial rule. John Chilembwe, the first Malawian freedom fighter, led an uprising in 1915 against forced recruitment of Malawians into the British Army during the First World War (1914–1919). He was also against the ill-treatment of Malawians who were forced to work in European estates without pay. He fought for respect for human dignity and human rights in Malawi.

Malawi was the first country in Southern Africa to free itself from colonial rule. It became independent on July 6, 1964, with Dr. Hastings Kamuzu Banda as its first president. The first democratic Constitution was adopted in 1964, and it promoted a Bill of Rights. However, in 1971, Malawi became officially a one-party state under President Kamuzu Banda, who declared himself president for life. Various repressive laws were instituted that significantly curtailed personal liberties until 1993. Malawi continued to suffer massive social, political, and economic injustices that characterized Dr. Kamuzu Banda's regime. Because of the autocratic and oppressive nature of his one-party rule, underground opposition sprang up.

This opposition against one-party rule took a new turn in 1992, when the Catholic bishops, for the first time in the postcolonial history of Malawi, issued a pastoral letter openly and publicly condemning one-party rule, the violation of human rights, and the lack of freedom of speech and democracy. The pastoral letter gave a strong impetus to the popular movement demanding political change. The pastoral letter of the bishops enabled the underground opposition to

President Kamuzu Banda's oppressive regime to become open, public, and vocal for the first time. Students and workers went to the streets to demonstrate, to protest, and to strike in support of the pastoral letter. At once, opposition to dictatorship became a popular mass movement, which could not be stopped by repression but only by democratization and rule of law.

Even though President Kamuzu Banda threatened the bishops with execution at first, he eventually gave in to the demands of the pastoral letter by proposing to have a referendum on multiparty democracy. The people chose multiparty democracy on June 14, 1993. In parliamentary elections, which took place on May 17, 1994, President Kamuzu Banda was defeated. Kamuzu Banda showed political common sense and maturity by gracefully accepting the defeat. This election marked a political milestone in Malawi because Bakili Muluzi, a Muslim, became the new president in a predominantly Christian country, after almost 30 years of one-man rule. That marked the end of an era of political repression and the beginning of a new, democratic era.

Since the remarkable Roman Catholic pastoral letter, Malawi has seen and experienced a redefinition of ethics, the birth of Christian ethics in Malawi. The aftermath of the pastoral letter was that Malawi became a free and democratic state. This development marked the beginning of a cultural liberalization, which has, however, ultimately undermined the preservation of the Malawian cultural integrity. Malawians are now busy trying to preserve their identity and to resolve ethical issues that arise in everyday life by restoring the dignity of our national cultural heritage—that is, our indigenous values, traditions, and morals. This chapter, therefore, attempts to discuss how we are working for the survival of our national cultural heritage, and the role bioethics plays in this. One key issue that the chapter discusses regarding the restoration of our cultural identity is the concept of *ubuntuology/uMunthuology* as an African ethical theory.

History of the Center for Bioethics in Eastern and Southern Africa (CEBESA)

The history of bioethics in Malawi is closely linked with the University of Malawi College of Medicine. It is at the College of Medicine where bioethics started. Today, the University Of Malawi College Of Medicine is one of the very few medical colleges in Africa that considers the subject of bioethics and research ethics as necessary and indispensable. It is one of the few medical schools in Africa to introduce a compulsory biomedical ethics curriculum, which covers all five years of training. All the initiatives in the area of bioethics at the college and in Malawi are spearheaded by the Center for Bioethics in Eastern and Southern Africa (CEBESA).

The Center for Bioethics in Eastern and Southern Africa (CEBESA) was established in 2001. CEBESA falls under the Division of Community Health at the College of Medicine. The center is committed to helping healthcare professionals, researchers, students, and policymakers in addressing ethical questions in Malawi. It seeks to promote the ethical practice of medicine and the ethical conduct of biomedical research in Malawi. The center also seeks to reach out to various institutions, projects, researchers, and communities, using various means. It also provides training to ethics committee members and researchers on research ethics, clinical trial monitoring and good clinical practice. In addition, it provides advice to various stakeholders including government, health practitioners, research ethics committees, hospitals, members of the public, and others on issues related to bioethics, research ethics and good clinical practice (GCP).

In order to achieve its goals, CEBESA has two main components, which include research and training. Below are some of the major activities carried out by CEBESA in the area of bioethics and research ethics:

- Teaching of bioethics to undergraduate students in all programs in the college from the first year up to the fifth year.
- Teaching of bioethics and research ethics to postgraduate students in the Master of Public Health Degree (MPH) and Master of Medicine (MMED).
- Training Fogarty Fellows from Eastern and Southern Africa in international research ethics, as part of the University of Malawi College of Medicine and Michigan State University Fogarty Training Program.
- Providing training to ethics committee members and researchers on research ethics, good clinical practice, and research methodology.
- Conducting research on various topics in the area of bioethics and research ethics.
- Advising various stakeholders including government, research ethics committees (RECs), hospitals, researchers, healthcare practitioners, students, members of the public, and others on issues related to bioethics, research ethics and good clinical practice.

Currently, CEBESA is running three projects funded by the Wellcome Trust Bioethics Research Project, the Fogarty International Research Ethics Training Program for Eastern and Southern Africa, and the European Union and Developing Countries Clinical Trials Partnership (EDCTP) projects on building and strengthening national capacities in ethical review and clinical trial monitoring in Malawi.

Bioethics is thus being championed by the Center for Bioethics in Eastern and Southern Africa (CEBESA) at the University Of Malawi College Of

Medicine, with financial investments from the United States, the United Kingdom, and the European Union. A related human rights initiative, which we will touch upon in our conclusion, is the Medical Rights Watch, which was born in a bioethics class and it is taking bioethics to the grassroots and making people aware of their rights and responsibilities. CEBESA is also championing the African moral theory of *ubuntuology/uMunthuology,* and urging medical students to apply it in their medical practice. The main goal of our chapter is to share this with the international bioethics community.

How the African Social and Cultural Context Influences the Emergence of African Bioethics

In the Malawian context, bioethics is seen as a relationship of a human being with himself/herself, with nature, and with other human beings. This relationship is based on cooperation and fairness, and it is rooted in the African moral thinking of *uMunthu,* or *ubuntu,* as it is commonly known in many Southern African countries. Ubuntu/uMunthu means *being humane.* It is a moral reflection or study of African humanism and moral systems. Malawian (African) bioethicists consider *ubuntuology/uMunthuology* as the main theory of African Bantu bioethics. The *ubuntuology/uMunthuology* theory starts with defining what African humanism is, and how one can become humane. The theory presupposes that not every human being is human. One becomes human through positive relationships and encounters which are based on beneficence, respect, trust, hope, and justice. To be good is to behave rightly, and to behave rightly is to relate well. Those who relate well are considered good and humane. Good people are those thought to have done good, right, and useful actions. "Useful" here ought to be understood in a wider context, and not limited to its materialistic meaning. The concept of goodness and rightness has biological, social, natural, supernatural, cosmological, and ethical dimensions. No one can declare herself or himself to be good and right. It is the other who can pass judgment on whether one is right or good. Moral goodness and rightness are not the same, but are interdependent. For instance, an action can be right but not good; e.g., killing in self-defense. Thus, morality is not individualistic but it is communalistic. In fact, African morality is characterised by the search for common good and truth (real facts) or *chowonadi* in the Chichewa language, which is something that can be seen or proven. Hence, personal ideologies and self interest are not part of African moral reasoning. The principle of flexibility for the sake of common good, common sense, or greater public good is always emphasized. This means both prejudice and bias are enemies of African moral reasoning, and conflict of interest in African morality is seen as conflict between personal interest against communal interest. Without willing communal good, one can not achieve personal goodness and common sense. Common goodness is also the source and goal of common sense and common interest. Here we need to note that common sense is indeed not common because not all humans or nations seek the common good or interest, but rather self interest. Therefore, a good decision should try to balance communal interest with self interest.

The common goodness is expressed through solidarity. Solidarity is understood as self-sacrifice or mutual sacrifice for the common good, instead of sacrificing the other for self interest. According to African bioethics, to be human is to be in relation, and to become human is to be constantly in right relation. Being in relation is an essential aspect of being human. "The concept of separate beings of substances, to use a scholastic term, which exist side by side, independent one from another, is foreign to African thought."[1] The African thought holds that created beings are interconnected, interdependent, and interrelated. A human person exists as a person in a family—not only as a family, but as part of the big extended human family. Our recognition of the human family to which we belong is extended yet further—beyond ideologies, the tribe, the community, the nation, or even the continent—to embrace the whole society of humankind. Speaking on the same theme, Kenneth Kaunda, an African humanist and former President of Zambia, once said, "let the West have its technology and Asia its mysticism! Africa's gift to the world culture must be in the realm of human relation."[2]

African humanity is defined in the context of the community. To be is to belong to each other; "no man is an island". The real esteem of the human being must be based on the assumption that no race, class, or group has a monopoly of all human gifts. It is through human interaction, and not rejection and projection, that the human being will achieve his potential. Marginalization and segregation, whether divine or human, deny the richness and variety of human heritage. For the humanist, "the fundamental human right is the right to love and to be loved."[3] Thus we are persons *in* a community and not *against* the community. Humanization and reconciliation processes find clear expression in the context of being in relation, in being in communion through communication and commitment to truth, justice, and mercy.

On the level of praxis, Africa stands on the crossroads between tradition and modernity. On this crossroads, according to our social analysis, there is a dialectic

---

1. Serequeberhan, T., *African Philosophy*, pp. 40–41.

2. Hilmer, O., *The Gospel and the Social Systems*, p. 103.

3. Shorter, A., *Evangelization and Inculturation*, p. 117.

between "*to be more*" and "*to have more*," a dialectic between "to relate to be" and "to relate to have"—a kind of *north–south conflict* on African soil among Africans themselves. The modern Africa, due to Western influence, tends to desire more to possess things rather than to relate, whereas the traditional Africa tends to desire more to relate than to possess.

The traditional African society is more life-centered, and the modern African society is more profit-minded. Why is the traditional life/community-centered Africa vulnerable to being dominated by the modern, profit-centered society? Which elements are there, in this African traditional culture, which make it easy to be dominated, manipulated, and exploited by power and money seekers? It is difficult to answer these questions, but what we have to understand is that both too much and too little material well-being are antihuman, antisocial, anti-culture, and that it hinders reconciliation based on truth and justice. Both overdevelopment and underdevelopment can undermine communitarianism and umunthu/ubuntu. Both hinder integration by destroying solidarity—the very basis of communitarianism and humanism.

The Implications of the African Concept of Ubuntu/uMunthu for African Bioethics

To bring out clearly the role of culture in African societies today, we proceed to give some examples of ubuntu/uMunthu in action. At funerals in Africa, all members of the community are welcome. Since an individual is a part of a broader community, there is no need to send formal invitations to others to attend. It is common to find more than a thousand people gathered at the funeral of an ordinary person, or even a child, and a beast has to be slaughtered so as to feed the multitudes. When it comes to marriage, the extended families from both sides are involved. On the day that the union is traditionally formalized, members from both sides gather over food and drink as a way of cementing the relationship between the two separate families, and the two families now become related.

In Malawi, among the Chewa, when one says *"uyu simunthu"* it means this human being is not human. *Uyu ndi munthu* means "this is a human being." According to a Malawian cultural understanding, that is the greatest compliment that can be said of a good, moral person. This Chichewa expression, *uyu simunthu,* seems to affirm that the biological condition of being man or woman is necessary, but it is not sufficient for being human. One is not born fully human, he/she must become human—that is, existence precedes essence. To be human is a process that begins with birth but does not end with birth. The child that has been born of a woman in flesh has to be born again in spirit, as a fully human person, in the community. To be born again, according to the Bantu bioethics, means that the child that has been born in flesh must undergo the painful and joyful process of becoming a full, corporate, human moral person (uMunthu).

Describing this process of becoming a moral human being, John Mbiti writes that "nature brings the child into the world, but the society (community) creates the child into a social being, corporate moral human person."[4] Here, Professor Mbiti seems to underline the fact that the human being must go beyond the biological level if he is to become a fully moral human being (Munthu) and fully alive (*umoyo*). The biological process ought to be complemented by a humanization process if one is to acquire uMunthu (reconciled moral identity). To be human is to have a heart of flesh (*mtima*)—a heart that cares (*woleza mtima*), a heart that is compassionate (*okoma mtima*), a heart that is patient (*mtima wofatsa*), a heart full of peace (*mtima wa mtendere*). Only the heart that has been reconciled with itself can reconcile or can be reconciled with other hearts.

There are so many other examples that can be used to show the close-knit quality of African societies. At the national levels, one can also see the role of uMunthu in the constitutions of Tanzania, Malawi, and South Africa, at the attainment of political independence. The constitutions emphasized reconciliation and unity between the oppressors and the oppressed, and there were some serious efforts toward building trust and acceptance between the two sides for the good of society in general. It was only because of uMunthu that the black people of these three countries were able to totally accept their oppressors, and did not even think about seeking retribution. Tanzania has emphasized welfare programs and cooperatives in line with the *Ujamaa* (community building-common good) concept championed by Mwalimu Julius Nyerere, one of the very important political figures in Africa.

Most African cultures do not share many of the assumptions implicit in the western autonomy-based approach to bioethical deliberations. On the contrary, the African cultures take a community-based approach rather than an individual, rights-based approach. Greater value and meaning rests in the interdependence of family, which transcends self-determination. This tradition emphasizes the value of a holistic view of a person that affirms the importance of the community, society, and the family. The community-based approach is opposite to the Western approach, with its emphasis on the individual. In African cultures, the community always comes first. The individual is born out of and into the community; therefore, he/she will always be part of the community. This is the ubuntu/uMunthu concept.

---

4. Muzorewa, G., *The Origins and Development of African* . . . p. 45.

With ubuntu, the individual's existence is relative to that of the community. This is manifested in anti-individualistic conduct in support of the survival of the community, if the individual is to survive. Ubuntu is seen as that which separates men and women from beasts, and actually offers the potential of being human. The notion of communalism is exemplified in proverbs such as "a single tree cannot withstand wind," or "knowledge is like the baobab tree—no single person can embrace it." These proverbs are used in day-to-day speech among the various Bantu languages in Africa. They discourage individualistic tendencies among Africans. In fact, individualistic people are looked down upon, and are characterized by labels meant to discourage individualism and selfish behaviors.

On the other hand, in the Western philosophical discourse, the "self" is characterized as a substantive inner agency, capable of taking a first-person standpoint, and human self esteem is seen as essentially independent of community. The individual is seen as an architect of his or her own personality. The individual is, therefore, seen as being self-contained, and children are socialized to be independent. An example is the infants in the Western world, who may be forced to sleep in their own bedrooms even after a few months, so as to train them to be independent and rely less on others. This Western idea of autonomy, with its emphasis on personal choice and individual rights, has culminated in present-day "democratic" society, which emphasizes the rights of the individual, and which has further culminated in a litigious society where individuals do not value harmony but trust in the quest to be individual and different from others. In present day Western societies, informed consent is now taken as a legal matter for protecting researchers and institutions associated with the focus on the signing of the document, which becomes a legal contract.

This notion of autonomy, just like any utopian idea, relies on several assumptions, including the wish that each and every person has the rational capacity to make decisions and is free from constraints. These assumptions can be challenged even in developed countries, where choices for persons are limited, and people are not totally autonomous. The assumptions become even more irrelevant in developing countries, because in some cases, people do not have even options to choose from, and there are many constraining factors such as oppressive governments, poverty, hierarchical societies, and even societal expectations. It is very important to realize how the ideas of people like Kant have impacted on bioethical deliberations in Western societies, as they have been important in defining personhood from the Western point of view. The important fact to note is that Kant was writing from a Western context that, even at that time, had already moved away from communitarian values to individual-centered values. Kant's ideas reflect what was happening in the Western societies during that time. The agricultural revolution, the famines, and the industrial revolution can be taken as useful matrices in the equation that seeks to explain the move from communal values to individualist values. Over time, the communal values have come to be viewed by Westerners as inappropriate to modern life. Indeed, the Western ethical concept of autonomy is antithetical to the African ethical concept of ubuntu/uMunthu. Descartes' *I think therefore I am* is in opposition to the African logical dictum according to John Mbiti, *I am because we are and since we are therefore I am.*

Conclusions and Reflections

To conclude, we would like to point out that reflections about ethics often arise when there are conflicts, or when human atrocities have been committed. In the Malawian context, ethics came about as a result of conflicts among indigenous people. People felt there was a need to have common rules of engagement that would bring harmony in society. Ethics was then redefined when violations of human rights and personal liberties were committed by the postcolonial government. This was championed by the Catholic Church, and it was the redefinition of Christian ethics in Malawi. Later on, academicians in the field of medicine felt there was need to introduce medical ethics (bioethics) at the College of Medicine due to the increase among healthcare providers of medical negligence, professional misconduct, and violations of patients' and research participants' rights. This saw the introduction of bioethics teaching at the College of Medicine. Through the work of the Medical Rights Watch (MRW) and some publications of the Centre for Bioethics, many people in Malawi are aware of bioethics, and patients and research participants are able to claim their rights.

The MRW was born in a Bioethics class in 2008 and was launched on April 11, 2008. The primary objective of the organization is to bring basic ethical values to the attention of all key health decision-makers at all levels, with the goal of transforming the health system into one that effectively applies justice, beneficence and autonomy. MRW[5] is achieving this through making basic bioethics

5. The MRW has laid down the following mechanisms in order to meet its goals and objectives: increasing awareness throughout Malawi about clients' (patients and research practitioners) and health practitioners' (and researchers) rights and duties, and patients' perspectives of healthcare, through public talks, drama performances targeting the general public and school children; conducting intensive training sessions on clients' and health practitioners' rights and responsibilities, targeting specific groups of people; influencing health rights policy by constant communication with public representatives, members of government departments, committees, regulatory bodies, and all other key health/human rights policy makers; being accessible to patients and healthcare practitioners, and to other representatives or bodies who speak on their behalf, for guidance in solving any ethical dilemmas and health rights issues; conducting research among patients or the general public, and within health care, in order to establish the extent and frequency of problems, or to enable comparisons to be made

knowledge available to all these decision-makers and giving them guidance on how to resolve ethical dilemmas, so as to achieve ethical decision making. The goal of MRW is to promote and protect the rights and responsibilities of patients, research participants, and health practitioners in Malawi. As the first and so far the only health rights organization in Malawi, MRW is fighting for safe, accountable health care that does not compromise the rights of patients. This work is extending to all parts of the Malawian healthcare system, including research and training institutions throughout the country.

We would also like to point out that that culture plays a very important role in bioethics. It influences bioethical thinking. It is with this conviction that we advocate for the broadening of the concept of Western bioethics in Africa, in the light of *ubuntuology/uMunthuology*. In other words, we feel bioethics needs to be contextualized. However, this does not mean that we are advocating for collective (communal) thinking only. We will never at any point advocate for the dumping of first-person informed consent. We acknowledge that individual informed consent serves as one of the best safeguards against exploitation of individuals, and hence it can and should never be done away with. The substantive principle of informed consent must apply. Here, it is worth noting that in the African context, community permission is prior to individual informed consent. Permission is first obtained from chiefs/village heads, who are regarded as gatekeepers. After obtaining permission from the gatekeepers, informed consent is obtained from individuals. In other words, permission from a gatekeeper does not substitute for individual informed consent.

Our main aim in this chapter has been to demonstrate the importance of looking at the person in Africa not as an agent in isolation, but also as part of a whole. Individuals in Africa value the common good and common sense, and their behaviors are aimed at maintaining social cohesion. The broadening of the concept of a "person" would also ultimately bring with it respect for multi-person involvement in the procedural implementation of consent, as well as the need for the endorsement of community leaders for one to enter a community, for instance, to do research. Western values and practices were not introduced in Africa in a vacuum, since Africa already had its own cultures and values, most of which are still in existence. The incorporation of these necessary steps is a sure way of respecting people's cultures. We also put forward that in order to avoid unnecessary conflict and debates, bioethicists should learn to appreciate the cultures, as well as the beliefs, of the people with whom they interact, so long as they are not oppressive, unfair and harmful. *Ubuntuology/uMunthuology* is a

---

concerning health rights, adequacy, effectiveness, or cost of health care; and organizing and participating in health rights conferences, seminars, and similar meetings.

practical philosophy that highlights the essential unity of humanity, and emphasizes the importance of constantly referring to the principles of empathy, sharing, and cooperation in our efforts to resolve our common problems. It forms the essence of our Malawian (African) identity. Obviously, Africa does not measure up in terms of the technological advancement and material prosperity of the West, but God bestowed on us a wonderful way of life, which is that of ubuntu/uMunthu. Ubuntu/uMunthu values and respects people the way they are. Someone's status is not a key determining factor in matters relational. Just because they are human and created by God, all people, despite their social standing, are regarded as worthy members of humanity—worthy to be treated with respect and dignity. Because of this outlook, in the ubuntu/uMunthu way of life, elements like loneliness, depression and unhappiness that are characteristic of individualism do not seem to find undue place. Thus, an *ubuntuology/uMunthuology* theory of bioethics is perhaps one of the precious gifts that Africans can share with the rest of the world. We believe it offers a unique paradigm for solving the cultural and social/economic problems confronting the world today, as it adopts a holistic approach in advancing human development and welfare. The main contribution of *ubuntuology/uMunthuology* as an African ethical theory is that a human being becomes more human through rightful relationships with other human beings and nature.

Glossary

Chowonadi the truth (real fact)
Mtima A heart
Mtima wa mtendere peace of mind
Mtima wofatsa a patient heart
Mudzi Village community
North-South Conflict the economic conflict between industrialized and developing countries; according to which industrialized countries use their economic power to strengthen the dependence of developing countries on them and to create cheap prices and wages in their own favor. The concept is "geographic" in origin, in that the majority of industrialized countries and earlier colonial powers lie on the Northern Hemisphere of the earth, while developing countries and earlier colonies are usually found in the Southern Hemisphere. This is likened to the situation in modern Africa, where the rich use the poor in their own favor.
Ubuntu/uMunthu Humane-*ubuntu* is a Bantu term for "humane" and it is widely used among Bantu people. However, in Malawi, it is commonly known as *uMunthu*
Ujamaa familyhood
Umodzi Unity

Umoyo to be fully alive
Woleza mtima a caring heart

References

Biko, S. *I Write What I Like*. London: Bowerdean Press, 1978.
Bonhoeffer, D. *Reality and Resistance*. Nashville: Abingdon Press, 1972.
Buber, M. *I and Thou*. Edinburgh: Charles Scriber's Sons, 1970.
Bujo, B. *Die ethische Dimension der Gemeinschaft. Das afrikanische Modell im Nord-Süd-Dialog*. Freiburg: Schweiz.Gilgamesch-Epos, 1993.
Buthelezi, M. Reconciliation and liberation in Southern Africa. In *African Challenge: Major issues in African Christianity*, edited by Kenneth Y. Best. Nairobi: David Philip Publications, 1975.
Chankanza, J. *Religions in Malawi*. Vol. 1, No. 1, December. Zomba, 1987.
Chinweizu, I. *Voices from Twentieth-Century Africa*. London-Boston: Faber & Faber edition, 1988.
Clinton, B. Remarks at Africa Trade Event, White House Briefing Room, June 17, 1997. Available at: http://www.africanews.org/specials/19970617-feat3.html, pp. 1–2.
Kamwambe, N. *The legacy of Malawians, Legacy of one-party rule*. Lusaka: Mojo Press, 1993.
Lwanda, J. *Kamuzu Banda of Malawi*. Glasgow: Bothwell, 1993.
Mandela, N. Autobiography, titled "Long Way to Freedom" available at: http://www.academic.sun.wits.ac.za/books/Mandela/Welcome.html.
Mazrui, A. *The African Condition*. New York: African World Press, 1980.
Mbiti, J. *Introduction to African Religion*. London: Heinemann, 1977.
Mfutso-Bengo, J. M. *In the Name of the Rainbow: Politics of Reconciliation as a Priority of Social Pastoral Care in South Africa and Malawi*. Frankfurt: Peter Lang, 2001.
Nzunda, M., Ross, K. *Church, Law and Political Transition in Malawi*. Balaka: Montfort Media, 1992.
Okolo, B. *African Synod: Hope for the Continent's Liberation*. Eldoret: Gaba Publications, 1994.
Patel, N., Svasand, L. *Government and Politics in Malawi*. Balaka: Montfort Media, 2007.
Powell, J. *Fully Human, Fully Alive*. Chicago: Resources for Christian Living, 1976.
Serequeberhan, T. *African Philosophy*. New York: Routledge, 1991.
Shorter, A. *Evangelization and Inculturation*. London: Maryknoll, 1994.
Tutu, D. Speeches on Truth and Reconciliation Commission, Documents and Hearings homepage. Available at: http://www.justice.gov.za/trc.
Vicenzo, C., Gruchy, J. *Resistance and Hope: South African essays in honour of Beyers Naude*. Cape Town: SCM Classics, 1985.
Vision of Malawi, Vision 2020: Available at: http://spicerack.sr.unh.edu/~llk/malawi/v2020.html.

11 REFLECTIONS ON BIOETHICS IN CHINA

THE INTERACTION BETWEEN BIOETHICS AND SOCIETY[1]

Qiu Renzong[2]

The Birth and Growth of Bioethics in China

In 2009, China marked the thirtieth anniversary of its annual National Conference on Philosophy of Medicine. This conference, first held in Guangdong in December 1979, was the first step toward the birth of bioethics in China. The conference brought attention to the various ethical issues inherent in scientific advancement, and focused on topics such as life-sustaining technologies, assisted reproductive technologies, organ transplantation, and genetics. One year later, in 1980, the journal *Medicine and Philosophy* was founded with help from the Chinese Society for Philosophy of Nature, Science and Technology, China's Association of Science and Technology. Articles focusing on bioethics also began to appear in the journal *Philosophical Problems in Natural Sciences*, which is sponsored by the Institute of Philosophy and the Chinese Academy of Social Sciences.[3] By 1986,

1. This article is a mix of narrative, explanatory, and prescriptive. Some contents are cited from the author's published articles, while others are from debates at meetings, workshops, and conferences. The Chinese, and Chinese scholars, don't publish everything they have debated, and are reluctant to publish anything criticizing their colleagues (including their scholarly opinions). For this reason, it is not possible to discuss the history or reality of bioethics in China solely through citation of publications. In any event, life and practice are much richer sources than the written word. However, the focus of this article is reflection.

2. Emeritus Professor at Institute of Philosophy and Honorary Director of Center for Applied Ethics, Chinese Academy of Social Sciences; Professor at the Department of Social Sciences and the Humanities & Center for Bioethics, Peking Union Medical College.

3. Professor Ru Xin, Vice-President of Chinese Academy of Social Sciences (CASS) at the time, argued that the effect of advances in science and technology on humans should be studied from a philosophical perspective. He was a strong supporter of bioethics in China. In 1979, the same year as the Guangzhou Workshop, a delegation from the Kennedy Institute of Ethics visited China. Professor Ru Xin acted as their host, and when his guests asked about other

China's Ministry of Education was sponsoring bioethics workshops for graduate students at Southeast University in Nanjing.[4] In 1987, the first book on bioethics by a Chinese bioethicist was published in China.[5] In 1988, bioethics moved beyond the scientific realm and entered the legal arena, as China saw its first litigation concerning euthanasia and assisted reproduction.[6] That same year, China held two conferences that focused on the intersection of science, ethics, and the law: the first National Conference on Social, Ethical and Legal Issues in Euthanasia, which took place in Shanghai in July 1988, and the first National Conference on Social, Ethical and Legal Issues in Assisted Reproductive Technologies, which took place in Yueyang, Hunan Province, in November 1988. In the space of nine years, the seeds sown at the 1979 conference in Guangzhou took root in the form of scholarly publications and graduate education in bioethics. In addition, the important role of ethics in scientific advancement and the law was realized, both through litigation and two national conferences specifically focused on this topic.

One might ask whether the birth and growth of bioethics in China was an indigenous development or a transplant from the West. Certainly, some Chinese scholars who studied bioethics in the West were enthusiastic to introduce this valuable field to China,[7] but China had already begun its own work in this area. The Chinese government had adopted a policy of reform and openness that created fertile soil and a strong root of bioethics, on which thoughts and ideas grafted from other countries and cultures could thrive. Indeed, the government's policy of reform and openness had led to widespread application of science and technology in many facets of life, and in health care in particular, which in turn raised a variety of ethical, legal and social issues. As a result, China needed critical

---

bioethicists in China, Professor Ru Xin said there weren't any. At that point, I had just moved to CASS from Peking Union Medical College, but had not yet met Professor Ru Xin.

4. Some individuals involved in these workshops became the backbone of bioethics in China, such as Zhai Xiaomei, who is now the Executive Director of the Center for Bioethics, Chinese Academy of Social Sciences/Peking Union Medical College; a member of the Ministry of Health's Ethics Committee; President of the Chinese Society for Bioethics; and a member of the HUGO Ethics Committee.

5. Qiu RZ, *Bioethics*, Shanghai: Shanghai People's Press, 1987; *Between Life and Death: Moral Dilemmas and Bioethics*, Hong Kong: Chinese Bookstore, 1988; *Between Life and Death: Moral Dilemmas and Bioethics*, Taipei: Chinese Bookstore, 1988.

6. See Qiu RZ: Morality in Flux, *Kennedy Institute of Ethics Journal*, 1: 16–27, 1991.

7. With the implementation of reform and openness, a number of scholars in the humanities and social sciences introduced new academic fields to China (bioethics is one example; philosophy of science—including the theories of Karl Popper, Thomas Kuhn, Imre Lakatos, and Paul Feyerabend—is another). Many journals and publishers expressed interested in publishing their work.

thinkers with expertise in bioethics to help address these new challenges. Interestingly, the government's policy on reform and openness, which created the need for bioethicists, also created an atmosphere in which discussion of various and competing viewpoints was tolerated and even promoted. Chinese bioethicists had the necessary environment in which they could consider, discuss, and debate ethical issues. In the next few paragraphs, I discuss some of the specific the changes the government made, and how those changes have influenced bioethics in China.

Each year since 1999, the Chinese government's financial investment in scientific research has increased by more than twenty percent. By December 2006, the Chinese government was funding more research than Japan, making China's monetary commitment to research the second highest in the world after the United States. In 2006, the Chinese government spent CNY (Chinese yuan) 71.6 billion *yuan* (Chinese dollars: Renminbi or RMB) on scientific research. This amounts to £4.7 billion, and exceeds the British government's expenditure of £3.2 billion during the same time period.

China spends a considerable portion of its research budget on biotechnology and biomedicine, and from 2005 through 2010, the Chinese government is expected to have invested between 500 million and 2 billion RMB ($63 million to $250 million USD) in stem cell science.[8] In addition, a significant effort has been made to create alliances between bio-industry, biotechnology, and education, in order to foster quick and efficient technology translation. As this occurs, however, a host of ethical issues arise. Let us take stem cell research as an example. In undertaking human embryonic stem cell research and contemplating the application of the resulting discoveries to humans, many serious ethical issues arise, such as: Should China permit human reproductive cloning or human therapeutic cloning? What is the moral status of a human embryo? How will scientists procure human embryos for stem cell research? Should this research require advance review and approval by an ethical review committee? Once stems cells have been extracted, what should happen to the human embryo? Should China require clinical trials of promising stem cell therapies before they are offered to the public? Should stem cell research and its clinical application be regulated and, if yes, how?

The Chinese government's positive attitude toward globalization has also had an impact, as China becomes an incubator for scientific research. In recent years, China has enjoyed an extended and dramatic upswing in its economy. At the same time, China's economic system, social structure, and the role of its

8. UK Stem Cell Initiative (2005). *Report and Recommendations*. Department of Health, London.

government have been changing and evolving. This transformation has forced innovation in virtually every facet of life in China, and, for example, market forces have become an increasingly pervasive and formidable power in medicine and scientific research. With its rich genetic resources and biodiversity, China is becoming a major research center.[9] China has also become one of the largest markets in the world for pharmaceuticals, and has surpassed India as host to the largest number of clinical drug trials in the world.[10] In some instances, however, scientists and pharmaceutical companies have acted in ways that ignore the welfare of both human and animal subjects. How can human and animal research subjects be protected in this rapidly evolving environment?

In 1985, China launched market-oriented healthcare reform. The government, upon the advice of liberal-minded economists, purposefully withdrew most of its financial support from the healthcare field to ease its financial burden. This subjected the healthcare field almost entirely to market forces, and public hospitals were forced into the open market as their government funding evaporated. This reduction of government funding was referred to as "cessation of lactation" (*duan nai*) or "cutting off grains" (*duan liang*). Currently, only 3% to 8% of a public hospital's funding comes from the government. In another words, at least 92% of its operating expenses must be derived from another source, which essentially means payments of patients for examinations and treatments.

When the government cut its funding to public hospitals, it softened the blow by allowing them to "sell drugs (and charge for medical examinations) to support public hospitals." (*yi yao yang yi*)[11] As a result, physicians and hospitals could sell drugs and medical services directly to patients. Since the Chinese government no longer provides free medical care, payment for medical services comes directly from patients, their employers, or a combination of the two. The consequences of market-oriented healthcare reform for patients have proven to be disastrous, as discussed below.

Market-oriented health care has resulted in improved medical diagnostics and treatment in China. China now possesses the most advanced technological means for providing the best possible care to patients. When the government introduced market-oriented health care reform, it also hoped to increase the

9. Some Chinese institutes claim to have built the largest base of experimental animals, including primates, in the world.

10. Jack A & Yee A: 2007 China Overtakes India in Drug Testing, *Financial Times*, August 28, 2007.

11. Qiu RZ: Bioethics in China (1990–2008): Attempts to Protect the Rights and Health of Patients, Human Subjects and the Public, *Asian Bioethics Review* v. 1, December 1, 2008.

earnings of medical professionals. That goal has been reached, but at a heavy, and even tragic, cost to patients.

With health care no longer subsidized by the government, many patients either cannot afford medical treatment or are reduced to poverty as they sell their belongings and even their homes to pay for it. As medical treatment technology has advanced, so have costs; however, the increased costs to patients are unbearable burdens that plunge them into poverty again in many cases. Some physicians have been intentionally overtreating patients in order to make more money. Unscrupulous physicians have prescribed unnecessary and expensive drugs, ordered unneeded special medical examinations, and otherwise disregarded their patients' best interests and welfare in favor of their wallets. Doctors who engage in this practice are known as "wolves in white," and in the 24 years since market-oriented healthcare reform was introduced, patient respect for physicians has plunged to its lowest point since medicine has been practiced in China. During the SARS epidemic and Sichuan earthquake disaster, however, physicians selflessly worked to save victims, putting their patients' interests before all other factors. These physicians showed true valor and altruism, and became known as "angels in white." Patients and the general public wondered why a physician would behave so differently during an emergency than during the day-to-day operation of her or his clinical practice. The answer is straightforward: in an emergency situation, there is no direct link between a physician's income and an individual patient's payment for medical services, but in a medical practice there is. Market-oriented healthcare reform has seriously eroded medical professionalism in China.[12]

These events raise concerns about the medical profession and how it might address the conflict between market-oriented health care and patient rights and welfare. What ought medical professionals (including biomedical scientists) do? It's clear that medical professionals cannot respond to this issue without the assistance of ethicists, and bioethicists in particular. Chinese bioethicists have already

12. Here is one sad incident: On November 21, 2007, a woman who was eight months pregnant died at the West Beijing Hospital. She presented with acute pneumonia and was also suffering from heart disease. The patient's doctor suggested a Caesarean delivery in order to save both her and her unborn child's life, but she slipped into a coma before she was able to provide consent. The patient's boyfriend refused to give his consent for the procedure. The hospital manager consulted an official at the municipal Bureau for Health, and the official reply was that the hospital should comply with the regulation governing medical institutions, which provides that "the conduct of medical practice should be done after obtaining written consent from the patient or her/his family." This was the official response, even though there, the guideline also states that a "medical institution should rescue critically ill patients immediately." (State Council, 1994). Based on the official reply, the Caesarean was not performed and the patient and the undelivered child died. This case evoked hot debate throughout the country. (Qiu RZ, 2007b).

been at the forefront of addressing similar issues in the past, sometimes working with medical professionals, sometimes offering an opposing view. For example, when worsening physician–patient relationships were attributed to patient ignorance of proper medical treatment and a sympathetic media,[13] bioethicists challenged those assertions as inaccurate. When the medical profession did not express concerns about the use of executed prisoners' organs for transplantation, bioethicists did,[14] and the government ended the practice.[15] In 1994, many of the world's geneticists viewed China's proposed Maternal and Infant Health Care Law as eugenic in nature, and threatened to boycott the 18th World Congress of Genetics, which was to be held in Beijing. As a result, Chinese geneticists asked bioethicists to help them analyze the proposed legislation to ensure it supported parental choice and did not permit a program of state-imposed eugenics. The collaboration was productive, and Beijing successfully hosted the World Congress of Genetics.[16] When medical and public health professionals teamed together to draft recommendations for an AIDS policy for China, they invited bioethicists to join them. The group's overall recommendations to the government included an Appendix of Ethical Framework for Evaluating Actions on AIDS. Eventually these recommendations were accepted by the government, and Chinese AIDS policy was improved as a result (Zeng, 2000). These examples are further demonstration of the level to which bioethics is becoming engrained in China, and that China has not adopted bioethics wholly from the West. Chinese bioethics has its roots in Chinese soil, and its stem, branches, and leaves, whether Chinese or Western, have flourished in the Chinese air.

The economic, scientific, social, and governmental transformation in China over the course of the past 24 years has benefited Chinese society in general, but has had an adverse impact on some vulnerable or marginalized populations, particularly women. Bioethicists have played a role in helping China to address these issues. For example, from 1993 through 2007, with sponsorship from the Ford Foundation and the Chinese Academy of Social Sciences, Chinese bioethicists focused on women's issues in concert with feminists/women's studies scholars, physicians, population study scholars, sociologists, and lawyers. Collectively, they discussed the ethical, legal, and social issues surrounding AIDS and other sexually transmitted diseases, including increased HIV testing and counseling;

13. Qiu RZ, 2005.

14. Qiu RZ, 1999.

15. According to the new regulation (The State Council: *Regulation on Organ Transplantation*, 2007), this practice is prohibited.

16. Qiu RZ: China: Views of a Bioethicist, in Wertz, D & Fletcher, J (eds.): *Genetics and Ethics in Global Perspective*, Dordrecht: Kluwer, 2004, pp. 187–207; and also see Qiu, R 2004b.

reproductive health; family planning; prostitution; domestic violence against women; women's health; sex-ratio at birth; sexual harassment; and the suicide rate among women. This group submitted draft recommendations on these issues to the government,[17] some of which received a positive response.[18]

In 2007 Chinese Society for Bioethics was established. This group of bioethicists has already organized two national conferences, each of which was attended by more than 140 enthusiastic participants. Attendees included philosophers, ethicists, medical professionals, humanities and social science faculty from several universities in China, scientists from the Academy of Science, and administrators from various medical schools and the Center for Applied Ethics at the Academy of Social Sciences.[19] The work of this Society is one of the latest leaves to spring from the fertile soil supporting bioethics in China. Clearly, while the growth of bioethics has not been without its challenges, it is increasingly recognized as a necessary component of biotechnological and biomedical advances, and is being nourished sufficiently to thrive and yield fruitful results.

Institutionalization of Bioethics

The regulation of biomedicine and biotechnology, and the institutionalization of bioethics, go hand in hand. In China, the institutionalization of bioethics began in 1997, when the paper on the cloned sheep Dolly was published in *Nature*. Upon publication of the article, the then Minister of Health, the late Professor Chen Minzhang, convened an unprecedented meeting at which scientists, physicians, bioethicists, and lawyers discussed the ethical, legal, and social implications of cloning. The consensus was that biomedical research and the application of biotechnology needed to be regulated by the government, and that China needed a national ethics committee.

Since 1998, the Chinese government has promulgated a number of regulations to protect the rights and interests of human subjects and patients.[20] Almost all of

---

17. See all these recommendations from 1993–1998, 2004–2007.

18. This project, called "Reproductive Health and Ethics," was initiated by a program officer of the Ford Foundation, Dr. Mary Ann Burris, in partnership with CASS. The PI on this project is a bioethicist. Qiu RZ.

19. Prior to 2007, the Chinese Society for Medical Ethics and Chinese Society for Philosophy of Medicine had organized conferences related to bioethics, but the participants were limited to faculty members from medical schools, and the topics were not sufficiently interesting to attract more participants.

20. See Laws and Regulations below after the text. These laws and regulations can be read on various websites, such as www.gov.cn; www.npc.gov.cn; www.most.gov.cn; www.moh.gov.cn; www.pop.gov.cn.

these governmental regulations were developed with the input of bioethicists, or were initiated by bioethicists working collaboratively with scientists. For example, in early in 1988, scientists and bioethicists jointly submitted recommendations on the regulation of assisted reproductive technologies (ART). The Minister of Health and the Minister of Family Planning at the time, the late Professor Chen Minzhang and Mrs. Peng Peiyun, respectively, were receptive to the ART recommendations, but felt that more urgent matters demanded the attention of their ministries. In 1999, scientists and bioethicists again joined forces and suggested the Minister of Health regulate ART. This time the recommendation resulted in action, and in 2001 China's *Regulation on ART* was promulgated. During this same time period, scientists and bioethicists in Beijing and Shanghai submitted recommendations regarding the regulation of human embryonic stem cell research. Both the Ministry of Science and Technology and the Ministry of Health accepted their recommendations, and in 2003 the Ministries issued joint guiding principles on the subject. As regulations of biomedical research and biotechnology are considered, two fundamental questions come to bear: Is it necessary and desirable to regulate biomedical research and biotechnology for the purpose of protecting human subjects? If yes, why not draft guidelines with Chinese cultural characteristics rather than adopting international guidelines that have been formulated based largely on input from Western ethicists? I will address the first question in this section, and respond to the second question in the next section (Universal Values and Traditional Culture).

After years of debate, China has reached a consensus that it is indeed necessary and desirable to regulate biomedical research and biotechnology for the purpose of protecting human subjects. Contemporary biomedicine and biotechnology provides, and promises to provide more advanced and effective diagnostic, therapeutic, and preventive methods for diseases that affect millions of people. On the other hand, there is general agreement that the development and commercialization of these advances tend to infringe upon the interests and rights of patients and human subjects, leading to frequent conflicts of interest for physicians and scientists. The purpose of regulating research in these fields is to ensure proper development of biomedicine and biotechnology so that millions may eventually reap the health benefits, while concomitantly protecting the rights and welfare of patients and human subjects who are involved during development phases. Some scientists in China have claimed that ethical norms intended to protect the rights and welfare of patients and human subjects would unduly impede scientific progress. These scientists argue that China is in the process of catching up to the most scientifically advanced countries, and until China is in scientific parity with them, Chinese scientists should not be hindered by the strict and stringent ethical norms those advanced countries use. This stance is wrong and dangerous. It is wrong because it opposes ethical norms in the development of science and technology. It is dangerous because it would put China's scientific and technological development at risk, since science without ethics loses its essential integrity and public support. The scandals of the Hwang Woo-suk case in Korea and the Chen Jin case in China[21] convincingly illustrate this point.

In 2007, China promulgated its "Regulation for Ethical Review of Biomedical Research Involving Human Subjects" (the "Regulation"). The Regulation clearly sets forth the rationale for regulating biomedicine and biotechnology while institutionalizing bioethics, stating that its purpose is "to protect human life and health, safeguard human dignity, respect and protect human subjects' legitimate rights and interests." The Regulation requires that each institution conducting biomedical research establish an Institutional Research Ethics Committee (IREC). The institution's IREC conducts an ethical review of any proposed biomedical and biotechnological research involving human subjects.[22] The Regulation is an exemplar. It stipulates that an IREC's ethical review must be consistent with China's laws and regulations, as well as related international principles. In addition, the Regulation states that an IREC's ethical review is to be independent, objective, just and transparent. The Regulation prescribes the composition of an IREC, the IREC's responsibility for ethical review, the principles of ethical review, the requirements for informed consent, the necessary elements of a research protocol involving human subjects, and the penalty for any violation of the Regulation. It also clearly states that the safety, health, rights, and interests of human subjects are to be given priority over scientific and societal interests. The Regulation establishes ethics committees at three levels: national, provincial and institutional (the IRECs). The provincial ethics committees have oversight of the IRECs, while the national ethics committees (such as the ethics committee of the Ministry of Health) have oversight of both the provincial ethics committees and the IRECS (Ministry of Health, 2007).

The Regulation is intended to build an infrastructure or framework that will protect human subjects. In building this infrastructure, the IRECs need to be established, proper regulations put in place, and training provided to those who

21. Mr. Chen Jin, the Dean of the School of Micro-Electronics, Shanghai Jiaotong University, fabricated a scientific innovation, integrated chips called "Han Xin" (Chinese chips), and fraudulently applied for more than a dozen patents and near CNY 100 million in research funds. See Yang JZ et al.: Lack of Transparency in Treating Scientific Misconduct in China, *Yulin Daily*, April 24, 2007.

22. Although assisted reproduction and organ transplantation have become relatively routine medical treatment, these practices still must be reviewed and approved by an ethics committee, and informed consent still must be obtained from patients and organ donors, because these technologies often raise ethical or legal issues of public concern.

need to be familiar with the Regulation's provisions (IREC members, ministry officials, principal investigators, etc.). There also need to be a sufficient number of capable bioethicists in the country as the Regulation is fully implemented and oversight is put in place.

A number of challenges have arisen during the course of implementing the Regulation. First, scientists and principal investigators sometimes misunderstand or are resistant to ethics. Some view the field of ethics as dogmatic, supercilious, or lacking in substance. Others believe that no area of scientific research should be subject to ethical constraints, and resist the concept that research should be conducted in conformity with social and moral norms, including protection of human subjects and animal welfare. Still others claim that it is not necessary to learn ethics, since science is constantly evolving while ethics chronically lags behind. These individuals do not appreciate that certain values that form the foundation of ethics—such as "nonmaleficence," "respect for person," and "justice"—are timeless and are never eclipsed by scientific or technological developments.

The second impediment to successful implementation of the Regulation concerns the malfunction of IRECs. Some IRECs comprise solely medical professionals or hospital managers, with no representation from nonscientists or laypersons. Ethicists serving on IRECs often lack experience and have not addressed ethical issues raised in the biomedical field, which can severely limit their impact and effectiveness. The members of an IREC may not have sufficient familiarity with international and domestic ethics guidelines to undertake an appropriate ethics review, or the committee may ignore ethics and conduct only with scientific review of the proposed research protocol. In some institutions, the IREC may function as a rubber stamp, never rejecting a protocol or requiring modifications before granting approval. Another concern is that IRECs cannot truly be independent when the director of the hospital serves as its chair, as can be the case. Furthermore, a principal investigator (PI) may not submit her or his research protocol to the IREC until after the research is concluded and s/he decides to publish the research findings in an international journal. When proposals are submitted before the research is conducted, they may be deficient in that they do not include information needed for ethical review, or the informed consent does not conform with ethical requirements.[23] While the

---

23. For example, in some hospitals the informed consent form was called "Notices for Human Subjects," stated there was no risk associated with the research, did not state that subjects could withdraw at any time for any reason, and the consent form did not include an article on compensation when a subject is harmed as a result of their participation in the research.

IRECs are an excellent step toward protection of human subjects, there is still work to do in increasing their effectiveness.

The third challenge in implementing the Regulation is about informed consent. Some PIs claim that informed consent is not appropriate, because human subjects are unable to grasp the information disclosed to them. Others worry that the informed consent process will slow down their research, or that potential candidates will refuse to participate in, or withdraw from, research when they learn what they are participating in is "research" As a result, some PIs deliberately withhold information regarding potential risks to subjects and exaggerate possible benefits. PIs may also rush to obtain a subject's signature without a valid informed consent process, or PIs may even evade informed consent, generally due to a conflict of interest or similar concern.

Although the Regulation has encountered some challenges, its development and implementation have further ingrained bioethics in scientific research. There is also a significant increase in the need for bioethics training. Since 2004, several entities have been working together to organize workshops that provide ethics training to PIs, ethics committee members, and healthcare administrators who are responsible for science and technology. These workshops have been offered in Beijing, Shanghai, Wuhan, Hangzhou, Chengdu, Xi'an and elsewhere in China. The organizations that have worked together to create and provide these workshops include the Center for Bioethics at Peking Union Medical College; Shanghai School of Medicine, Fudan University; the Center for Bioethics at Central China (Huazhong) University of Science and Technology; the Health Science Center at Peking University; the World Health Organization (Alex Capron); and their counterparts at the Harvard School of Public Health (Richard Cash and Daniel Wilker), the University of California–San Francisco (Bernard Lo), University of Minnesota (Jeff Kahn), the University of Chicago (Mark Siegler), Yale University (Robert Levine), University of Bergen (Reidar Lie), the Department of Clinical Bioethics, NIH (Ezekiel Emanuel), and the University of Singapore (Alastair Campbell). This collective effort was undertaken with sponsorship from the Fogarty International Center and Department of Bioethics of the National Institutes of Health (NIH), the Chinese Medical Board, and the Directorate-General for Research, European Commission.[24] These training workshops have increased understanding of bioethics and improved the environment in which the Regulation is being implemented. This, in turn, will facilitate the protection of human subjects and foster additional progress in this area of bioethics.

In terms of future work in bioethics in China, there are still a number of regulatory gaps and new challenges that have yet to be addressed. First, patients,

---

24. Qiu RZ: Bioethics in China (1990–2008*), Asian Bioethics Review*, vol. 1, December 1, 2008.

physicians, PIs, and healthcare administrators tend to confuse clinical trials with medical care. To make matters worse, some physicians/PIs intentionally disguise clinical trials as medical care, which allows them to circumvent ethical review and informed consent. Such physicians/PIs are focused more on the money to be made from uninformed patients than on their patient's/research subject's best interests. These physicians/PIs are the biomedical research version of the "wolves in white" discussed above. Another issue that deserves attention is consistent application of existing regulations. Although the Ministry of Health has the authority to regulate all forms of clinical trials and research with human subjects, not everybody involved in such research adheres to the Ministry's regulations. Even within the Ministry, not all bureaus or high-ranking officials recognize the difference between clinical research and medical care, resulting in inconsistent enforcement of relevant regulations. A third area that needs to be addressed concerns the ethical issues that arise out of cutting-edge research in biotechnology involving human subjects, such as clinical application of stem cell therapy, gene therapy, nanotechnology, and others. These ethical issues either have not been addressed, or have not been addressed adequately. Still another issue deserving of attention is the continued lack of regulation of the conflict of interest inherent in certain relationships between drug and equipment manufacturing companies and physicians, PIs, and IREC members. And finally, a very controversial ethical issue that remains to be addressed within China is whether advances in traditional Chinese medicine (TCM) should be subject to clinical trials.

In response to the first of the two questions I posed above, China recognizes that it must regulate biomedical research and biotechnology for the purpose of protecting human subjects, and has taken strides toward doing so. Despite this progress, bioethics, like science, is not a static field, and as each challenge is addressed a new challenge takes its place.

Universal Values and Traditional Culture

When China decided that biomedical research and biotechnologies needed to be regulated, it prompted a second question: Why not draft guidelines with Chinese cultural characteristics, rather than adopting international guidelines that have been formulated based largely on input from Western ethicists? Underlying this question is a subject of everlasting controversy in China: Are there values that are truly universal?

Lee Kuan Yew first put forward the concept of Asian values.[25] Logically speaking, if you agree there are Asian values, you must also agree that there are

25. Sen, 1997.

universal values. Throughout Asia, there are diverse cultures and subcultures, with some subcultures crossing national boundaries. Religion is one example of a subculture that can cross national boundaries, and within Asia one finds Confucianism, Daoism, Buddhism, Hinduism, Christianity, and Islam, among others. In some countries, a particular religion may have a strong, even inextricable, connection to the nation's culture, such that they are identified as one and the same thing. Those who believe in "Asian values" argue that irrespective of nation, religion, or other subculture, there are certain values that are common to every Asian country. If they think so, then along this line of reasoning it should be believed that other regions across the world, such as Europe, Africa, and Latin America, share common values, and that when common values from various regions around the world are compared with Asian values and with one another, certain commonalities emerge. Those common values, which appear across regions, nations, and even religions, could be labeled "universal values." Some Chinese Marxists have argued against universal values, believing that class-based societies cannot share the same values as societies with flat class structures. Even in a class-based society, however, there are common human needs that transcend class, meaning that values can be shared between countries with quite different social configurations. Another argument against universal values is that some values identified as "universal," such as democracy, liberty, and human rights, are actually Western values and are not truly universal. While this argument is offered in opposition to the concept of universal values, it is inapt for that purpose except to the extent it supports the contention that perhaps democracy, liberty, and human rights are not universal values. Chinese Confucians also argue against universal values, stating that China's values are uniquely Confucian, although they believe Confucian values will eventually become universal within the world.[26]

In the field of bioethics, some Chinese ethicists have claimed that international ethical guidelines are Western in nature, and that China should use guidelines that are consistent with Confucianism and Confucian values instead. Those who make this argument do not realize that many international ethical guidelines were developed with the participation of, and input from, Chinese representatives,

---

26. For the debate on universal values see Zhen Y: Some epistemic issues on universal values, *Beijing Daily*, June 16, 2008; Li M: Respect universal values and achieve scientific development, September 17, 2008, http://news.xinhuanet.com/theory/2008-09/17/content_10032093.htm. Both are proponents of universal values. Critics include Chen Kuiyuan, the President of the Chinese Academy of Social Sciences, Hou Huiqin, the Deputy Director of the Institute of Marxist Studies, Research Group on Deng Xiaoping Theory and The Thought of Three Representatives, the Ministry of Education, See http://news.163.com/08/1120/10/4R6EV5ME00012Q9L.html.

along with representatives from other countries, other continents, and other cultures. As such, how can one argue that international guidelines are Western? Furthermore, the fundamental values these international ethical guidelines represent, such as nonmaleficence/beneficence, respect, and justice, are recognized by all countries and cultures that were involved in developing the guidelines. In that sense, they truly are universal values. Mencius said: "To do no harm is the art of *ren*." (*Meng Zi,* chapter on King Lianghui I, paragraph 7). Xunzi said: "The man with *ren* must respect person" (*Xun Zi,* Chapter 13 on Chen Dao, paragraph 7). And Confucius said: "Human nature is similar, only the practice makes them apart" (*Lun Yu,* Chapter 17, paragraph 2). These values are found in Confucianism, Hinduism, Islamism, Christianity and other religions. No cultural values ever claim that we should disrespect human life, cause injustice, or cause harm to others, unless such "values" are imposed through a government or other political mechanism.

Eventually, after much discussion, the consensus in China is that although China has unique cultural traditions, it is imperative to comply with international ethical guidelines on biomedical research involving human subjects. This consensus is in part due to the fact that international guidelines have resulted from communication and negotiation among experts from different countries and different cultures from all over the world, including China. While China takes its own culture into account when implementing international guidelines and their underlying principles, there is no valid basis upon which to reject their general applicability within China (Zhai, 2008).

Even with the acceptance of international ethical guidelines, ethical issues cannot be addressed in a vacuum in which local culture and values play no part. I propose the view of "ethical issue is local," in which the ethical issue is viewed within the sociocultural context in which it arises. As such, the issue is assessed not only with the assistance of universal values supported by international ethics guidelines, but also with consideration of the cultural values operating *in situ.* This ensures that international guidelines are followed while simultaneously showing respect for the values of the immediate stakeholders and local community. For instance, in China, the Confucian concept of personhood has a great impact upon bioethics. The Confucian concept of personhood is monistic, gradualist, and relational. From the Confucian monist view, a person is a psychosomatic unity: *xing* or *ti* (body, form) and *shen* (psyche, spirit), both of which come from *qi* (vital energy) and are related to each other. When the two basic forms of *qi* (*yin* and *yang*) are united, a human being is formed. So, in contrast to the dualism observed in Western medicine, in which medicine and psychiatry/psychology are practiced separately, this dichotomy has never existed in traditional Chinese medicine. The Confucian gradualist view also has an impact on the Chinese view of bioethics. The Confucians view a human embryo as a product of the interaction of *yin* and *yang*. There are many transformations in the process from embryo to newborn, and the human embryo will develop or transform into a human person. The human embryo is not viewed as human person yet, although it is recognized as having inherent teleology or self-actualization to develop into human person. "Person begins with birth and ends with death. Human *tao* lies in good beginning and good end." (*Xun Zi*, chapter 19 Li Lun, paragraph 10 *Xun Zi*, chapter 19 Li Lun, paragraph 10) Even after birth, Confucians do not consider a newborn to be a person, because although all three aspects of a person are present [the psyche (*shen*), the vital energy (*qi*), and the physical body (*ti*)], they are imperfect. The newborn is waiting to be cultivated and perfected, which is what creates a person. In Confucianism, no one is born a moral person. Such a person is created though the effort of person-making (*zuo ren*), which is a lifetime process. This is the reason Confucians emphasize:

> Cultivate life (*yang sheng*) via diet, exercise, deep breath, drug, etc.;
> Cultivate senses (*tao ye qing cao*) via music, painting, calligraphy, sightseeing, etc.; and
> Cultivate character (*yang xing*) to be a moral person.

Another aspect of Confucian thought is to view individuals relationally. Individuals are not thought of as existing independently or being separate from any other being. On the contrary, in Confucian thought, human beings are distinguishable from animals because of their relational/social capacity. A person is never seen as an isolated individual, but is always conceived of as a part of a network of relations. The "effort of person-making" undertaken as one strives to become a real (moral) person, is a process that is carried out in and through a social context and for the purpose of fulfilling social responsibility, rather than self-actualization *per se*.[27]

This concept of Confucian personhood may pose a barrier in implementing the principle of informed consent. In China, individuals are not as independent as in the West, and are closely tied to their families and/or community. For this reason, individuals must be considered in terms of these relationships rather than as individuals who make decisions for themselves without regard for, or the close involvement of, others. In China, when a person needs medical attention, families are actively involved in providing care as well as emotional and financial support. As a result, the family, and sometimes even the community, becomes involved in the process of informed consent. In a pure research context,

27. Hui, 2004.

the subject is expected to make a decision her/himself and without family or community involvement, although family may be consulted. However, when the prospective subject is a medical patient being considered for experimental treatment, or the research is being conducted in rural areas, the family and/or community must be allowed to be involved in the informed consent process. In these cases, consent may not come from the individual who will be participating in the research but, rather, from the head of the family or clan, head of the village, chief of the tribe, or similar leader. These cases are sometimes referred to as "family consent" or "community consent." In these situations, is the self-determination of the individual who is the prospective subject denied? Do "family consent" or "community consent" meet the ethical requirements for informed consent? Does the inherent authority of family and community leaders compromise the principle of informed consent and its implementation?

Another Chinese cultural issue that may affect informed consent is the higher value that is placed on verbal agreements, in the sense that an oral commitment is more sacred than one that is written. A research subject might fully comprehend the informed consent document and be willing to serve as a research subject, but still refuse to sign the written informed consent form for this reason. Similarly, research subjects who are illiterate may agree to participate in research but refuse to sign an informed consent form because they have signed written contracts in the past only to find themselves the victims of fraud when the explanations provided to them and the written contract were not in accord.[28]

There are three potential approaches for addressing the tension between international guidelines and local culture during the informed consent process:

(1) Traditionalist Approach

In the "traditionalist" approach, precedence is given to the beliefs and values of the traditional native culture of the country where the scientific research is being conducted. If one were to take this approach in addressing the tension between the principle of informed consent and local culture, it would likely violate international guidelines on research ethics and result in an inability to protect the rights and welfare of human subjects. Using family as an example, in a culture in which individuals do not make decisions independent of their family unit, a family may infringe upon a vulnerable family member's individual rights and freedom, and also may not allocate family resources in a fair manner. Under a traditionalist approach, that cultural value would be upheld, even to the extent

28. See Zhu, 2009; Zhai, 2009.

that it operated to the detriment of a research subject. This approach is not ethically justifiable, and therefore not acceptable.

(2) Modernist Approach

In the "modernist" approach, precedence is given to the beliefs and values in Western culture that are embodied in ethical guidelines of Western countries. The values and beliefs of the native culture would be disregarded. Such an approach would likely increase the tension between local culture and international ethics guidelines. Native culture is not monolithic; rather, it can be divided into positive elements, which may benefit native people, and negative elements, which may harm them (such as the example of family provided in the discussion of the traditionalist approach). Again using family as an example, in a culture in which individuals do not operate independently of their families, the family may provide much needed support during times of crisis, providing immense assistance to an individual and preserving or even improving his or her well-being. To act in a manner that discounts family involvement, or actively discourages it, may operate to the detriment of the subject. Thus, as was the case with the traditionalist approach, the modernist approach of completely disregarding native values is not ethically justifiable or acceptable.

(3) Reconciliation Approach

A "reconciliation" approach applies international ethical guidelines while respecting the beliefs and values of the native culture, and in some cases even assimilating its positive elements into informed consent procedures. This approach allows China and other countries to address the tension between native culture and effective protection of the rights and welfare of human subjects. In order to reconcile the two, one must strictly adhere to the "hard core" of informed consent, and be flexible with the less essential "periphery".[29]

The "hard core" of the informed consent principle includes: (1) faithful disclosure of clear and accurate information that is sufficient to allow patients/human subjects to make an informed decision; (2) actively assisting patients/subjects to understand the information contained in the informed consent; and (3) ensuring consent (either from a competent patient or subject, or from a

29. The terms "hard core" and "periphery" are borrowed from Lakatos. See Lakatos, I. (1970). Falsification and the Methodology of Scientific Research Programmes, In Lakatos, I. & Musgrave, A. (eds.). *Criticism and the Growth of Knowledge*. Cambridge: Cambridge University Press, pp. 91–196.

guardian in the event of an incompetent patient or subject) is obtained without inappropriate inducement or coercion. These core principles must not be compromised when reconciling informed consent procedures with local culture.

Aside from these "hard core" aspects, there are peripheral aspects of informed consent that can be modified to suit local cultures. These peripheral aspects of informed consent include: (1) the manner in which information is disclosed (a written document *versus* verbal or audiovisual presentation); (2) the manner in which patients or subjects express their consent (a signature *versus* a verbal commitment in the presence of a witness); (3) the wording of the consent form (whether to use the term "research" or "experiment"); and (4) the extent to which others, such as a family or community leader, are involved in the consent process.

In implementing the reconciliation approach, there are several issues that must be addressed:

(1) The difference between scientific research (including clinical trials) and medical care must be made clear to prospective human subjects in order to prevent misunderstandings between established medical treatment and experimental procedures/research; however, if a prospective subject fully comprehends the clinical trial and is willing to participate, but objects to the use of the terms "experiment," "drug research," or "genetic research" in the informed consent document, it would be appropriate to replace those terms with an equivalent term than isn't problematic for the subject, such as "observing a new drug's safety and efficacy" or "studying the relationship between genes and diseases." This is only appropriate when the prospective human subject has already received clear and accurate information regarding the clinical research trial, and has agreed to participate, but prefers to sign a form with alternate but equally descriptive language.

(2) When family or community involvement is a known cultural value, the family or community should be involved in the informed consent process. This means that prior to any contact with any prospective human subject, the research project should first be discussed with the head of the family or community in order to obtain their approval for family or community member involvement. This does not mean, however, that the family or community leader has the power, or should be given the power, to decide who should participate in the research. That decision must rest with the individual. Although the terms *family consent* and *community consent* are used to describe this process, they are somewhat misleading, and might be more accurately described as "informed consent with the aid of family/community."

(3) Some research subjects prefer oral agreements to those that are written. If the prospective human subject has been provided clear and accurate information about the clinical trial, understands it, and has voluntarily expressed a desire to participate in the research, but has a cultural aversion to written agreements, an oral agreement should be permitted. In such instances, the oral agreement should be formalized through the use of a third-party witness who has no connection to the subject, the PI, or PI's institution. This witness, upon verifying that the subject understands the information in the informed consent document and consents to participate in the research, should sign the consent form in the subject's stead. The witness should also indicate that a witness was used due to the subject's preference for verbal agreements.

The result of the reconciliation approach will be, to use Confucius' words, "*he er bu tong*" (*Lun Yu*, chapter 13, paragraph 23), which means "harmonized, but not identical" or "harmonized as well as diversified." Such is the end result when both China's values and international bioethics standards are treated with the respect each deserves.

Acknowledgment

Kind thanks to Professor Zhai Xiaomei for her more than ten years' collaboration on basic ideas underlying this chapter, to Professors Qi Guoming and Yu Xiucheng for their efforts in bioethics institutionalization, to Professor Hu Chingli for his hard work on establishing a research ethics framework in China, and finally to Pam Heatlie, JD & Catherine Myser, PhD, for their invaluable English language editing throughout this chapter. The chapter could not have come to fruition without their contributions and generous assistance.

Glossary

Bioethics In China, bioethics is a branch of applied normative ethics, which addresses substantive and procedural ethical issues (what ought to be done and how) in life sciences/biotechnologies and health care. Bioethical study begins with an ethical issue, and identifies possible solutions. Arguments for and against each potential solution are assessed, and the solution that best balances risks with benefits, respect for persons, and justice, is selected. The selected solution is implemented, but subjected to continued study and replaced with an improved solution should one be identified. Bioethics is not to be confused with biolaw or biomedical sociology. Bioethics is a rational endeavor based on evidence and reasoning, and is not subject to religious influence.

Bioethicist In China, a bioethicist is a professional with training in philosophy. Many bioethicists are employed as faculty in departments of philosophy, or departments of the humanities and social sciences, at the center for bioethics or center for applied ethics of a university or college, or at the academy of science or social sciences. Bioethicists may be employed to teach courses in philosophy, philosophy of science, ethics, applied ethics, medical ethics, or bioethics. Bioethicists may also study ethical issues in life sciences/biotechnologies or healthcare fields. Bioethicists are working as members of institutional ethics committees, provincial ethics committees, or the national ethics committee of MOH, as well as other committees providing expertise on relevant policies. Bioethicists do not perform the same work as lawyers, who address legal issues in life sciences/biotechnologies or healthcare fields, or sociologists, who conduct sociological study in these fields. While anybody can become a bioethicist, not every person who offers an opinion on an ethical issue actually is a bioethicist.

CASS Chinese Academy of Social Sciences: In parallel with Chinese Academy of Science (CAS), CASS is a state research institution that focuses on the study of the humanities and social sciences. CASS is established and supported by the State Council, central government; in addition, there are provincial academies of social sciences that are established and supported by the respective provincial governments.

IREC Institutional research ethics committee, which is similar to an IRB in the United States. According to the 1999 *Regulation for Drug Clinical Trials* and the 2007 *Regulation for Ethical Review of Biomedical Research Involving Human Subjects*, each institution that conducts biomedical research or clinical trials involving human subjects is required to establish an institutional research ethics committee, for the purpose of reviewing and approving or disapproving research protocols involving human subjects.

MOH Ministry of Health.

MOST Ministry of Science and Technology, which is responsible for the programming and financing major scientific and technological innovation projects in China.

NPC The National People's Congress, China's legislature.

Qi This Chinese character means air; however, in Chinese culture it refers to a kind of physico-psychic entity or vital energy, which is the origin of all things in the universe. Its counterpart may be something like *pneuma*. The *qi* has two basic forms: *yin* and *yang*. All things in the universe, including human beings, are the product of *yin-yang* interactions.

Ren Humaneness and humanness. The basic concept of Confucianism. *Ren* requires a person to care for, and do good toward, others.

SFDA State Food and Drug Administration. Its functions are similar to the FDA in the United States. Prior to 2008, the SFDA was directly under the State Council, but it is now affiliated with MOH.

Shen This Chinese character means mind, soul, psyche, god.

The State Council China's central government.

Ti This Chinese character means *soma*, body.

Xing This Chinese character means shape, body, form.

Zuoren person-making. In Confucianism, a human being is born only biologically. To become a moral agent or person, one should make efforts of *zuo ren* (person-making).

Chinese Classics

Lun Yu The title of this book in English is *Analects of Confucius*. This book contains the collected dialogue of Confucius and his disciples.

Men Zi This book contains Mencius' collected statements and speeches. Mencius, or Meng Zi, is the second greatest Confucian after Confucius.

Xun Zi This book contains the collected statements and speeches of Xun Zi, the third greatest Confucian after Confucius.

References

Articles and Books

Bai J. (2006). Can Organ Trading Be Permitted? *Chinese Medical Ethics, 19*(5), 14–16.

Bai J. et al. (2008). Ethical Considerations on Exchange of Living Donated Organs between Family. *Chinese Medical Ethics, 21*(5), 25–28.

Cao N. (2004). *Updating Statute and Idea after Technology–Advance in Organ Transplantation in China.* Presented at Beijing International Conference on Bioethics, January 1998, see www.chinaphs.org/bioethics.

CASS (Chinese Academy of Social Sciences)/Ford(the Ford Foundation). (1993). *Ethical Guidelines on the Policy of Prevention and Treatment of AID/STDs*. Expert Workshop on AIDS/STDs: Social, Ethical and Legal Issues, March 15–18, 1993. In Qiu RZ (ed.). (1996). *Reproductive Health and Ethics*, Vol. 1. Beijing: Beijing Medical University & Peking Union Medical College Joint Press, pp. 52–64.

CASS/Ford. (1994). *Ethical Principles and Action Recommendations on Promoting Reproductive Health and Safeguarding Women's Rights*. Expert Workshop on Reproduction, Sexuality, Ethics and Women's Rights: Feminist Perspectives, February 25–March 1, 1994. In Qiu RZ (ed.). (1996). *Reproductive Health and Ethics*, Vol. 1. Beijing: Beijing Medical University & Peking Union Medical College Joint Press, pp. 166–174.

CASS/Ford. (1995). *Ethical Principles and Action Recommendations on Family Planning.* Expert Workshop on Family Planning, Ethics and Human Values, April 23–27, 1995. In Qiu RZ (ed.). (1996). *Reproductive Health and Ethics*, Vol. 1. Beijing: Beijing Medical University & Peking Union Medical College Joint Press, pp. 307–315.

CASS/Ford. (1996). *Consensus and Recommendations on HIV and Prostitution.* Expert Workshop on HIV and Prostitution: Social, Ethical and Legal Issues, October 29–31, 1996. In Qiu RZ. (ed.) (2006) *Reproductive Health and Ethics*, Vol. 2. Beijing: Peking Union Medical College Press, pp. 137–142.

CASS/Ford. (1997). *Consensus and Recommendations on Preventing and Combating Domestic Violence against Women.* Expert Workshop on Combating Domestic Violence against Women: Social, Ethical, and Legal Issues, October 29–31, 1997. In Qiu RZ. (ed.) (2006) *Reproductive Health and Ethics*, Vol. 2. Beijing: Peking Union Medical College Press, pp. 245–253.

CASS/Ford. (1998). *Policy Recommendations on Women's Health in China.* Expert Workshop on Cairo-Beijing Conferences and Reproductive Health in China: Social, Ethical and Legal Issues, November 28–30, 1998. In Qiu RZ. (ed.) (2006) *Reproductive Health and Ethics*, Vol. 2. Beijing: Peking Union Medical College Press, pp. 340–349.

CASS/Ford. (2004). *Action Recommendations on Correcting the Birth Sex Ratio Imbalance.* Expert Workshop on Ethical, Legal and Social Issues of Birth Sex Ratio Imbalance in Mainland China, 27–June 28, 2004. In Hu L & Qiu RZ. (eds.) *Reproductive Health and Ethics*, Vol. 3. Beijing: Peking Union Medical College Press, forthcoming.

CASS/Ford. (2005). *Action Recommendations the Fight against Sex Harassment at Work.* Expert Workshop on the Fight against Sex Harassment at Work: Ethical, Legal and Social Issues, September 24–25, 2005. In Hu L & Qiu RZ. (eds.) *Reproductive Health and Ethics*, Vol. 3. Beijing: Peking Union Medical College Press, forthcoming.

CASS/Ford. (2006). *Recommendations on Preventing Women's Suicide in Rural Areas.* Expert Workshop on Ethical, Legal and Social Issues of Women's Suicide in Rural Areas, 16–December 17, 2006. In Hu LY & Qiu RZ. (eds.) *Reproductive Health and Ethics*, Vol. 3. Beijing: Peking Union Medical College Press, forthcoming.

CASS/Ford. (2007). *Guidelines and Action Recommendations on Scaling up HIV Testing and Counseling.* Expert Workshop on Ethical, Legal and Social Issues in Scaling up HIV Testing and Counseling in Mainland China, 22–December 23, 2007. In Hu L & Qiu RZ. (eds.) *Reproductive Health and Ethics*, Vol. 3. Beijing: Peking Union Medical College Press, forthcoming.

Center for Development Research, the State of Council. (2005). *Evaluation and Recommendations on the Reform of Chinese Health System* (Summary). Available at: http://www.sohu.com.

Chen X. et al. (2007). Remarks on the Regulation of Organ Transplantation. *Law and System Daily*, April 17.

Chen Y. et al. (2003). *Biomedical Research Ethics*. Beijing: PUMC Press.

Du ZZ. (2005). Health Care Services, Markets and the Chinese Moral Tradition: Establishing a Humanistic Health Care Market. In Tao, J (ed.) 2008 *China: Bioethics, Trust, and the Challenge of the Market*, New York, Springer, 2008, pp. 137–150.

Hui E. (2004). *Personhood and Bioethics: Chinese Perspective*. In Qiu, R. (ed.). *Bioethics: Asian Perspectives: A Quest for Moral Diversity*. Dordrecht: Kluwers, pp. 29–44.

Ma YH. (2006). Can Organ Trading Be Permitted: Challenges from Deontological and Consequential Perspectives. *Chinese Medical Ethics, 19*(5), 11–13.

Minutes of the First National Workshop on Ethical and Legal Issues in Limiting Procreation, Beijing, November 11–14, 1991. *Chinese Health Law, 5*, 44–46.

Proceedings of the Symposium on Health Care and Development, November 16–18, 1998. Beijing: Chinese Health Economics Press.

BIONET Workshop on Ethics and Governance in Clinical Trials/Research in Europe and China, Xi'an, *9–September 12, 2008.* http://www.bionet-china.org/workshop_pages.htm#generated-subheading4.

Qiu RZ. (ed.). (1996). *Reproductive Health and Ethics, Vol. 1*. Beijing: Beijing Medical University & Peking Union Medical College Joint Press.

Qiu RZ. (1998). Health Care Reform from Ethical Perspectives. In *The Proceedings of the Symposium on Health Care and Development, November 16–18, 1998.* (pp. 61–62). Beijing: Chinese Health Economics Press.

Qiu RZ. (1999). Can the Use of Organs from Executed Prisoners Be Justified? *Medicine & Philosophy, 3*, 22–24.

Qiu RZ. (2003). Ethical and Policy Issues raised in the Epidemic of SARS in China. *Studies in Dialectics of Nature, 6*, 1–6.

Qiu RZ. (2004a). *Bioethics: Asian Perspectives*. Dordrecht: Kluwers.

Qiu RZ. (2004b). Does Eugenics Exist in China? Ethical issues in China's law on maternal and infant care. In: Qiu RZ (ed.). *Bioethics: Asian Perspectives*. Dordrecht: Kluwers, pp. 185–196.

Qiu RZ. (2005a). Where Are Vitals of the Serious Worsening of Physician–patient Relationship? *Medicine and Philosophy, 6*, 5–7.

Qiu RZ. (2005b). Human Cloning: Arguments For and Against. *Journal of Huazhong University of Science and Technology, 19*(3), 108–118.

Qiu RZ. (2006). *Reproductive Health and Ethics*, Vol. 2. Beijing: Peking Union Medical College Press.

Qiu RZ. (2007a). Ethical Issues in the Frontier of Life Sciences. *Wenhui Daily*, October 14. p. 8.

Qiu RZ. (2007b). Physician's Choice in Moral Dilemmas. *Science Times*, December 14, p. 3. http://www.sciencenet.cn/htmlnews/20071214832523431967728.html.

Qiu RZ. (2008). On the Reform of Health Care Reform. In Tao, J (ed.) *China: Bioethics, Trust, and the Challenge of the Market*, New York, Springer, 181–192.

Sen A. (1997). Human Rights and Asian Values: What Lee Kuan Yew and Le Peng Don't Understand about Asia. *The New Republic, 217*(2–3), 33, 38.

Wang CS. (2006). The Third Approach to the Procurement of Transplanted Organs. *Chinese Medical Ethics, 19*(5), 17–19.

Zeng Y. et al. (2000). *A Call for Effectively Containing HIV Pandemic in China*. Chinese Academy of Science, pp. 4–12, 45–48.

Zhai XM. et al. (2005). *An Introduction to Bioethics*. Beijing: Tsinghua Press.
Zhai XM. et al. (2008). Capacity Building in Ethical Review in China in an International Context: Ideas and Practices. *Chinese Medical Ethics*, *2*, 3–6.
Zhai XM. (2009). Informed Consent in the Non-Western Cultural Context and the Implementation of Universal Declaration of Human Right. *Asian Bioethics Review*, *1*(1), 5–16.
Zhou YL. (2003). *Fairness, Efficiency and Economic Growth: A Study in Health Care Investment in China in Transition*. Wuhan: Wuhan Press.
Zhu W. (2006). Arguments against Living Organ Transplantation. *Chinese Medical Ethics*, 19(5), 7–10.
Zhu W. (2009) *Informed Consent in Bioethics*. Shanghai: Fudan University Press.

Laws and Regulations

Minister of Health (MOH): Regulation on Assisted Reproductive Technologies, 2000, 2003.
MOH: Regulation on Ethical Review of Biomedical Research Involving Human Subjects, 2007.
MOH: Regulation on Clinical Application of Organ Transplantation Technology, 2005.
Ministry of Science and Technology (MOST)/MOH: Protecting Human Genetic Resources, 1998.
MOST/MOH: Ethical Guiding Principles for Human Embryonic Stem Cell Research, 2003.
National People's Congress (NPC): Maternal and Infant Health Care Law, 1994.
NPC: Family Planning and Population Law, 2001.
People's Congress, Gansu Province: Regulation on Prohibiting Procreation of Mentally Retarded, 1988.
People's Congress, Heilongjiang Province: Regulation on Maternal and Infant Health Care, 2005.
People's Congress, Liaoning Province: Regulation on Preventing Inferior Births, 1990.
State Council: Regulation on Medical Institutions, 1994.
State Council: Regulation on Marriage Registry, 2003.
State Council: Regulation on AIDS Prevention and Control, 2006.
State Council: Regulation on Organ Transplantation, 2007.
State Food and Drug Administration (SFDA): GCP for Clinical Trials, 1999, 2003.

III

BIOETHICS AS A MEANS FOR NEGOTIATING SOCIAL, REGIONAL, AND/OR NATIONAL IDENTITY, AND BIOETHICS AS NATION-BUILDING

12 THE DOMINION OF BIOETHICS

NATIONALISM AND CANADIAN BIOETHICS

Andrea Frolic, Michael D. Coughlin, and Bernard Keating

Introduction

Canadians are preoccupied with questions of national identity. When comparing ourselves to other countries, Canadians articulate both a longing for a stronger national identity, and a suspicion of this impulse.[1] Our preoccupation with (and ambivalence toward) national identity might itself be called a defining national characteristic. In casual conversation, Canadians generally begin any definition of their national identity in negative terms. In any foreign context, English-speaking or Anglo-Canadians will hastily clarify, "We are not American." French-speaking or francophone Canadians, though usually less concerned about mistaken identity, will also make it known that, "We are not French."[2] However, defining exactly what we *are* is more difficult. Anxiety over what makes Canada unique among nations, and what defines Canadian culture, is fueled by three major challenges. The first is our geographical proximity to the economic, military, and cultural superpower of the United States of America. The second is the official

1. Canada has the second largest land mass of any country globally, with a current population of 33.5 million. It is a federation composed of ten provinces and three territories. These are often grouped into regions: Western Canada consists of British Columbia, and the three Prairie provinces (Alberta, Saskatchewan, and Manitoba); Central Canada consists of Québec and Ontario; Atlantic Canada comprises the three Maritime provinces (New Brunswick, Prince Edward Island, and Nova Scotia), along with Newfoundland and Labrador. The three territories (Yukon, Northwest Territories, and Nunavut) make up Northern Canada.

2. Canada's two official languages are French and English. According to the 2006 census, 65.9% of Canadians speak English at home, 21.2% speak French at home, while another 11.1% speak a non-official language at home. Most Francophones live in Québec and New Brunswick; outside of those two provinces only 4.1% of the population have French as their mother tongue. (See Statistics: Canada's 2006 Census Data Products on Language: http://www12.statcan.ca/english/census06/data/highlights/language/Table402.cfm).

policy of multiculturalism, which fosters diverse cultural identities within Canada, as well as the competing nationalist discourses of Québécois and aboriginal peoples. A third is Canada's geographic vastness and diversity, and the resulting regionalism which is reinforced by a relatively weak federal (i.e., national) government that delegates regulation of most social services to the provinces and territories.

In an increasingly globalized world, all nations are confronted with questions of national identity,[3] and challenged to define or redraw their national character and borders (both literal and virtual). Some have argued elsewhere that bioethics has served as an instrument of globalization by elevating (so-called) universal principles that transcend and transgress borders and cultures, or that it serves as an instrument of modernization or secularization.[4] However, the authors of this paper[5] argue that Canada provides a counter-example of a country in which bioethics explicitly serves to reinforce and inform nationalist aspirations. Three features of the Canadian cultural/political landscape create fertile ground for synergy between bioethical and nationalist discourses and practices: (1) the recent shift toward a knowledge- and innovation-based economy; (2) the role of health care and health policy in the Canadian national psyche; and (3) the perceived centrality of values and principles to our national character.

While the national identity of the United States is closely linked to its economy (as global champion of the free market and technological innovator), Canada's nationalist discourses historically were detached from its economy. Since its origins as a source of fish and fur for European markets, Canada's economy has remained dependent upon the extraction of natural resources and commodities (through mining, oil and gas exploration, logging, fishing, and farming). However, over the past decade, federal and provincial governments[6] have begun

---

3. McQuaig, 1998.

4. See Englehardt, 2003; this volume, Introduction by Myser.

5. Andrea Frolic (ANF) hails from Saskatchewan; she received a BA and MA in religious studies in Ontario, undertook doctoral education in anthropology and clinical ethics in the United States, and returned to Canada to take up a clinical ethics position in a teaching hospital in Ontario. Bernard Keating (BK) is a Québécois bioethicist with a PhD in theological ethics, who holds faculty appointments in departments of theology, pharmacy, and dental medicine, and is a member of the *Conseil du Medicament* for the province of Québec. Michael Coughlin (MDC) is an American with graduate training in theology, and a PhD in neuroscience, who immigrated to Canada in 1981 and has enjoyed a 25-year career as a university researcher and a clinical ethicist at a hospital in Ontario.

6. The recent rise in commodity prices has caused an economic boom for the extractive economies of Saskatchewan and Alberta, while the deepening U.S. recession has hit the manufacturing heartland of Canada—Ontario and Québec—very hard. In response, these two provinces have made strategic investments to grow the research-based sectors of their economies. For example, Ontario's provincial government includes a cabinet post (Minister of Research

to invest public resources to enhance Canada's competitiveness in a global knowledge economy through research, innovation, and knowledge-transfer activities.[7] Funding for research has increased by 93 percent from 1992–2007[8] leading to an astonishing number of Canadians participating in research (1 in 10, according to some estimates).[9] Given that Canadian bioethicists have made significant contributions to the field of research ethics and regulation at international, national, and local levels,[10] the strategic growth of the research and innovation sectors of the economy provide fertile ground for examining the link between the discourses and practices of bioethics, and Canadian national identity.

Secondly, the Canadian healthcare system is intrinsically linked to Canadian national identity. This system is in reality not a single system, but rather a network of ten provincial and three territorial healthcare systems, founded on and governed by the Canada Health Act (1984), and funded through a combination of general tax revenues (70%) and private contributions (30%).[11] The Canada Health Act (CHA) enshrines core principles of comprehensiveness, universality, accessibility, portability, and public administration, to which all provincial and territorial governments must adhere in order to receive access to general tax revenues (through federal transfer payments) to pay for health care and other social services.[12] Canadians have never perceived health care as a "market good" (as in the United States) but as a "public good." Our general devotion to a publicly administered healthcare system is founded on the principles of equity (defined as

---

and Innovation) dedicated to promoting an "aggressive innovation agenda" as a pillar of Ontario's economic growth strategy. See Ontario Ministry of Research and Innovation, http://www.mri.gov.on.ca/english/programs/oia/program.asp. The Québec government, in partnership with AstraZeneca, Pfizer Canada, and Merck Frosst, recently announced the creation of the Québec Consortium for Drug Discovery (CQDM) to stimulate pharmaceutical research and to foster synergy between university and industry research.

7. The federal government's "Advantage Canada" economic plan—dedicated to "creating the best-educated, most skilled, and most flexible workforce in the world" (http://www.fin.gc.ca/n06/06-069-eng.asp)—has increased funding for university-based research, and attracted and retained high-profile academics through funding Canada Research Chair positions (Association of Universities and Colleges of Canada, 2008; Canadian Institutes of Health Research, 2007; Lewkowicz & Schellenberg, 2006).

8. Association of Universities and Colleges of Canada, 2008.

9. Munro, 2004; Davey et al., 2004.

10. Kenny, 2003.

11. Kenny, 2004, p. 70.

12. "Universality: all citizens and permanent residents are covered. Accessibility: to 'medically necessary' hospital and doctor care. Comprehensiveness: a full package of healthcare services is provided. Portability: any Canadian requiring health care outside her or his home province is covered (at the provincial rate, not for full cost). Public administration: of a single payer, not-for-profit system" (ibid, p. 72).

the treatment of persons equally, taking in to account substantial differences) and solidarity (the obligation to respond to health need without consideration of the ability to pay). While Canada's commitment to universal access and public administration have been challenged on a number of fronts over the past thirty years,[13] Canadians remain fiercely proud of their healthcare system, and often cite it as a distinguishing feature of Canadian identity, especially in contrast to the two-tiered (and predominantly for-profit) health insurance system of the United States. Given that bioethics chiefly concerns itself with health care and health policy, bioethics in Canada may have more synergy with nationalist aspirations than in other countries.

In addition, Canadians most frequently (and passionately) refer to Canada's *moral* character as our most distinctive (and unifying) feature.[14] Canadians tend to position themselves ideologically between the communitarian ethics of European nations, and the individualism of the United States, which Canadians perceive as a "middle way" that is morally superior to both extremes. Canadians generally perceive their country as peaceful and peace-making,[15] progressive and tolerant of diversity, with a strong commitment to solidarity with all citizens, as expressed through general public support for "social safety nets" such as public education, public health, old-age pensions, employment insurance, and other social programs. While recent commentators have questioned Canada's claim to moral superiority over its neighbor to the south,[16] nevertheless, the emphasis on the *moral* character of Canada (as expressed in its public policies) remains a cornerstone of Canadian national identity. As a field that is substantively concerned with ethics and public morality/policy, we postulate that Canadian bioethics is significantly influenced in its discourses and practices by nationalism.

Methods

True to our Canadian character, we begin with a disclaimer, defining what this paper is *not*. It does not advocate for a particular vision of what bioethics in

13. For example, in the late 1980s, seven provinces attempted to introduce extra billing to patients to cover charges exceeding what the national health insurance system plan allowed (this ceased when the federal government stopped transfer payments to these provinces). As well, the CHA only covers physician and hospital services, making more people more reliant upon private health insurance for other necessary treatments, such as dentistry, long-term care, and medications.

14. Adams, 2003.

15. Canadian Prime Minister Lester B. Pearson is considered the father of the modern concept of peacekeeping, and won the Nobel Peace Prize in 1957.

16. Griffiths, 2008.

Canada should be or do; it is not prescriptive. It is not a comprehensive literature review of Canadian bioethics, or a history of bioethics in Canada,[17] or even a catalog of the most important bioethical issues in Canada.[18] Rather, this paper makes a unique contribution by exploring how questions of Canadian identity and national character are expressed in the discourses, practices, and products of Canadian bioethics. We argue that Canadian bioethics is strongly influenced by nationalist discourses, and that the Canadian bioethics community consciously engages in the project of nation-building. We build this argument through the analysis of several data sets.

First, a literature review was conducted using the search terms "bioethics" or "ethicist" *and* "Canada" or "Canadian."[19] One literature search was conducted in English, another in French, to capture literature in both official languages. Second, the archive of the Canadian Bioethics Society (CBS) was analyzed, with particular attention paid to the themes of CBS annual conferences, minutes of general meetings, taskforce reports, newsletters and strategic planning processes. Third, the websites of the major bioethics research centers in Canada were reviewed to identify relevant themes in their research, education, and outreach activities. These data sets were chosen because they represent the "public face" of bioethics in Canada.[20] They were analyzed with one key question in mind: *How do current discourses regarding Canadian nationalism (and perceived challenges to Canadian national identity) influence Canadian bioethics?*

This chapter constitutes a critical descriptive treatment of the national character of Canadian bioethics as a field, and as a community of practitioners and scholars. Our analysis is organized around three themes representing the major challenges to Canadian national identity in public discourse: (a) Canada's official commitment to multiculturalism and bilingualism, (b) regionalism, and (c) American cultural dominance. Because Canadian national identity is so ambiguous and contested (and usually begins with a description of what we are *not*), these challenges function as lenses enabling us to focus on the unique character of Canadian bioethics and its relationship to the project of nation-building.

---

17. Kenny, 2003.

18. Breslin et al., 2005.

19. The databases used for this literature search were Medline and the Philosopher's Index.

20. Each author took primary responsibility for gathering the data and conducting the initial analysis of a particular data set, which were then presented to and deliberated among all three authors.

National Identity and Canadian Bioethics

Diverse Ethics: Québec and Multiculturalism in Canadian Bioethics

Canada is one of the world's main immigrant-receiving nations; this fact, along with the recognition of the distinctive cultures of Canada's "two founding peoples" (British and French)[21] prompted the creation of a series of policies promoting bilingualism and multiculturalism starting in the 1970s. "Multiculturalism" is used in at least three senses in Canadian policies: to refer to a society that is characterized by ethnic or cultural heterogeneity; to refer to an ideal of equality and mutual respect among a population's ethnic or cultural groups; and to refer to specific government policies that support bilingualism and multiculturalism,[22] namely the Canadian Constitution (1982) and the Multicultural Act (1988). The Multicultural Act purports (among other goals): to support the freedom of Canadians to preserve their cultural heritage; to promote equitable participation in public life and equal protection under the law; and to foster the recognition and appreciation of the diverse cultures of Canadian society.

Criticisms of specific policies, as well as the philosophical and sociological premise of multiculturalism, have been leveled from both the right and left sides of the political spectrum, and from minority and majority ethnic groups alike. Multiculturalism has been particularly contentious in Québec, as these policies are perceived by some as a direct challenge to Québec's identity as a distinct society.[23] However, Canadians generally support the concept of tolerance of diversity as an expression of Canada's moral commitment to creating a peaceful and just society for all. Many also perceive multiculturalism as a distinctive cultural characteristic in comparison to the U.S. immigration policies, which promote assimilation to the dominant culture. Multiculturalism has significantly influenced the Canadian bioethics community, as demonstrated in recent attempts to recognize and support the distinctive cultural identities of Québécois and aboriginal peoples in bioethics practice and policy.

---

21. The notion of Canada's "two founding peoples" references the two colonial powers (France and England) that settled Canada and created the political infrastructure of this new nation. Canada's aboriginal peoples were largely marginalized in this political process; however, recently Canadians have begun to speak of "three founding peoples" to acknowledge the important economic and cultural contributions aboriginal peoples have made to this nation-building process.

22. See the Canadian Encyclopedia, "Muliculturalism," http://www.thecanadianencyclopedia.com/index.cfm?PgNm=TCE&Params=A1ARTA0005511.

23. In 2007, the Québec government created the Consultation Commission on Accommodation Practices Related to Cultural Differences, chaired by sociologist Gérard Bouchard and philosopher Charles Taylor, to examine how provincial policies can better reflect the secular, pluralistic reality of contemporary Québec. See Bouchard & Taylor, 2008.

Québec Nationalism and Bioethics

In Québec, bioethics is perceived as the child of American pluralist culture. As such, it has been embraced over the past 30 years to support Québec's transition to a secular society in the wake of the *révolution tranquille* (in English, "quiet revolution") of the 1960s, when the province rapidly transitioned from a traditional society to a modern, liberal democracy. Bioethics provided a new, open forum for discussing ethical questions arising in medicine and the biological sciences, debates that were previously dominated by Roman Catholic authorities.[24]

In preparing this chapter, the authors sought to articulate the specific contributions of Québécois bioethics to Canadian bioethics. We began with the question: "How is Québécois bioethics different from Anglo-Canadian bioethics?" In attempting to answer this question, BK undertook a review of Québécois bioethics literature. This inquiry revealed a somewhat distinctive philosophical genealogy in Québécois bioethics. For example, in a recent bioethics handbook published (in French) by Guy Durand,[25] the "standard" English and American philosophical traditions are cited, with additional references to continental philosophers (specifically the works of Ricoeur, Levinas, and Habermas). Québec intellectuals, reading in both English and French, tend to draw upon a wider range of philosophical influences from both Europe and North America. Nevertheless, the framing of most bioethical issues and debates does not appear to differ substantially between Québécois scholars and their Anglo-Canadian counterparts.

Instead, we discovered that the primary distinguishing feature of Québécois bioethics is its high degree of integration into governmental and health policy initiatives and institutions. Québécois people view Québec as a nation;[26] this view is not merely the vision of the separatist party, but is shared by all the parties in the province's *National* Assembly. As such, Québec politicians take seriously their constitutional (and moral) authority to develop provincial programs and regulations to serve the people of Québec.

The political latitude afforded to provinces under the Canadian constitution, combined with Québec's identity as a distinct society within Canada, have prompted the Québec government to address the societal and cultural challenges

---

24. Paradoxically, however, the leading pioneers of bioethics in Québec were Roman Catholic theologians (David Roy, Guy Durand, Hubert Doucet, and Guy Bourgeault).

25. Durand, 2005.

26. The metaphor of "two solitudes," commonly used to describe anglo-franco relationships in Canada, was popularized by John Hugh MacLennan's 1945 novel of the same title. The vision of Canada as the product of a pact between English and French founding peoples is constitutive of Québec's vision of the country. It gives legitimacy to Québec's claim to special status as a linguistic minority in North America, requiring special protection to ensure its cultural survival.

posed by emerging bioethical issues through the creation of several advisory committees and commissions, whose role is to deliberate ethical issues and generate policy recommendations. The role of the state in addressing and organizing debate regarding emerging societal issues, through consultative processes and legislative intervention, is also rooted in Québec's French legal tradition; while English Canada uses a common law system, Québec is the only province with a civil law system, known as the Civil Code.

For example, in 1998 Québec's *Ministère de la santé et des services sociaux* (Ministry of Health and Social Services) adopted a plan of action[27] for the regulation of research ethics, through a consultative process directed by Pierre Deschamps, a lawyer with ethics training.[28] The plan provides directives for the implementation of *Comités d'éthique de la recherche* (in English, "research ethics boards" or REBs) by virtue of Article 21 of the Civil Code of Québec. The plan authorizes REBs to approve and monitor research involving minors and incapable adults, and supports the Ethics Unit, whose mandate is policy development and implementation related to research ethics.[29] In addition, in 2001, the government of Québec created the Science and Technology Ethics Commission (CEST) as a forum for reflection and deliberation on major ethical issues raised by scientific and technological progress. Its task is not to provide answers to ethical questions but to promote discussion and public education, to foster reflection, and examine options as "a forum for the development and expression of collective choices." The CEST has published reports on topics such as nanotechnology, genetically modified organisms, and genetic databases.[30]

In 2005, Québec's government created a new entity, the Health and Welfare Commissioner,[31] whose mandate is to evaluate health and social services systems and provide the public with information regarding the government's plans to address issues and problems such as the use of medications and technology in

---

27. *Gouvernement du Québec, Ministère de la Santé et des Services sociaux, Plan d'action ministériel en éthique de la recherche et en intégrité scientifique. Direction générale de la planification et de l'évaluation.* http://ethique.msss.gouv.qc.ca/site/fr_pam.phtml.

28. *Gouvernement du Québec, Ministère de la Santé et des Services sociaux, Rapport final du Comité d'experts sur l'évaluation des mécanismes de contrôle en matière de recherche clinique au Québec* (Rapport Deschamps). http://ethique.msss.gouv.qc.ca/site/download.php?db8ed61de92e77ed49b5f93c94f95108.

29. Ibid.

30. For details, see: *Commission de l'éthique de la science et de la technologie, Gouvernement du Québec,* 2008, "Informing Reflecting Proposing. 2001–2007 Activity Report and Future Prospects," http://www.ethique.gouv.qc.ca/IMG/pdf_CEST2001-2007Activity-Web.pdf.

31. *Gouvernement du Québec, Commissaire à la santé et au bien-être,* http://www.csbe.gouv.qc.ca

health care.[32] To achieve this mandate, the Commissioner committed to extensive use of public and expert consultation.

Thus, while the authors don't find substantial differences between Québécois and Anglo bioethical debates in Canada, Québec is distinctive in its extensive use of state-sponsored consultative processes to address controversial issues and generate policy recommendations, and its integration of bioethics into health-related government agencies. Many Québécois bioethicists who were trained during and shortly after the Quiet Revolution serve on these commissions and consultative bodies. The pluralistic orientation of bioethics, in the context of the strong cultural motivation within Québec to shape its own destiny, has arguably enabled bioethics to be more influential in the formation of public policy than in any other Canadian province.

Aboriginal Issues in Canadian Bioethics

Canada continues to have a large and growing aboriginal[33] population, totaling over 1,100,000 in the 2006 census (roughly 3% of the population). However, aboriginal communities continue to bear the scars of colonialism, in spite of the official policies of multiculturalism and significant federal efforts to understand and respond to the needs of these communities.[34] In June 2008, Prime Minister Stephen Harper formally apologized in the House of Commons for the tragedy of the residential school system which systematically removed aboriginal children from the custody of their parents for education in publicly-funded boarding schools, often run by Christian organizations. The express purpose of this policy was cultural genocide: to "kill the Indian" inside these children, forcing them to assimilate the language, religion, and manners of the majority culture by removing them from their aboriginal communities. In addition to the psychological trauma this system inflicted on children and their families, these children were subjected to widespread physical, emotional, and sexual abuse. The scars of the residential school system,[35] as well as the failure of the Canadian government to uphold the conditions of their treaties with aboriginal peoples and improve the

---

32. An Act Respecting the Health and Welfare Commissioner. R.S.Q., chapter C-32.1.1, art. 2 http://www.canlii.org/en/qc/laws/stat/rsq-c-c-32.1.1/latest/rsq-c-c-32.1.1.html.

33. *Aboriginal* refers to the descendants of the original inhabitants of North America, including persons who identify themselves as North American Indian, Métis, and Inuit. (Indian and Northern Affairs Canada. "Terminology" http://www.ainc-inac.gc.ca/ap/tln-eng.asp).

34. These efforts include the Royal Commission on Aboriginal Peoples, which engaged in wide consultation with aboriginal communities across the country in the early 1990s, and the creation of Nunavut as a new territory in 1999, to preserve and protect its distinctive Inuit culture.

35. Castellano M., Archibald, L. & DeGagne, M., 2008.

living conditions on reservations, are frequently blamed for the significant social and health issues that plague the aboriginal population, described by many as a public health emergency as well as a national embarrassment.

The Canadian bioethics community's primary response to the plight of aboriginal peoples has been to support the creation of regulations governing research in aboriginal communities. The source of ethics standards governing research with human subjects in Canada is not legislation (as in the United States) but rather a policy established by three Canadian granting agencies that provide the majority of public funding for research. This policy is called the "Tri-Council Policy Statement: Ethical Conduct for Research Involving Humans" (TCPS, or "Tri-Council Policy").[36] The TCPS was originally promulgated in 1998 (after many years of wide consultation), and contains a specific section on research with aboriginal peoples. After years of further consultation, the 2010 revised 2nd edition of the TCPS has expanded the recognition and authority of aboriginal peoples in the research process.[37] In the spirit of multiculturalism, the policy recognizes a "distinct place" for aboriginal peoples in society and in the research sphere. The policy also recognizes the "parallel codes of ethics" of aboriginal communities in reviewing research, and accepts that research results and data belong both to the aboriginal community and the researchers, such that communities "consider that their review and approval of reports and academic publications is essential to validate findings."[38] While the response of the Canadian bioethics community to the public health crises faced by the aboriginal population has been disappointingly uneven, respect for the distinct moral codes of aboriginal communities (in the spirit of multiculturalism) is supported by Canadian research ethicists and policies.

Regional Bioethics: Fragmentation and Cohesion

A vast country, Canada's multiculturalism not only embraces the distinctive cultures of Québec, new immigrants, and aboriginal peoples, but also regional cultures—from the fishing villages of Newfoundland and Labrador, to the

36. Canadian Institutes of Health Research, Natural Sciences and Engineering Research Council of Canada, Social Sciences and Humanities Research Council of Canada, *Tri-Council Policy Statement: Ethical Conduct for Research Involving Humans, 2nd Edition,* 2010. Available at: http://www.pre.ethics.gc.ca/eng/policy-politique/initiatives/tcps2-eptc2/Default/.

37. Interagency Advisory Panel on Research Ethics, Aboriginal Research Ethics Initiative, http://www.pre.ethics.gc.ca/eng/archives/policy-politique/reports-rapports/arei-iera/; see also Canadian Institutes of Health Research, CIHR Guidelines for Health Research Involving Aboriginal People, May 2007, http://www.cihr-irsc.gc.ca/e/29134.html.

38. Ibid.

manufacturing heartland of Ontario, to the agrarian culture of Saskatchewan, to the Alberta oil patch and the mixed economy of mountainous British Columbia. The Canadian Bioethics Society (CBS) has struggled to meaningfully integrate multiculturalism, regionalism, and bilingualism into its practices and policies since its inception. Canadian bioethicists frequently articulate anxiety over the predominantly white membership of the CBS, and the paucity of minority voices at its annual meetings.[39] Nevertheless, throughout its history, the CBS has made conscious efforts to integrate diversity into its structures and practices. This is most obvious in the by-laws of the CBS, which include several provisions to ensure the inclusion of diverse regional and linguistic perspectives in the governance of the CBS:

- The CBS Executive must include members with both French and English language preferences.
- The Executive must include representatives from the various geographical regions of Canada—Atlantic, East (Québec), Central (Ontario), and West—with the addition of a Northern representative in June 2008.
- Executive membership must include diverse disciplines, including philosophy/theology, health law, medicine, nursing, and other health professions, as well as students.
- The presidency of the CBS must alternate between clinical and normative bioethicists, and between Francophone and Anglophone bioethicists.
- Annual meetings rotate among the four geographic areas.

In addition, the annual meetings must provide simultaneous translation in both official languages for all plenary sessions. Although this constitutes a significant financial burden, CBS members accept this cost out of a sense of solidarity, to honor the bilingual and multicultural character of the country, and to promote collaboration across the different regions.

Sleeping with an Elephant: Canadian and American Bioethics

Sharing a border and a language with the United States makes Canadians (feel) vulnerable to the overpowering influences of American popular culture, economic policies, and political moods.[40] Canadian bioethics has struggled since its inception to define its unique voice and contribution to the field, in part because

39. Roy, Williams, & Baylis, 2004.

40. Canadian Prime Minister Pierre Trudeau famously compared Canada's relations with the US to "sleeping with an elephant. No matter how friendly and even-tempered is the beast,

our neighbor to the south is globally recognized as the birthplace of bioethics, and currently produces the most bioethics research, publications, and leading practices. While Canadian and American bioethicists share many of the same research questions and are frequent collaborators, so ingrained in our national character is this comparative impulse that any reflection on Canadian bioethics always (consciously or unconsciously) entails comparison with American bioethics. In this section, we examine some features of Canadian bioethics that distinguish us from our U.S. counterparts: (1) the research agenda of bioethics centers in Canada; (2) the vision of the Canadian Bioethics Society; (3) Canada's collaborative approach to creating health policy; and (4) the Canadian bioethics community's leadership in defining the distinctive roles and responsibilities of bioethicists.

Canadian Bioethics Research Centers

Canada has a form of weak federalism, whereby the federal government devolves responsibility for many public services to the provinces and territories, including health care. Each province has its own distinct history, immigration patterns, and economic base, all of which influence its approach to public policy. Because the administration of health care is a provincial responsibility, and because many provinces over the past decade have devolved healthcare resource management and planning to regional authorities within provinces, health policy in Canada is becoming more local in nature.

As in Québec, bioethicists across the country are increasingly participating in the creation of health policy at the regional and local level, as key stakeholders or consultants. As Nuala Kenny writes, "Public policy is a manifestation of public values," a statement of identity and character.[41] Bioethics, she argues, has a significant role to play in public policymaking by virtue of its commitment to identifying the values and interests underlying options, and the field's capacity to reflect on the ends or goals of social institutions and the virtues they ought to embody.[42]

An analysis of the activities of major bioethics research centers supports the impression that one of the primary concerns of the Canadian bioethics community is to articulate and examine the ethical dimensions of health policies and

if I can call it that, one is affected by every twitch and grunt." (Speech to the National Press Club in Washington, DC, on March 25, 1969.)

41. Kenny, 2004, p. 67.

42. Ibid., p. 68.

health systems, at various levels of government.[43] Dalhousie is one institution that identifies health policy ethics as one of its key research areas, focusing on the importance of policy in setting the overarching principles that shape the experience of health care: "In Canada, health policy ethics is concerned specifically with the ethical foundations of Canadian medicine; justice and equity implications of health reform strategies; issues across the full continuum of health and health care; and the reform and revitalization of public health."[44]

To this end, CIHR has created a program in Health Law, Ethics & Policy to address the "acute shortage of experts in law, ethics and policy able to address significant health care challenges, such as measuring the effectiveness of regulation of private health insurance, assessing the impact of tort law on patient safety, and formulating ethical means to distribute scarce health care resources."[45] This program emphasizes the importance of maintaining the credibility and feasibility of Canada's health sector, by equipping the next generation of researchers and decision-makers to meet these ethical challenges.

The role of bioethics in the endeavor to articulate national values and advocate for the Canadian healthcare system is also evident in the University of Toronto's Joint Centre for Bioethics (JCB) Canadian Priority Setting Research Network (CPSRN): "The CPSRN's vision is to strengthen the Canadian health system by improving the politics and processes of healthcare priority setting and enhance research capacity in regard to priority setting."[46] This vision, and the associated research projects of the CPSRN, advance Canadian values such as collaboration and public consultation in setting public policy;[47] social justice,

43. ANF conducted this analysis by examining the websites of the major bioethics research centers across Canada, including: the Department of Bioethics at Dalhousie University; the Biomedical Ethics Unit at McGill University; the Joint Centre for Bioethics (JCB) at the University of Toronto; the John Dosseter Centre at the University of Alberta; and the W. Maurice Young Centre for Applied Ethics at the University of British Columbia (UBC). (Accessed between May 1 and July 22, 2008). This analysis focused on identifying relevant themes by examining the centers' (1) predominant research topics and questions, (2) annual reports, and (3) mission and vision statements.

44. Dalhousie University Faculty of Medicine, Health Policy Ethics, http://www.bioethics.medicine.dal.ca/research/healthpolicy.php.

45. CIHR Training Program in Health Law, Ethics & Policy, www.healthlawtraining.ca/About.asp. The affiliated institutions for this program include: Faculté de droit de l'Université de Sherbrooke, Faculty of Law, University of Alberta, Faculty of Law, University of Toronto and Schulich School of Law, Dalhousie University.

46. Canadian Priority Setting Research Network, http://www.utoronto.ca/cpsrn/html/home.html.

47. As in one CPSRN project: *Evaluating Interventions to Improve Priority Setting: Public Beliefs about Priority Setting Criteria,* which aims to describe the Canadian public's preferences for priority-setting criteria in the areas of patient type and services.

solidarity, and multiculturalism;[48] and the principles underlying the Canadian healthcare system.[49]

Finally, the role of the bioethics community in describing and reinforcing national values in health policy is evident in some recent GE³LS research projects (GE³LS=**G**enomics and **E**thical, **E**nvironmental, **E**conomic, **L**egal and **S**ocial issues), funded by Genome Canada and its various genome centers across the country. For example, one project out of UBC, entitled "Building a GE³LS Architecture," addresses three questions:

> What social norms do Canadians use to make judgments about genome research and applications (how do Canadians make moral decisions about a policy)? What are the leading moral perspectives on genomics (and what makes different judgments understandable)? And, finally, what is the relevance for policy development and implementation (how are worldviews and norms incorporated into policy)?[50]

Thus, while Canadian bioethicists and bioethics centers conduct research on a wide range of topics—including "traditional" bioethical issues, such as clinical decision making at the end of life, research ethics, consent and reproductive technologies—three of the major bioethics research centers in the country (UBC, the JCB, and Dalhousie) have specific research programs dedicated to health policy ethics. These programs and projects position bioethicists as crucial players in articulating national norms, in safeguarding the Canadian healthcare system through principled reform, in engaging in public consultation and including minority voices in health policy development, and in aligning our ambition to be competitive in the global innovation economy with fundamental Canadian values. In these research endeavors, bioethics is portrayed (in part) as a nation-building activity.

The Vision of the Canadian Bioethics Society

The Society for Health and Human Values (SHHV) pioneered bioethics collaboration in the United States from the late 1960s, and the Society for Bioethics Consultation (SBC) was created in the mid 1980s as a specific forum for those

---

48. As in another CPSRN project: *Exploring the Role of District Health Authorities and Community Health Boards: Attending to the Health Needs of African Nova Scotians.*

49. As in the CPSRN project : *Priority Setting and Health System Reform*, the goal of which is to examine three recent reports on health system reform in Canada (Mazenkowski, Kirby, & Romanow) and explore ways of strengthening the health system through improved priority setting.

50. Genome Canada, http://www.genomecanada.ca/en/portfolio/GE3LS.aspx.

working in clinical ethics. Canadian bioethicists participated in both of these societies; however, by the mid 1980s many recognized that the Canadian context gave rise to different issues and challenges, and that a distinctive forum was needed to deliberate Canadian bioethics.[51] Interestingly, Canadian bioethicists started out by forming (in exactly the same time and place) two separate societies (one for medical professionals and one for academic ethicists),[52] which quickly amalgamated in 1988.[53] *Collaboration* was the theme of the first two meetings of the new Canadian Bioethics Society (CBS), a theme that is present in many Canadian bioethical endeavors and that echoes national collaborative discourses and practices.[54] The amalgamation also prompted a change in vision, expanding from education and the professional exchange of ideas, to a more practically and politically oriented society to assist "in solving the problems of daily practice," and to "develop long-term solutions to broader social questions."[55]

The preoccupation with health policy and with social issues such as multiculturalism, social justice, and the influence of market forces on the Canadian healthcare system, is seen in many of the themes of CBS meetings over the past 20 years, including:

- Money, Power and People: Social Dimensions of Bioethics (1992)
- Ethical Choices, Economic Realities: the Health Care System in Flux (1994)
- Health Care in a Multicultural Society (1995)
- Deciding for Others: Power, Politics & Ethics (1996)
- Changing the System: Interprofessional and Interdisciplinary Approaches (1997)
- Money, Money, Money: Bioethic$ Confront$ Dollar$ & ene (2005)
- Just Evidence? (2009).

These themes reflect the unwavering commitment of the Canadian bioethics community to the principles of the Canada Health Act and to the shared vision

51. Lynch, 1998.

52. Keyserlingk, 1996; Kenny, 2003.

53. This amalgamation foreshadowed the union of the various societies in the United States (SSHV, SBC, American Association for Bioethics-AAB) ten years later, into the American Society for Bioethics and Humanities in 1998.

54. Kenny, 2002.

55. Lynch, 1998.

that one of the functions of the field is to advocate for a just, accessible, and equitable healthcare system as a crucial component of our national identity.[56]

In the mid 1990s, and again in 2007, the CBS went through a process of "re-visioning" to update the mission, vision, and strategic goals of the society. The 2007 consultation process resulted in the following vision statement for the CBS: "To be the leading bioethics collaborative forum in Canada working towards *advancing the health and well-being of people in Canada* and other countries" (emphasis added).[57] The mission statement also identifies one of the five strategic goals of the CBS as "public engagement and policy development around bioethics issues"[58] by promoting public consultation, and encouraging ethical reflection on existing health policies and the use of explicit ethical frameworks in the development of new health policies.[59] The CBS' current vision thus situates the bioethics community squarely within the project of nation-building.

"The Canadian Way" of Policymaking: The Development of DNR Orders

Throughout North America, the development of new technologies was (and is) a driving force behind the creation and expansion of the field of bioethics. After the development of cardiopulmonary resuscitation (CPR) in the late 1960s, many physicians felt they were legally obligated to provide CPR to everyone dying from any cause, regardless of their ability to benefit from CPR. In 1984,

---

56. This vision was evident in Nuala Kenny's acceptance speech for her Lifetime Achievement Award at the 2008 CBS meeting. Dr. Kenny's research has focused on Canadian health policy, and is founded on her deep personal commitments as a physician and ethicist to equity and public health. In her speech, she chastised the Canadian bioethics community for paying too much attention to technological innovation and individual clinical cases, and not enough to defending the fundamental principles of the Canadian healthcare system.

57. CBS Vision 2012: Strategic Plan at http://www.bioethics.ca/vision-ang.html. In contrast, the mission statement of the ASBH is more education- and research-focused: "The purpose of the ASBH is to promote the exchange of ideas and foster multidisciplinary, interdisciplinary, and interprofessional scholarship, research, teaching, policy development, professional development, and collegiality among people engaged in all of the endeavors related to clinical and academic bioethics and the health-related humanities." (American Society for Bioethics and Humanities, Purpose of the ASBH, http://www.asbh.org/about/purpose.html).

58. "*Our Mission:* The Canadian Bioethics Society (CBS) is a collaborative national member-driven organization that is committed to building bioethics capacity through the promotion of: 1) interdisciplinary and inter-professional networks of individuals (including students) and organizations; 2) excellence in bioethics education, research, & policy; 3) the advancement and dissemination of leading practices in bioethics; 4) the examination of professional issues in bioethics; 5) and public engagement and policy development around bioethics issues." (http://www.bioethics.ca/vision-ang.html).

59. This mission and vision stands in sharp contrast to that of the American Society for Bioethics and Humanities (ASBH), whose membership has refused to allow the ASBH to take any stand or advocate for any position of a substantive ethical or political nature, with the exception of issues directly related to academic freedom.

the Canadian Nurses Association, the Canadian Medical Association, and the Canadian Hospital Association, with input from the Catholic Hospital Association of Canada, the Law Reform Commission of Canada, and the Canadian Bar Association, met together to develop a "Joint Statement on Terminal Illness" which articulated the ethical rationale for not doing CPR in certain situations, and formulated a process for making decisions around CPR.[60] The insurance lawyers for physicians (the Canadian Medical Protective Association) endorsed this Joint Statement, arguing that it established DNR as a standard of practice that would now be defensible in court. This health policy innovation was done without resorting to the courts, or awaiting a legislative response, but rather through a consultative process with key stakeholders, resulting in a consensus on the issue. This represents a paradigmatic example (along with the Tri-Council Policy Statement) of how much of Canadian health policy is developed through collaborative dialogue and consensus-building outside of formal legislative or judicial bodies.

Creating an Identity for Canadian Bioethicists

Controversies around the roles of bioethicists and the professionalization of the field have given rise to a growing body of literature over the past two decades,[61] most notably the ASBH report, *Core Competencies for Health Care Ethics Consultation*,[62] which many now consider the professional standard for ethics consultation competencies. It is often forgotten, however, that much of the groundbreaking work that laid the foundation for this report was done in Canada and appeared in the 1994 book, edited by Françoise Baylis, entitled, *The Health Care Ethics Consultant*. The book resulted from a two-year collaborative dialogue between a number of ethicists (including one of the authors, MDC) representing diverse disciplines. The key chapter in that work is the "Profile of the Health Care Ethics Consultant."[63] This article describes (rather than defines) the clinical ethicist, creating a profile of the required knowledge, skills, and character traits. This prescient attention to the need to clearly articulate the identity of the ethics consultant might itself have arisen from the Canadian preoccupation with identity creation and articulation. The particular attention paid to the character traits

60. Canadian Medical Association, 1984.

61. For reviews, see especially Churchill, 1999; Agich, 2005; Dubler & Blustein, 2007; Scofield, 2008.

62. American Society for Bioethics and Humanities, 1998.

63. Baylis, 1994.

required in an ethics consultant[64] also reflects Canadians' perception of moral character as a defining feature of identity.[65]

This emphasis on moral character traits, especially integrity and courage, has created within the Canadian bioethics community an expectation that bioethicists have a duty to "speak truth to power." Some Canadian bioethicists have done so within their organizations, and as a consequence have lost their jobs or had their jobs threatened.[66] No current empirical data exists regarding the prevalence of bioethicists working in Canadian healthcare institutions on a contract basis (rather than occupying tenured academic positions).[67] However, it is the perception of the authors that this cohort of bioethicists has grown substantially over the past ten years, due in part to the ethics requirements of Accreditation Canada (the organization that accredits healthcare organizations). Recognizing the inherent vulnerability of these roles, the CBS established a working group to establish standards for working conditions for bioethicists. Over the past 15 years, the CBS has supported several projects intended to clarify the roles and obligations of bioethicists, and to develop structures for professional support, including:[68] a model code of ethics for bioethicists; a peer support network for members who feel vulnerable when speaking out on matters of conscience within their organizations;[69] a model role description for clinical ethicists (intended to clarify expectations during the hiring process); and an empirical study of experiences of conflicts of interest within the Canadian bioethics community.[70] These projects arise from (and reinforce) the Canadian preoccupation with questions of identity, and the centrality of moral character in the practice of Canadian bioethics.

---

64. Subsequent work by Benjamin Freedman and George Webster continued to highlight the moral character of the bioethicist. (Freedman, 1996; Webster & Baylis, 2000).

65. Interestingly, the emphasis on character was significantly diluted in the ASBH "Core Competencies," reflecting a more instrumental view of the role in the American context.

66. The potential for problems in this area had already been anticipated in Freedman, 1994.

67. The most recent study of this kind was carried out over 15 years ago; see Coughlin and Watts, 1994.

68. Canadian Bioethics Society, Publications, Working Conditions for Bioethics in Canada, http://www.bioethics.ca/publications-ang.html - The section on Working Conditions includes the "Draft Code of Ethics" and a "Model Role Description of the Bioethicist."

69. See also Freedman, 1996.

70. Frolic & Chidwick, 2010a and 2010b.

Conclusions and Reflections

During her dissertation research—an ethnographic study of the practices of clinical bioethicists in the United States and Canada—ANF discovered (to her surprise) that health policy and resource allocation were central preoccupations for Canadian clinical bioethicists, but not for American clinical bioethicists. Even when confronted with an individual patient situation, Canadian clinical bioethicists are keenly aware of the healthcare needs of the broader community, and the impact that individual treatment decisions (such as offering an ICU bed to a patient with little chance of recovery) can have on the whole system (such as the need to divert ambulances to another regional hospital if there are no ICU beds available to accept an incoming trauma victim). The Canadian bioethics community's commitment to the principles enshrined in the Canada Health Act, and to playing a visible role in public engagement and health policy development, makes Canadian bioethics a rich and multilayered field. However, the goal of advancing the public good can also prove to be a moral minefield, as bioethicists juggle competing obligations (to individual patients and to the healthcare system). In addition, our commitment to solidarity, public consultation, and consensus decision-making can curtail substantive debate about pressing policy issues, such as healthcare rationing and the goals of health care.

Similarly, another author (MDC) sees the Canadian bioethics community as striving for the "middle path," which he sees as a quintessentially Canadian trait. Rather than being driven by law and the assertion of individual rights, Canadians prefer to develop health policy through consultation, negotiation, and compromise. This commitment to inclusive decision-making processes undoubtedly stems from the relatively small population of the country, with its "small town" feel. This is particularly true in the Canadian bioethics community, which boasts only about 500 members (of the CBS). Almost everyone in the Canadian bioethics community knows everyone else. This intimacy can enable rapid and inclusive decision-making processes, but it can also result in "groupthink," hurt feelings, and ugly accusations from bioethicists who believe their colleagues are not living up to the vision of the field as the champion of social justice, the public good, and Canadian values.

One example of how the lofty goals and principles espoused by the Canadian bioethics community can backfire is seen in the CBS' commitment to bilingualism. One author (and former CBS executive member, BK) pointed out in his presidential addresses at two successive CBS meetings that Anglo bioethicists generally refuse to attend French panels and presentations, or to wear headsets to enable simultaneous translation during French plenary addresses, even if they don't understand French. The availability of simultaneous translation at its annual meeting is intended to enable the CBS to function as a fully bilingual (and thereby culturally inclusive) professional society (at great expense to the membership). However, the refusal of Anglo-Canadian bioethicists to avail themselves of this resource is perceived by some Québécois bioethicists as a *de facto* boycott of their presentations, and an indicator that Anglos believe Québécois research and innovations in bioethics are not of interest to the rest of the country. Thus, a tactic intended to facilitate multicultural engagement serves (unintentionally) to reinforce historical divisions between these two communities.

All the authors agree that the intertwining of nationalist discourses and the project of nation-building with the research agenda, discourses, and practices of Canadian bioethicists provides an interesting counterpoint to the "globalizing" or "homogenizing" effect that bioethics may have in other countries. We also recognize that this unique situation has both positive and negative dimensions. On the positive side, it opens the possibility (or mandate) to enable Canadian bioethicists to openly engage in the process of health policy development and system reform at various levels of government, thus expanding the traditional roles of bioethicists as educators, researchers, and clinical consultants. However, there is also a risk that Canadian bioethics could be hijacked by nationalist values and discourses, and lose its critical, reflective, and creative voice.[71] Nevertheless, the Canadian propensity to reflect on questions of identity and moral character has helped Canadian bioethics to make significant contributions to global bioethics, particularly in our groundbreaking work in defining the roles and ethical obligations of bioethicists as individuals and as emerging professionals.

Glossary

Aboriginal: Aboriginal refers to the descendants of the original inhabitants of North America, including persons who identify themselves as North American Indian, Métis and Inuit.

Anglo or Anglo-Canadian: English-speaking Canadian; often used to refer to those living in Canada outside of Québec.

Bilingual: In Canada, bilingual refers to speaking both English and French.

Bilingualism: A social policy that recognizes Canada's two official languages (English and French) and encourages use of both languages. While the federal government is officially bilingual, the only province that is officially bilingual is New Brunswick.

71. Given the distinctive regional cultures and policy environments across the country, a fruitful area for future research would be to examine the extent to which local cultures influence the analysis and articulation of bioethical issues and principles, within and between provinces.

Canadian: This term normally refers to any citizen of Canada; however, it is alternatively used by people in Québec to refer to English-speaking Canadians or to citizens of the "rest of Canada" (other provinces and territories).

Francophone: In Canada, this term refers to French-speaking Canadians both within and outside of Québec.

Ministry/Minister: The various major departments or sections of government and the elected head of that section.

Multiculturalism: Refers to a society that is characterized by ethnic or cultural heterogeneity; or to an ideal of equality and mutual respect among a population's ethnic or cultural groups; or to specific government policies that support bilingualism and multiculturalism.

Province (provincial): Provinces (similar to the states in the U.S.) have a defined jurisdictional autonomy from the federal government. The provinces are responsible for most of Canada's social programs (such as health care, education, and welfare). Using its spending powers, the federal government can initiate national policies in provincial areas, such as the Canada Health Act; the provinces can opt out of these, but rarely do so in practice. Equalization payments are made by the federal government to ensure that reasonably uniform standards of services and taxation are kept between the richer and poorer provinces. All provinces have elected legislatures headed by a Premier.

Québec: A province in east central Canada; it was settled by the French in 1608, ceded to the British in 1763, and became one of the original four provinces in the Dominion of Canada in 1867. Québec is also the name of this province's capital city.

Québécois: Used to denote French-speaking residents of the province of Québec, usually descendants of French colonists.

Québecer or Québecker: In English, used to denote any resident of Québec, of any origin or language preference, including French, English, and Aboriginal residents, as well as allophones (persons, usually recent immigrants, whose mother tongue is neither French nor English).

Research Ethics Board (REB): This is the Canadian equivalent of the IRB (Institutional Review Board) in the United States, or IEC (Independent Ethics Committee) in Europe, charged with reviewing and approving research studies, with the aim of protecting research subjects.

Reserve/Reservation: An area of land set aside for the use of a specific group of Aboriginal people.

TCPS (Tri-Council Policy Statement: Ethical Conduct for Research Involving Humans): This policy statement is the primary national document that defines the roles and ethical obligations of researchers and REBs in Canada.

Territory: A region of Canada which has not been admitted as a province and which is governed by a federally appointed commissioner and an elected legislative assembly. There are three territories: Yukon, Northwest Territories and Nunavut.

References

Adams, M. (2003). *Fire and Ice: The United States, Canada and the Myth of Converging Values*. Toronto: Penguin.

Agich, George J. (2005). What kind of doing is clinical ethics? *Theoretical Medicine and Bioethics 26,* (1): 7–24.

American Society for Bioethics and Humanities. (1998). *Core Competencies for Health Care Ethics Consultation*. Glenwood, Illinois: ASBH.

American Society for Bioethics and Humanities. *Purpose of the ASBH*. Available at: http://www.asbh.org/about/purpose.html (Accessed July 22, 2008).

Association of Universities and Colleges of Canada (2008). *Momentum: The 2008 report on university research and knowledge mobilization*. Available at: http://www.aucc.ca/_pdf/english/publications/momentum-2008-primer.pdf.

Baylis, F.E. (1994). The Profile of the Ethics Consultant. In Baylis (ed.). *The Health Care Ethics Consultant*. New Jersey: Humana Press.

Bouchard, G., & Taylor, C. (2008). Commission de consultation sur les pratiques d'accommodement reliées aux différences culturelle. Building the Future. A Time for Reconciliation, Abridged Report. Québec.

Breslin, J.M., MacRae, S.K., Bell, J., Singer, P.A., and the University of Toronto Joint Centre for Bioethics Clinical Ethics Group. (2005). Top 10 health care ethics challenges facing the public: views of Toronto bioethicists. *BMC Medical Ethics 6*:5. Available at: http://www.biomedcentral.com/1472-6939/6/5.

Canadian Bioethics Society, Publications, Working Conditions for Bioethics in Canada. Available at: http://www.bioethics.ca/publications-ang.html (Accessed July 18, 2008).

Canadian Encyclopedia. "Muliculturalism." Available at: http://www.thecanadianencyclopedia.com/index.cfm?PgNm=TCE&Params=A1ARTA0005511 (accessed July 19, 2008).

Canadian Hospital Association, Canadian Medical Association and Canadian Nurses Association. (1984). Joint statement on terminal illness: a protocol for health professionals regarding resuscitative intervention for the terminally ill. *Can Med Assoc J 130*:1357.

Canadian Institutes of Health Research. (2007). CIHR Guidelines for Health Research Involving Aboriginal People. Available at: http://www.cihr-irsc.gc.ca/e/29134.html (Accessed February 23, 2011).

Canadian Institutes of Health Research, Natural Sciences and Engineering Research Council of Canada, Social Sciences and Humanities Research Council of Canada. (2010). *Tri-Council Policy Statement: Ethical Conduct for Research Involving Humans, 2nd Edition*, 2010. Available at: http://www.pre.ethics.gc.ca/eng/policy-politique/initiatives/tcps2-eptc2/Default/ (Accessed February 23, 2011).

Canadian Priority Setting Research Network, http://www.utoronto.ca/cpsrn/html/home.html (Accessed February 23, 2011).

Castellano M., Archibald, L. & DeGagne, M. (2008). *From Truth to Reconciliation: Transforming the Legacy of Residential Schools.* Ottawa: Aboriginal Healing Foundation.

Churchill, L.R. (1999). Are we professionals? A critical look at the social role of bioethicists. *Daedalus 128*(4): 253–274.

Coughlin, M., & Watts, J. (1994). What Does a Health Care Ethics Consultant Look Like? Results of a Canadian Survey. In *The Health Care Ethics Consultant* (F. Baylis, ed.). New Jersey: Humana Press.

Dalhousie University Faculty of Medicine, Health Policy Ethics, http://www.bioethics.medicine.dal.ca/research/healthpolicy.php (accessed July 21, 2008).

Davey, K., McGillivray, B., & Carpentier, R. (2004). Protecting human research participants in Canada. *Royal College Outlook 1*(2): 21–23.

Dubler, N.N., & Blustein, J. (2007). Credentialing Ethics Consultants: An Invitation to Collaboration. *The American Journal of Bioethics 7*(2): 35–37.

Durand, G. (2005). *Introduction générale à la bioéthique - histoire, concepts et outils*, 2nd ed. Montréal: Fides.

Engelhardt Jr., H.T. (2003). Introduction: Bioethics as a Global Phenomenon. In: Peppin, J., & Cherry, M. (eds.). *Annals of Bioethics*, Vol. 1, Regional Perspectives. Lisse: SWETS & Zeitlinger.

Freedman, B. (1994). From Avocation to Vocation: Working conditions for clinical health care ethics consultants. In *The Health Care Ethics Consultant* (Ed. F. Baylis), 109–132. New Jersey: Humana Press.

Freedman, B. (1996). "Where are the Heroes of Bioethics?" *J Clinical Ethics 7*(4): 297–299.

Frolic, A. & Chidwick, P. (2010a). "A Pilot Qualitative Study of 'Conflicts of Interests and/or Conflicting Interests' Among Canadian Bioethicists. Part 1: Five Cases, Experiences and Lessons Learned." *HEC Forum* 22: 5–17.

Frolic, A. & Chidwick, P. (2010b). "A Pilot Qualitative Study of 'Conflicts of Interests and/or Conflicting Interests' Among Canadian Bioethicists. Part 2: Defining and Managing Conflicts." *HEC Forum* 22: 19–29.

Genome Canada, http://www.genomecanada.ca/en/portfolio/GE3LS.aspx (accessed July 21, 2008).

Gouvernement du Québec. Ministère de la Santé, des Services sociaux. Juin 1998. Plan d'action ministériel en éthique de la recherche et en intégrité scientifique. Direction générale de la planification et de l'évaluation. http://ethique.msss.gouv.qc.ca/site/fr_pam.phtml (Accessed July 2, 2008).

Gouvernement du Québec, Ministère de la Santé, des Services sociaux, Rapport final du Comité d'experts sur l'évaluation des mécanismes de contrôle en matière de recherche clinique au Québec (Rapport Deschamps). http://ethique.msss.gouv.qc.ca/site/download.php?db8ed61de92e77ed49b5f93c94f95108 (Accessed July 2, 2008).

Gouvernement du Québec. Ministère de la Santé, des Services sociaux, Avril 2008, Unité d'éthique, mecanisme multicentrique, http://ethique.msss.gouv.qc.ca/site/fr_mecanismemulticentrique.phtml (Accessed July 2, 2008).

Gouvernement du Québec, Commission de l'éthique de la science, de la technologie, 2008, Informing Reflecting Proposing. 2001–2007 Activity Report and Future Prospects, http://www.ethique.gouv.qc.ca/IMG/pdf_CEST2001-2007Activity-Web.pdf (Accessed July 2, 2008).

Government of Québec, Public Health Act, R.S.Q., chapter S-2.2, http://www2.publicationsduquebec.gouv.qc.ca/dynamicSearch/telecharge.php?type=2&file=/S_2_2/S2_2_A.html (Accessed July 2, 2008).

Gouvernement du Québec, Commissaire à la santé, au bien-être, http://www.csbe.gouv.qc.ca (Accessed July 2, 2008).

Griffiths, R. (2008). *American Myths: What Canadians Think They Know About the United States*. Toronto : Key Porter Books.

Indian and Northern Affairs Canada, "Terminology" http://www.ainc-inac.gc.ca/pr/info/tln_e.html (Accessed July 18, 2008).

Interagency Advisory Panel on Research Ethics, Aboriginal Research Ethics Initiative, http://www.pre.ethics.gc.ca/eng/resources-ressources/reports-rapports/arei-iera/ (Accessed July 18, 2008).

Kenny, N.P. (2002). *What Good is Health Care? Reflections on the Canadian Experience*. Ottawa: Canadian Health Association Press.

Kenny, N.P. (2003). Bioethics in Canada. In: Peppin J, Cherry M (eds.). *Annals of Bioethics*, Vol. 1, Regional Perspectives, pp. 3–20. Lisse: SWETS & Zeitlinger.

Kenny, N.P. (2004). The Continental Divide: A Modest Comparison of American and Canadian Values in Healthcare. *Organizational Ethics: Healthcare, Business, and Policy*, *1*(2): 65–80.

Keyserlingk, E.W. (1996) The Birth of the Canadian Bioethics Society (CBS). *Canadian Bioethics Society Newsletter*, *1*(2): 12–June 13, 1996.

Lewkowicz, A., & Schellenberg, P. (2006). Research Chairs: A Systematic Change in Ontario's Universities. *COU Colleagues Working Paper Series* 5(3): 18–23.

Lynch, A. (1998). Canadian Bioethics Society: Time for "Back to the Future." *Canadian Bioethics Society Newsletter*, v.3 (2): October 7, 1998.

MacLennan, J.H. (1945). *Two Solitudes*. Toronto: Collins.

McQuaig, L. (1998). *The Cult of Impotence*. Toronto: Penguin Books.

Munro, M. (2004). The privacy myth: One in 20 Canadians take part in a secretive industry that cries out for oversight, experts say. *National Post*, February 23, A13.

Ontario Ministry of Research and Innovation, Ontario Innovation Agenda, (http://www.mri.gov.on.ca/english/programs/oia/program.asp. (Accessed July 18, 2008).

Canada's New Government Releases Advantage Canada, An Economic Plan to Eliminate Canada's Net Debt and Further Reduce Taxes. (2006). http://www.fin.gc.ca/n06/06-069-eng.asphtml.

Roy, D., Williams, J., & Baylis, F. (2004). Canada. In *Encyclopedia of Bioethics*. 3rd edition. Stephen G. Post (ed.) Vol 3. New York: Macmillan, 1540–1547.

Scofield, G. (2008). What is Medical Ethics Consultation? *J. Law, Medicine & Ethics* 36(1) (Spring 2008): 95–118.

Webster, G., & Baylis, F. (2000). Moral Residue In *Margin of Error* (Susan B. Rubin and Laurie Zoloth, eds.), 217–230. Hagerstown, MD: University Publishing.

13 NEGOTIATING ISLAMIC IDENTITY IN EGYPT THROUGH BIOETHICS

CONTESTING "THE WEST" AND SAUDI ARABIA

Thomas Eich and Björn Bentlage

Introduction

A North African country with a population of approximately 70 million, Egypt is the most populous country in the Middle East/ North Africa region. The population is growing at a rapid 2% per annum, and the religious breakdown is roughly 90% Sunni Muslim, with the remaining 10% predominately Christian. In recent decades, Egypt's economy has suffered from large deficits. A high inflation rate posed enormous challenges in the 1980s and 1990s, but has more recently been on significant decline. Offically, Egypt is a presidential democracy. The country has been led by military officers since the 23rd of July revolution in 1952, with president Hosni Mubarak holding office from 1981 until 2011. Parliamentary elections are routinely criticized by opposition political forces, as well as by international organizations, for being illiberal and unfair. Still, Egypt's multiparty parliament is far from a mere puppet in the president's hands. Paired with an increasingly important modern mass media, parliamentary plurality placed constraints on Mubarak's political power. Therefore, it had become increasingly important for Mubarak to present his political decisions as *legitimate* to Egypt's large population. Although socialist/secularist ideologies have heavily influenced the military government since the 1952 revolution, governments have swayed back and forth between attempts to exert control over religious life via funding, appointment, cooptation, and nationalization of its institutions, and granting influence and independence in return for legitimization. Egypt's legal system is based on the *šarīʿa*, as declared by an amendment to the constitution in 1981. The conformity of laws to the *šarīʿa* is usually certified by the leading religious institutions, and mosques and the al-Azhar's religious education system play a determinant role in social life.[1]

We will show that bioethics functions as *the* place for Egyptians to freely negotiate their values and vision of Egyptian society.[2] It is true that other issues, such as the recent constitutional changes—most likely intended to prepare the transferral of the presidential office from Hosni Mubarak to his son, Gamal—are also fervently contested by Egypt's public. However, until recently, issues directly related to Mubarak's position and power cannot really be discussed freely as a means of negotiating and *shaping* Egyptian identity.

First, we will briefly characterize the key actors in the field of Egyptian bioethics (without any claim to completeness, of course). In the second part, we present two case studies to show how institutions and individuals interact. These cases are public debates about medical personnel wearing face veils (*niqāb*) and female genital mutilation (FGM). These cases are not meant to represent bioethics in Egypt as a whole. Bioethics as a discipline in its own right is just beginning to emerge in Egypt. As in many other Muslim-majority countries, bioethics is largely considered a branch of the ethical reasoning inherent to Islamic law. Hence, Egyptian bioethics effectively "functions" by treating individual issues in order to identify specific rules, rather than "developing independent reflection with respect to the clinical decision-making phase."[3] Therefore, we have chosen to present some of the most recent and public debates relating to bioethics at large, in order to illustrate the many possible ways in which the key actors of Egyptian bioethics interact. The fact that they both relate to sexuality, and the role of women in society, certainly limits the scope of observations we were able to make in this article. However, we think that this common link appears to be an important point in the current development that ought not to be neglected.[4]

We will argue that the social functions of bioethics in Egypt, by and large, provide powerful symbols in public debates to negotiate what it means

---

1. Moustafa, 2000.

2. Many bioethical discussions in the Middle East are similar to debates in Europe and the United States, because certain assumptions and concepts questioned by scientific and medical developments are common to both regions, as can be seen in the debates about the brain death criteria for example. Other discussions clearly differ because they arise particularly from concepts, beliefs, or regulations in the Islamic faith—whether Muslims may receive organs transplanted from a non-Muslim, for instance—or from developments and factors special to the regional or national history, like the importance of prenatal diagnosis due to a relatively high percentage of marriage among relatives.

3. Atighetchi, 2007: 19.

4. There are other currently hotly debated issues in Egyptian bioethics, such as the government's plans to reform the health insurance system, or organ transplantation, which are not genuinely linked to gender issues.

(or should mean) to be Egyptian today. As we will show, Egyptians' reactions to these changes do not create a binary paradigm of secularism or even laicism versus a religiously oriented society. Alternatively, it is largely agreed upon that the fundamental referential framework for defining Egyptian identity is Islam. Therefore, Egyptians do not negotiate "how Islamic do we want to be?" but rather "in any given situation, what does it mean to act as a good Muslim?"

The Actors

Government Religious Actors

Ministry of Religious Endowments *(wizārat al-awqāf)*

The Ministry of Religious Endowments (*awqāf*) is the state's most important instrument to centralize authority over the religious sector. The Ministry channels state funding, and is involved in licensing and appointing preachers and deciding the topics to be covered in state-controlled mosques.[5] The current minister of *awqāf* is Dr. Maḥmūd Ḥamdī Zaqzūq (often also rendered as Zakzouk). He is a multilingual theologian and philosopher by training, holding a PhD in philosophy from the University of Munich.

National Fatwa Office (*dār al-iftā'*)

The *dār al-iftā'*, the office of the Grand Muftī, is Egypt's principal institution for the issuance of religious expertise, or *fatwās*. Appointed by the *wizārat al-awqāf*, the Grand Muftī is routinely addressed by the government to establish conformity of laws, regulations, or public policies to the *šarīʿa*. The current Muftī, Dr. ʿAlī Ǧumaʿa has held office since September 2003. Unlike many religious scholars at al-Azhar, Ǧumaʿa didn't initially devote himself to Islamic studies, but rather began his religious scholarship only after receiving a BA degree in commerce. In polemics against him, this is often used as a pretext to question his competence on issues of Islamic law.[6] Both he and his predecessor in office, the recently deceased Šayḫ al-Azhar Muḥammad Sayyid Ṭanṭāwī, are often criticized for serving the government's interests too freely.[7]

5. After a wave of nationalization under President Mubarak, 71% of Egypt's mosques were state-owned by 1994. Moustafa: 2000

6. *Rūz al-Yūsif*, 2007/06/16 (No. 4123)c.

7. *al-maṣrī l-yawm* 2007/05/16a; 2007/07/07a; 2007/07/11b; and 2007/10/19; *al-iḫwān al-muslimūn*: 2008/08/011.

al-Azhar

Al-Azhar today stands for an entire religious education system, from kindergarten to universities all over Egypt, encompassing subjects from theology to medicine and engineering. The al-Azhar university is praised as arguably the most prestigious institute of Islamic scholarship in the world.

Since 1952, the state has made increasing efforts to control and subdue al-Azhar, culminating in a 1961 law which put al-Azhar under direct government regulation. It now stands under the jurisdiction of the Ministry of *awqāf*, and its highest ranking religious scholar is the appointed Šayḫ al-Azhar. While al-Azhar has lost independence and legitimacy with the people, it gained access to more government funding, allowing the institution to extend its role in society. In 1996, President Mubarak appointed the pro-government Muḥammad Sayyid Ṭanṭāwī as Šayḫ al-Azhar, a move leading to tensions with the state and within al-Azhar.[8] In 2010, after Ṭanṭāwī died unexpectedly, Aḥmad al-Ṭayyib followed him in office. Like the Grand Muftī, the Šayḫ al-Azhar is often asked by the government for expertise regarding legislation and public issues.

The *maǧmaʿ al-buḥūṯ al-islāmiyya*

Al-Azhar's Council for Islamic Studies, the *maǧmaʿ al-buḥūṯ al-islāmiyya*, is directed by the Šayḫ al-Azhar and is largely composed of Egyptian Islamic scholars. Legally, the *maǧmaʿ* is the binding authority in all questions regarding Islamic dogma, and has a loosely defined obligation to watch over public discourse, which can, and has, bordered on censorship.

New members to the *maǧmaʿ* must be nominated for election by at least one member of the *maǧmaʿ* and receive a majority of votes from its members. Only the Šayḫ al-Azhar and the Grand Muftī are members qua office.[9] According to the Azhar law of 1961, members must hold a diploma from al-Azhar.[10]

The relations between these religious institutions are not always cordial. The appointed Grand Muftī and the Šayḫ al-Azhar have both criticized each other on several issues, and the *maǧmaʿ* sometimes openly opposes the two other institutions.[11] In January 2007, it claimed for itself the exclusive right to criticize *fatwās* by the *dār al-iftāʾ* and tried to set rules for issuing *fatwās* in the media.[12] Since the

---

8. Moustafa: 2000; Kienle: 2000: 113f.

9. *Rūz al-Yūsif*, 2007/06/16 (No. 4123)a; *Rūz al-Yūsif*, 2007/06/16 (No. 4123)c, where it is also claimed that the election process is manipulated at times.

10. Skovgaard-Petersen: 1997: 187.

11. *al-maṣrī l-yawm*: 2007/12/20

12. *al-maṣrī l-yawm*: 2007/02/21.

Šayḫ al-Azhar heads the *maǧmaʿ*, of which the Grand Muftī is only an "ordinary" member, the position of the Šayḫ al-Azhar in the religious hierarchy of Egypt has to be viewed as higher than the Grand Muftī's. This is also accounted for in official protocol, where the Šayḫ al-Azhar is in the ranks of ministers, whereas the Muftī—since he is essentially working *for* a ministry—is ranked below that.[13]

Nongovernment Religious Actors

These are primarily individual actors whose influence stems mainly from their use of modern mass media. A prominent example in Egypt is Dr. Suʿād Ṣāliḥ, former dean of the women's branch of the faculty for Islamic studies at al-Azhar. Dr. Ṣāliḥ is one of the few female religious scholars who appear regularly in the mass media, and is usually consulted on questions involving religion and women. She has made repeated attempts at proposing organizational reforms in the largely male-dominated religious establishment of the country.[14]

Ṣāliḥ is part of a larger trend, present since the 1980s, in which non-state religious scholars have by and large marginalized the state *ʿulamāʾ* in the Egyptian mass media.[15] One example is the relatively new and extremely popular TV channel, al-Nās ("The People," shut down in late 2010), which features non-state scholars with obvious links to Saudi Arabia exclusively offering religious advice and guidance. In addition, telephone *fatwā*-enterprises, which offer religious consultation over the phone within 24 hours of request, are now a growing industry. The result is an increasing number of contradictory *fatwās*, which all claim to be authoritative.[16]

Another type of individual nongovernment religious actor is the member of parliament Yūsuf Badrī, a religious scholar with Islamist leanings. Badrī campaigns

---

13. *Rūz al-Yūsif*, 2007/06/16 (No. 4123) a; *Rūz al-Yūsif*, 2007/06/16 (No. 4123) c.

14. For example, she tried to get elected as first female member of the *maǧmaʿ*. See *Rūz al-Yūsif*, 2007/06/16 (No. 4123)c.

15. It has to be reiterated that Suʿād Ṣāliḥ, as a female religious scholar, is really exceptional in this context. The overwhelming majority of independent preachers and scholars are male, like the late Šayḫ ʿAbd al-Ḥamid Kišk (having died 1996, his influence rested largely on audiotapes), ʿAmr Ḫālid and Yūsuf al-Qaraḍāwī (only the latter is a religious scholar by training, and both have extremely popular TV shows).

16. *al-Aḥrār*, 2007/02/26; *al-maṣrī l-yawm*: 2007/02/07 and 02/21; *aš-šarq al-awsaṭ*: 2007/05/25; *al-ǧazīra*: 2006/05/31; *Rūz al-Yūsif*, 2007/06/16 (No. 4123)b. The repeated emphasis of the *maǧmaʿ* on its role as the highest religious institution of the country and its attempts to establish itself and the *dār al-iftāʾ* as the only *fatwā* bodies in Egypt must be interpreted within this context.

for his cause mainly by means of litigation against institutions and individuals on issues pertaining to public mores and Islam.[17]

Government Nonreligious Actors

Founded in 1988, the National Council for Children and Motherhood (NCCM) is composed of several ministers, an advisory committee of experts, prominent public figures, and the office of the general secretary. Its decisions are binding for all ministries and institutions of state in matters related to motherhood and the welfare of children. The Council aims to lay out a national plan in order to achieve the goals set by international conventions on children's rights, and is also obliged to prepare for all international conferences in this respect.[18]

In bioethical discussions involving medical issues, the Ministry of Health and Population (MOHP) is the most important state actor. Directly administrating state clinics, the MOHP watches over the quality of treatment generally, and can immediately influence the entire health sector with executive decrees. In addition, the MOHP is responsible for family planning and related services, frequently cooperating with the NCCM, of which the MOHP minister himself is a member, and is involved in international conferences.[19]

Not a state actor in the strict sense, but an intermediate, is the doctors' syndicate. In line with the nature of Egyptian corporatism, the doctors' syndicate is as much a tool to control the medical sector as it is a functionary for members to communicate and even enforce their interests. The syndicate is to be consulted in all legislation involving the medical sector, and represents its members vis-a-vis the state. It also watches over professional regulations, has provided binding ethical guidelines, and has the legal capacity to take disciplinary action against its members that can lead to an effective employment ban.

The syndicate, just like medical faculties and individual doctors, may play an important role in debates as a source of both expertise and moral authoritiy. In the case studies given in this article, however, they hardly play a role on the debate level. Nevertheless, one should bear in mind that actual, practical decision making

17. *Al-Ahram Weekly Online*: 2006/04/13; *islamonline*: 2006/11/17; *islamonline*: 2007/08/8.

18. NCCM 2005a-c; *Al-Ahram Weekly Online*: 1998/11/19.

19. MOHP 2007; *al-maṣrī l-yawm*: 2006, February 18; 2007/07/2; Huntington: 2003.

and ethical reasoning is often bestowed upon doctors and medical faculties by both legislators and by religious experts.[20]

Non-Egyptian Actors

Egypt is regarded a key state for the MENA region. Because the government is conscious of its dependency on good international relations, Egypt has become the field for activities of a vast variety of local and international NGOs. According to Law no. 83, of 2002, all the 16,000 NGOs active in the country must register with the Ministry of Social Affairs and secure its permission for foreign funding.[21] In context with international agreements, the state works alongside NGOs willingly, as long as its immediate political interests are not harmed, and the NGOs' activities steer clear of the most divisive issues. NGOs are often attacked for serving a foreign agenda.[22]

The same holds true for the government, which, as legislation shows time and again, strives to implement provisions directly inspired by international agreements. This occurs despite the fact that Egyptian public debates often follow patterns of argument different and at odds with the secular rhetoric of international conferences. Egypt routinely cooperates with organizations of the United Nations and hosts several regional and cluster offices in Cairo. It established a National Bioethics Committee in accordance with the UNESCO's bioethics program, and the first regional meeting of national bioethics committees was held in Cairo in May of 2007.[23]

The Media

Despite the autocratic nature of the country's political regime, the Egyptian media enjoys a high degree of freedom and independence. While state-owned

20. See, for example, Hamdy: 2006: 268–316. Much the same can be said about the International Islamic Center for Population Studies, situated at Azhar University and headed by Gamal I. Serour, a gynecologist. The Center regularly arranges conferences on (bio)ethical issues, and serves as a communication platform between religious scholars and scientists.

21. *Al-Ahram Weekly Online*: 2003/06/12; *baheyya*: 2005/09/3.

22. Walker: 2004; *al-maṣrī l-yawm*: 2006/11/21; *Al-Ahram Weekly Online*: 2003/06/26; Ercevik Amado: 2004; *al-iḫwān al-muslimūn*: 2003/11/7; 2007/07/11 and /08/21; 2008/02/25 and March 26.

23. To the best of our knowledge, the Egyptian National Bioethics Committee does not play a significant role in the public debates about bioethical issues.

newspapers and TV channels[24] may still be predominant, the advent of each new technology (cheap audiotapes, satellite TV, the Internet) has led to further media diversification, with which the state's formerly strict censorship program could not keep up. In an age of Internet and widely available international satellite programs in Arabic language, censorship on the national level seems out of date. Nevertheless, transnational players have not diminished the role of Egyptian local media. The number of local and national newspapers has risen to over 500, due to partial liberalization since the 1980s, the majority of which are independent. Even relatively small papers have displayed a capacity to trigger national debates.[25] Egypt's movie industry and print media market remain the largest players in the Arab world, widely consumed at home and abroad. With regard to public discussions, and even political consequences, the art and entertainment sectors play a role no less important than producers and presenters of hard news, especially when it comes to hot topics that border on the taboo.[26]

The Cases

The following two short case studies illustrate the interactions of the described actors. We aim to show how bioethical debates in Egypt have to be situated in their wider sociopolitical context, in order to grasp their deeper implications that turn them into loci of negotiating Egyptian identity at large. The first case study can be seen as the result of a friction between different orientations of and in Egyptian society, namely toward international and scientific standards on one side, and notions labeled "Islamic" and often identified with a Saudi Arabian influence on the other.

The Niqāb Debate

The *niqāb* is a veil, either covering the face beneath the eyes or the whole face, usually worn by women. It is generally combined with a head scarf (*ḫimār*

24. As of 2008 there were two national and six regional channels owned by the state; the same holds true for the country`s biggest newspapers, news agency and radio stations, BBC News 2008/04/18.

25. Pintak: 2007; Lynch: 2007.

26. For example the seemingly non-issue (*Al-Ahram Weekly Online*: 2007/1018; *al-maṣrī l-yawm*: 2005/12/05) of abortion that was taken up by at least three major cinema productions in 2006 (*al-maṣrī l-yawm*: 2006/07/12; *Al-Ahram Weekly Online*: 2006/02/22 and /06/29) and a Ramadan series in 2007, setting off a heated discussion among religious scholars and probably leading soon to the first major legal change regarding abortion since 1937 (*al-maṣrī l-yawm*: 2007/10/11 and 2008/02/01; *al-iḫwān al-muslimūn*: 2007/12/31).

or *ḥiǧāb*) to cover the hair, and sometimes gloves, in order to cover every part of the body in public.

In November 2007, the Egyptian magazine *Rūz al-Yūsif* published several articles (Edition 4144, November 16, 2007) documenting the increasing trend among nurses to wear the *niqāb* during their working hours in hospitals, which was criticized for several reasons.[27] The basic problem of the whole situation would be that no official document whatsoever explicitly regulated and defined the nurses' dress code. This made it impossible to forbid the niqāb (p. 24).[28] In this context, several nurses and medical doctors were cited, terming the *niqāb* a question of personal freedom (pp. 19, 24f). Against this, authors of *Rūz al-Yūsif* reiterated that hospital personnel had to conform to global standards of their profession. Consequently, the *niqāb* was not a question of personal freedom in this context (pp. 17, 27f). This last opinion was also stated in a short article describing the Muftī ʿAlī Ǧumaʿa's stance on the issue, who added that the detailed regulations had to be spelled out by the organizations of the respective professions (p.29).

This *Rūz al-Yūsif* issue provoked public debate in other forms of media, and the MOHP promised to issue a decree by 2008.[29] In addition, *Rūz al-Yūsif* devoted several lengthy articles to the issue in the following weeks. In early 2008, a decree standardizing dress code for medical personnel and prohibiting the *niqāb* was announced, to be put into effect by June of the same year.[30]

The Background

The *niqāb* is considered by those endorsing it, as well as those opposing it, as a kind of "religiously loaded part of a woman's way of dressing."[31] The difference

27. For the different points, such as security and hygiene issues, see *Rūz al-Yūsif*: 2007/11/16 (4144), pp. 19, 20f, 24f. In what follows, we will mostly simply refer to certain pages in the respective issues of *Rūz al-Yūsif*. Only the most important articles from the journal's *niqāb* campaign in Fall 2007 are referenced in the bibliography.

28. This statement was modified in the following issue (*Rūz al-Yūsif*: 2007/11/23 (4145), p. 20). The health ministry's decree 140 from 1997 would regulate standardized clothing for medical doctors and nurses. In addition, there were several decrees and laws from the 1970s to the same effect.

29. *Rūz al-Yūsif*: 2007/11/23 (4145), p. 4.

30. *Rūz al-Yūsif*: 2008/03/17 (4171), pp. 59ff.

31. This is also true, though to a much lesser extent, for the *ḥiǧāb*. For example, critical comments about the *ḥiǧāb*, from Egypt's minister of culture in 2006, caused some public debate to that effect (see *al-maṣrī l-yawm*, 2006/11/20 and /12/02). For reasons of space we leave the *ḥiǧāb* debate aside.

between the two opinions is whether wearing the *niqāb* is a custom (*ʿāda*) without genuine connection to the religion of Islam, or an Islamic obligatory religious act (*ʿibāda*). The latter view was expressed explicitly several times, by the medical personnel supporting the *niqāb,* in *Rūz al-Yūsif.* The former view was taken by Egypt's *awqāf*-minister Zaqzūq, *Rūz al-Yūsif,* and Suʿād Ṣāliḥ.

The interaction of these two opposing views can be illustrated with several public debates that have taken place in Egypt since 2006, and illustrate how the debate about the *niqāb* in hospitals is not restricted to bioethics, but serves as a locus to negotiate Egyptian Islamic identity. For example, in 2007, Zaqzūq took several measures against female religious tutors (*muršidāt*), working for the *awqāf* ministry, who wore *niqābs*,[32] with the Šayḫ al-Azhar publicly expressing disagreement.[33] Also, in 2006, Suʿād Ṣāliḥ had caused some debate by stating on TV that she considered the *niqāb* to be un-Islamic, and expressed that she felt contempt for women wearing it. (Later, she apologized publicly for the latter part of her statement.) Yūsuf al-Badrī replied by accusing Ṣāliḥ of intolerance, stating that in his eyes the *niqāb* was a religious duty, and he threatened to sue the TV channel in court if they did not offer space for voices to express this view.[34]

The difference between the two views of the *niqāb,* being either *ʿāda* or *ʿibāda,* is fundamental in Egypt: especially in the court decisions, it was mentioned explicitly that the Egyptian constitution described the *šarīʿa* as the major source for Egypt's legal system. If the *niqāb* is termed *ʿibāda*, a religious duty, it has to be considered as a central part of the *šarīʿa.* The opposite is the case if it is seen as *ʿāda.* This is essential, because nobody wants to deny that Egypt's identity is largely Islamic. Therefore, those opposing the *niqāb* have to argue that it is not pivotal to Islam.

One important aspect to this is the repeated observation that the spread of the *niqāb* in Egypt would be a comparatively recent development, with origins

32. For example, at a meeting in January 2007, he ordered a *muršida* either to take off her *niqāb* or to leave. (See lakii.com/vb/archive/index.php/t-257427.html, accessed March 2008). In March 2007, he canceled a competition between *muršidāt* in order to avoid giving *munaqqabāt* a public arena. (See okaz.com.sa/okaz/osf/20070315/Con2007031595247.htm; accessed March 2008). Zaqzūq reiterated his opinion of the *niqāb* being *ʿāda* and not *ʿibāda* several times (for example, *al-maṣrī l-yawm*2007/08/13a).

33. See, for example, okaz.com.sa/okaz/osf/20070315/Con2007031595247.htm; accessed March 2008. Another example was a widely reported court case between the American University of Cairo (AUC) and a *munaqqaba* student, who was forbidden entrance to the campus.

34. See his interview in *al-maṣrī l-yawm*, 2006/10/23.

in Saudi Arabia.[35] This line of presenting the issue is further elaborated in a *Rūz al-Yūsif* piece, which was obviously intended to close the media campaign on the issue in December 2007,[36] and portrayed the preacher Abū Isḥāq al-Ḥuwaynī, whose teachings are said to be linked to the spread of the *niqāb*.[37] Al-Ḥuwaynī is characterized as being well connected to conservative religious circles in Saudi Arabia, as well as the *an-Nās* Channel. In this way, wearing the *niqāb* is depicted as not being genuinely Egyptian but of Saudi Arabian origin.[38]

This case illustrates how a bioethical debate (nurses wearing the *niqāb*) is based on the understanding that Egyptian identity is basically Islamic, and thus can be turned into a discussion about national identity. Therefore, the argument that medical personnel dress code has to be in accordance with international standards, and would thus supersede personal religious beliefs, has to be legitimized by a religious scholar. The example also shows that negotiating Egyptian identity as an Islamic identity is not to be described in a neat binary of Islam vs. the West. Rather, this debate is about asserting Egyptian Islamic identity in the face of strong influences from Western countries as well as from Saudi Arabia. For this reason, religious actors can be found on both sides of the debate.

FGM

Our second case study, about Female Genital Mutilation (FGM),[39] is bioethics backwards, as it were. Rather than asking for the ethical application of a

35. *Rūz al-Yūsif*: 2007/11/16 (4144), p. 21; 2007/11/23 (4145), pp. 24f. In this context Rūz al-Yūsif also covered a Saudi debate between the liberal author ʿAlī al-Barāk and the conservative, high-ranking religious scholar Ṣāliḥ al-Fawzān about the *niqāb* in hospitals, which followed the same lines as in Egypt (No. 4147 (2007/12/01), p.23). This debate had taken place already in 2006. See *Ǧarīdat ar-Riyāḍ*, Nos. 14009, 14016, 14021, 14024 (all from November 2006).

36. *Rūz al-Yūsif*: 2007/12/01 (4147). In the first of three extended articles on the *niqāb* in this issue, *Rūz al-Yūsif* looks back on the past weeks and sums up the results of the campaign.

37. *Rūz al-Yūsif*: 2007/12/01 (4147), pp. 28–31.

38. It is also interesting to see how the *niqāb* debate is sometimes directly linked to FGM, since al-Ḥ uwaynī is said to support both in order to set Christians and Muslims apart from each other. For other examples, where the *niqāb* and the FGM issues are presented in connection to each other, see *Rūz al-Yūsif*: 2007/11/23 (4145), p.28, Rūla Ḫarsa's critical analysis of patriarchal discourse in *al-maṣrī l-yawm*, 2007/07/11c or Zaqzūq's statement that FGM and the *niqāb* both had nothing to do with the religion of Islam (*al-maṣrī l-yawm*2007/08/13a).

39. Female Genital Mutilation (FGM) is the general term for all procedures that partially or completely remove the external female genitalia for nontherapeutic reasons. Procedures range, according to the classification of the World Health Organization (WHO), from the excision of the prepuce (1st degree) to the excision of all the external genitalia and stitching or narrowing of the vaginal opening (3rd degree). See "Female Genital Mutilation..." in *JAMA,* 1995;

new technology against a specific cultural background, it presents a prominent example of a widespread custom at odds with medical findings. However, the question of what is the right thing to do in this situation is not one of medicine vs. Islam. The dominant referential framework is Islam. Rather, the question is whether the procedure is ascribed a status within that framework, which allows medically proven harmfulness to be an argument.

On June 22, 2007 the Egyptian daily newspaper *al-Maṣrī l-Yawm* reported the death of a teenaged girl, Badūr, who died in the course of an FGM operation,[40] the article marking the beginning of a national campaign against FGM that finally led to its legal prohibition in Egypt.[41] The newspaper's efforts were immediately joined by the NCCM, who played a leading role in coordinating the state's actors throughout the ensuing action against female circumcision. At that time, the NCCM was preparing a draft for a new childrens' law that intended, accordant with international agreements, to outlaw FGM.[42]

The weeks following Badūr's death witnessed a quick procession of actions against FGM. The doctors' syndicate started investigating against the doctor who had operated on Badūr, and, on grounds of existing regulations, warned its members against pursuing female circumcision.[43] A few days later, the Ministry of Health and Population, urged by the NCCM, issued a decree banning FGM from all public and private clinics, and announced that an overall prohibition within the penal code, independent of the ban already entailed in the draft for a new childrens' law, would follow during the next parliamentary season. The Ministry of Justice started to prepare the according draft in July.[44] All the while, NGOs, the Ministry of Health, and the NCCM conducted various activities to raise awareness about FGM,[45] such as conferences, demonstrations, or a hotline

WHO study group, 2006; Seif El Dawla, 1999. For statistics about the spread of FGM in Egypt see: *al-maṣrī l-yawm*: 2007/06/26c and /07/02 . For FGM in European countries: *al-maṣrī l-yawm*: 2007/07/14; Gamble, 1995; *NZZ Online*: 2008/07/04).

40. *al-maṣrī l-yawm*: 2007/06/22a.

41. *al-maṣrī l-yawm*: 2007/06/28a; 2008/06/18; *Al-Ahram Weekly Online*: 2008/03/13.

42. *al-maṣrī l-yawm*: 2007/06/22b, and 2007/05/18.

43. *al-maṣrī l-yawm*: 2007/06/24; *al-maṣrī l-yawm*: 2007/06/28b.

44. *al-maṣrī l-yawm*: 2007/06/23b; /06/29; 07/03; 07/23 and 07/29.

45. Some of these had been going on for quite some time, but only now came to the public's awareness (*al-maṣrī l-yawm*: 2007/06/26a and b; 2007/07/3 and 2007/04/10).

to report FGM-related cases,[46] while reports of new cases and investigations kept the public interest alive.[47]

The public rhetoric employed throughout the campaign focused to a large extent on the question of religious permissibility of FGM; i.e., *fatwās* prohibiting or allowing the procedure.[48] Only one day after the initial report, ʿAlī Ǧumʿa confirmed on TV that FGM was forbidden in modern times.[49] An official *fatwā* by the *dār al-iftāʾ* and the Šayḫ al-Azhar soon followed.[50]

The *fatwā* by the *dār al-iftāʾ* recognizes FGM not as a religious issue (*qaḍīya dīniyya taʿabbudiyya*) but as a matter of custom (*ʿāda*), in which the judgment of medical doctors ultimately prevails. However, the main arguments against FGM note the lack of any authoritative text obligating FGM even in its mildest form, the lack of reports that the Prophet Muḥammad had his daughters circumcised, and the fact that FGM is not practiced in other Arabic countries, especially Saudi Arabia.[51] These *fatwās* were a crucial element in the campaign. The Minister for Endowments demanded that Imāms refer to them in Friday prayers.[52]

The *maǧmaʿ* acted differently. It soon admitted that female circumcision wasn't a duty in Islamic law,[53] but after long discussions decided not to issue a *fatwā* on the ban of FGM. It stated that no person within the *maǧmaʿ*—headed

---

46. *al-maṣrī l-yawm*: 2007/06/26b; /10/28 *Al-Ahram Weekly Online*: 2007/09/16; *al-maṣrī l-yawm*: 2007/08/4 (conferences); *al-maṣrī l-yawm*: 2007/07/19 and 2007/07/6 (demonstrations); *al-maṣrī l-yawm*: 2007/08/13c (hotline). Other activities included workshops and public discussions (*al-maṣrī l-yawm*: 2007/08/17b.), theatre plays (*al-maṣrī l-yawm*: 2007/07/7b), special training for youths, nurses, doctors, and preachers, as emissaries to the provinces (*al-maṣrī l-yawm*: 2007/07/3), a plan to supervise the ban in hospitals, TV spots (*al-maṣrī l-yawm*: 2007/07/12 and 2007/07/2), and a special council with members of the Ministry of Health, the doctors' syndicate, and the NCCM, to develop an overall strategy (*al-maṣrī l-yawm*: 2007/08/10; *Al-Ahram Weekly Online*: 2007/11/23)

47. For example: *al-maṣrī l-yawm*: 2007/06/25c; 07/29; 07/29; 08/11; 08/13b; 08/15; 08/16; 08/17a; 08/20; 08/23; 08/26; 09/02; 09/04b; 09/07; 11/09.

48. The NCCM had been trying for some time to win over the Islamic authorities for a religious ban of female circumcision, but only succeeded after Badūr's death. (*al-maṣrī l-yawm*: 2006/11/21; 11/26; 12/04; 2007/05/16b and 23; *al-iḫwān al-muslimūn*: 2006/11/23; *al-gumhūriyya*: 2007/07/4).

49. *al-maṣrī l-yawm*: 2007/06/23a; *al-maṣrī l-yawm*: 2007/06/25b.

50. *al-maṣrī l-yawm*: 2007/07/4; Dār al-Iftāʾ "Fiqh al-Marʾa. Ḫitān al-Ināṯ".

51. The latter argument was sometimes referred to as an indication that FGM is not an Islamic custom (*al-maṣrī l-yawm*: 2007/08/13a and 12/19).

52. *al-maṣrī l-yawm*: 2007/08/13a; August 14; August 17b;/12/17.

53. *al-maṣrī l-yawm*: 2007/06/29.

by the Šayḫ al-Azhar—had the right to either forbid or obligate FGM on religious grounds, due to lack of normative texts.[54]

Of course, opponents of the FGM ban exploited this dissent.[55] Apart from individual preachers,[56] it was mainly the Muslim Brotherhood who publicly denounced the prohibition in the media, as well as in parliament. They doubted the formal validity of the involved legislative procedures and of the financing of the campaign, explicitly questioned the authority of the Grand Muftī's and the Šayḫ al-Azhar's *fatwās*, and called for an independent body of Azhar scholars to assess the permissibility of FGM—which, according to studies presented by the Brotherhood's members of parliament, was not necessarily harmful, and for them was a valued part of the Islamic tradition. Yet, the Muslim Brotherhood's main argument was that female circumcision was a minor issue, neither forbidden nor obligatory, while the real problems of Egypt and Egyptian women were left unattended, that the ultimate motive of the campaign was Westernization and the weakening of Islam—as attested by international funding and the involvement of Western NGOs.[57]

Fears of Westernization were easy enough to arouse in this case, mainly because of the prohibition campaign's ties to international agreements, which are often suspect of a hidden agenda. The NCCM and its higher staff are, in fact, strongly committed to the secular and rights-oriented framework set by international conferences, declarations, and relations, and previous as well as the current program against FGM are partly funded by UN organizations.[58] Additionally, the childrens' law prepared by the Council did indeed have its background in

---

54. *al-iḫwān al-muslimūn*: 2007/09/4; see also *aš-šarq al-awsaṭ*: 2007/07/19. See also *al-iḫwān al-muslimūn*: 2008/03/26 and *aš-šarq al-awsaṭ*: 2008/04/24.

55. *al-iḫwān al-muslimūn*: 2007/09/04 and 2008/03/26.

56. Yūsuf al-Qaraḍāwī and Yūsuf Badrī filed a lawsuit against the health minister's ban of FGM (*aš-šarq al-awsaṭ*: 2007/07/19; *al-maṣrī l-yawm*: 2007/12/13; and 2007/09/4a). And, of course, there were other *fatwās* contradicting the grand muftī's and the Šayḫ al-Azhar's judgments (*al-maṣrī l-yawm*: 2007/07/7a), while anonymous pamphlets printed out previous rulings by the Šayḫ al-Azhar contradicting his current stance on FGM (*al-maṣrī l-yawm*: 2007/10/14).

57. *al-iḫwān al-muslimūn*: 2008/03/26; 2007/08/21; 2007/06/27; 2007/07/11; 2007/07/25; 2006/12/04; and 2006/12/5; *al-maṣrī l-yawm*: 2007/08/27; 2008/06/8.

58. This shows, for example, in an article by Dr. Vivian Fu'ād of the NCCM, shortly after Badūr's death, in which she blames patriarchy, conservative and religious politics, medical doctors, and the education sector's failure to further the "scientific and civilized" awareness of the Egyptian people (*al-maṣrī l-yawm*: 2007/06/25a). See also *al-maṣrī l-yawm*: 2007/04/10 and for the funding by UN organizations *Al-Ahram Weekly Online*: 2003/06/19; *Al-Ahram Weekly Online*: 2007/09/16; *al-maṣrī l-yawm*: 2007/09/16.

international agreements, and followed through on some of Egypt's obligations resulting from these agreements.[59]

The childrens' law was passed after heated discussions in June 2008. It is the first comprehensive legal prohibition of FGM in Egypt.[60]

The Background

Of course, that FGM is medically harmful has been known for decades. The first moves against this practice took place in the 1950s. However, the background for the first encompassing public discussion arose from the confrontation with rights-oriented notions maintained on the international level. The current debate about FGM has its roots in the 1994 International Conference on Population and Development in Cairo, where, besides abortion,[61] FGM was the most divisive topic. The discussion was started by NGOs, but erupted on a larger scale only when CNN aired a documentary that graphically showed the circumcision of a young girl. The government immediately promised to prohibit FGM, yet, once the conference was over, faced a wide alliance opposing all attempts to ban this practice.[62] It took until 1997 to come up with a ministerial decree prohibiting FGM. But the decree left a loophole and permitted the operation if medically indicated, which rendered the decision rather useless.[63]

However, as the topic of FGM was raised during the conference, and put under attack by international NGOs and the Egyptian government itself,

---

59. *al-maṣrī l-yawm*: 2007/06/22b; *Al-Ahram Weekly Online*: 2008/03/13. Other than the FGM ban it entailed stipulations to raise the minimum age for marriage to 18 years, gave children born out of wedlock the right to a birth certificate with the family name of the mother, and enhanced protection from physical abuse and child labor.

60. *Al-Ahram Weekly Online*: 2008/03/13; *al-maṣrī l-yawm*: 2008/05/16; 2008/06/18; and 2008/06/13; *Al-Ahram Weekly Online*: 2008/06/12.

61. *al-ḥayāt*: 1994/09/4;/09/05; 1994/09/7; 1994/09/06; and 1994; Lee Bowen: 1997 and 2003)

62. The most prominent opponent was the Šayẖ al-Azhar Ǧād al-Ḥ aqq, who used this issue to confront the government and achieved concessions important for the interests of al-Azhar. He even issued a *fatwā* permitting FGM, and stating that uncircumcised girls would be subject to situations that would lead them to immorality and corruption. See Moustafa 2000: 13ff.; Ǧād al-Ḥ aqq: 1981.

63. Dār al-Iftā' "Fiqh al-Mar'a. ẖitān al-ināṯ"; Seif El Dawla: 1999; *al-maṣrī l-yawm*: 2007/07/11a; the first survey by the Ministry of Health in 1995, shortly before the ministerial ban, showed that 97% of married women aged 15–49 were circumcised. Another survey in 2005 showed a decline among women younger than 18 years old, of whom only 75% were circumcised. The ratios shouldn't be compared directly, though, because of the different age groups (*al-maṣrī l-yawm*: 2007/07/2). In 2007 approximately 70% of FGM operations took place in clinics (*al-maṣrī l-yawm*: 2007/07/26), and large portions of society still support FGM (*al-maṣrī l-yawm*: 2007/11/20).

Islamic activists and some scholars defended what they saw as a valuable tradition. Just like abortion, FGM was turned into a symbolic issue, a border marker of the Egyptian Islamic identity vs. Western influence.[64]

Its defenders claim that circumcision would limit women's sexual urges, thus safeguarding the chastity of women and society. But above all, it's part of an Egyptian tradition with some Islamic justification.[65]

This case shows again the importance of Egypt's media, this time even successfully aiming at the introduction of a new law—forming a contrast to the *niqāb* debate, which merely aimed at the enforcing of already-existing codes. It is most likely for this reason that it was not sufficient in the FGM case to muster only the Muftī's public support. Rather, it was also important to at least secure the Šayḫ al-Azhar's consent, and although the attempt to also integrate the *maǧmaʿ* failed, it is clear that it was considered useful to at least *try* to bring it into the coalition supporting the new law. Also, the pattern shows again how debating a bioethical issue quickly develops into negotiating Egyptian Islamic identity at large. This pattern is constructed not so much as a binary of Islam vs. West, but rather as a multilayered process in which the identity of the Self is contrasted to a variety of markers of Muslim and non-Muslim Others alike.

Conclusion

How, then, can the contents of these debates, and thus of Egyptian bioethics, be characterized? First, with the exception of organ transplantation, the most fervently contested bioethical issues in Egypt are usually related to sexual mores and the role of women in society—often focusing on questions of how to control female sexuality.[66] Therefore, these debates are not perceived as issues of a sort of "compartmentalized ethics," being of interest only to a select group of ethicists or researchers, but rather as societal ethics at large. Bioethical issues thus become symbolic issues, which are used to promote one's own values and vision of society.

64. Seif El Dawla, 1999: 130–133.

65. ibidem: 1999, 129; Ǧād al-Ḥaqq: 1981.

66. Other examples are the abortion debate (see above Fn. 27) or the public discussion about hymenorraphy (see Eich, 2010).

Second, this society, and therefore Egyptian identity, is perceived to have faced significant challenges in recent years. On a socioeconomic level, these challenges can be swiftly described by pointing to high unemployment rates, low wages, scarcity of housing, and an education crisis.[67] On a value-oriented level, these challenges can be depicted as a fear of Westernization on the one hand, and of "Saudification" on the other.[68] Bioethical discussions in Egypt, then, are public negotiations about Egyptian identity.

Third, Islam—often in the sense of *šarīʿa* as Islamic law—is the general framework of all these debates. This is because the Egyptian consitution identifies *šarīʿa* as the main source of legislation, and because Egyptians see their country's identity as largely shaped by Islam. Consequently, for Egyptians, the question of how to react to these changes does not present itself as a choice between secularism or laicism versus a religiously oriented vision of society. It is largely agreed that the fundamental referential framework for what it means to be Egyptian is primarily the religion of Islam. Therefore, Egyptians do not negotiate their "Egyptianness" as "how Islamic they want themselves to be," but rather as "in such-and-such situation or issue, what does it mean, concretely, to act as a good Muslim?" For this reason, the opposition of essentially religious issues (*ʿibāda*) versus those pertaining to fields open for nonreligious arguments (*ʿāda*) is most determinant and most contested in the process of reducing complex topics to a narrow spectrum of talking points (agenda-setting). It seems noteworthy that conceptions of local identity also contribute to the classification of *ʿibāda* and *ʿāda*: While the somehow-foreign *niqāb* was quite easily termed *ʿāda*, in the case of indigenous FGM, the perception of the practice as an Islamic tradition was hard to counter.[69] Since Islam is seen as the main component of Egyptian identity, claims to the Islamic nature of a custom in question focus on the potential consequences of its abandonment; i.e., that the entire Islamic order of society would cease to function. Theories of conspiracy against Islam are common in this context. On the other hand, exclusion of an issue from the religious sphere (opting to refer the

---

67. For example, in the Rūz al-Yūsif-issues of the *niqāb* campaign, the deplorable state of the education system for nurses repeatedly became an issue.

68. See for example *al-maṣrī l-yawm*: 2006/10/2, where the author terms the growing number of Egyptian women wearing the *ḥiǧāb* a "Wahhābī [i.e., Saudi-Arabian] razzia on Egypt."

69. Saudi Arabia served as a focal point against which to contrast the Egyptian identity in both cases, highlighting the foreignness in one case and signifying the original Islam in the other.

final decision to the medical profession, for example) seems to give more leeway to adapt to new situations, but must be legitimized by religious institutions.

Glossary

ʿāda custom; the term is used to label habits as having no genuine connection to the religion of Islam

Al-Azhar University The leading university in Egypt; pronouncements by the religious head of al-Azhar have substantial authority in the Sunni Muslim world

al-Maṣrī l-Yawm Egyptian daily newspaper

al-Nās TV channel which features non-state scholars with obvious links to Saudi Arabia

Awqāf (sg. Waqf) Religious endowments

dār al-iftā' Office of the grand muftī of Egypt

fatwā (pl. fatāwā) a non-binding legal opinion, rendered by a mufti

ḥarām forbidden; one of the five values of legal action

ḥiǧāb Islamic headscarf

ʿibāda Islamic obligatory religious act

ICPD International Conference on Population and Development

iftā' the giving of legal opinions (fatwas) by muftis

laicism absence of religious involvement in government affairs and of government involvement in religious affairs

maǧmaʿ al-buḥūṯ al-islāmiyya Al-Azhar's Council for Islamic Studies

munaqqaba pl. munaqqabāt Woman wearing the face veil

muršidāt female religious tutors, primarily working at Egyptian, state-run mosques

MENA Middle East and North Africa region

MOHP Ministry of Health and Population (Egypt)

muftī a jurisconsult; authoritative person who renders a legal opinion (fatwā) in response to a query

NCCM National Council for Children and Motherhood (Egypt)

niqāb face veil

Qur'ān God's revelation to the Prophet Muhammad; the most authoritative document in Islam

Rūz al-Yūsif Egyptian weekly

Šayḫ al-Azhar religious head of al-Azhar University

šarīʿa Islamic law; the correct path of action as determined by God

Sunni the majority sect of Muslims, as opposed to Shiite

ʿulamā' religious scholars; lit. the people of knowledge

wizārat al-awqāf Ministry of Religious Endowments in Egypt. The minister of awqāf appoints the country's grand muftī and also controls the state-run mosques of the country. By 1994 71% of Egypt's mosques were run by the state.

zinā illicit sex in Islamic Law

References

al-Ahrām, 2007/04/16. Hibā ʿAbd al-ʿAzīz: "al-ǧamīʿ tuwāǧih ḥarb az-zawāǧ al-ʿurfī."

Al-Ahram Weekly Online, 1998/11/19. Shahine, Gihan: "Better, not more."

Al-Ahram Weekly Online, 2003/06/12. Tadros, Mariz: "Judges rule out comliance."

Al-Ahram Weekly Online, 2003/06/26. Ezzat, Dina: "Putting down the scalpel."

Al-Ahram Weekly Online, 2006/02/22. Marzouk, Waleed: "Abortion Moral."

Al-Ahram Weekly Online, 2006/04/12. Ezzat, Dina: "Take it down."

Al-Ahram Weekly Online, 2006/06/29. El-Assyouti, Mohamed: "To balance the scales."

Al-Ahram Weekly Online, 2007/09/16. Leila, Reem: "Challenging tradition."

Al-Ahram Weekly Online, 2007/11/23. Leila, Reem: "Drop the knife."

Al-Ahram Weekly Online, 2008/03/13. "Child shield."

Al-Ahram Weekly Online, 2008/06/12. Essam El-Din, Gamal: "Children accorded greater rights."

al-ǧumhūriyya, 2007/07/04. ʿAbd al-Ǧawwād, ʿUmar: "dār al-iftāʾ: ḫitān al-ināṯ muḥarram šarʿan."

al-ḥayāt, 1994/09/04. Ibrāhīm, Saʿd ad-Dīn: "iġlāq al-aql al-ʿarabī. muʾtamar ad-duwalī li-s-sukkān wa l-ġawġāʾīyāt al-arbaʿ (1 min 4)."

al-ḥayāt, 1994/09/05. Ibrāhīm, Saʿd ad-Dīn: "iġlāq al-aql al-ʿarabī. al-muʾtamar ad-duwalī li-s-sukkān: ʿayyinat arāʾ wa-rudūd (2 min 4)."

al-ḥayāt, 1994/09/06. Ibrāhīm, Saʿd ad-Dīn: "iġlāq al-aql al-ʿarabī al-muʾtamar ad-duwalī li-s-sukkān: masʾalat 'waqf numūw al-bašar' (3 min 4)."

al-ḥayāt, 1994/09/07. Ibrāhīm, Saʿd ad-Dīn: "iġlāq al-ʿaql al-ʿarabī. muʾtamar as-sukkān: Mao... ʿAbd an-Nāṣir... al-Ḫumaynī! (4 min4)."

al-iḫwān al-muslimūn, 2003/11/07. al-Ḫalafāwī, Ǧīhān: "kalimat al-aḫawāt fī ḥafl ifṭār al-iḫwān al-muslimīn (ramaḍān 1424 h)."

al-iḫwān al-muslimūn, 2006/11/23. Muḥammad, Tasnīm: "al-ʿulamāʾ al-mušārikūn rafaḍū taḥrīm ḫitān al-ināṯ wa-ḥašd iʿlāmī ġarbī kaṯīf."

al-iḫwān al-muslimūn, 2006/12/04. al-Ḫaṭīb, Muḥammad ʿAbdallāh: "aš-šayḫ al-ḫaṭīb yaktub: al-ḫitān min sunan al-fiṭra wa-makrama li-n-nisāʾ."

al-iḫwān al-muslimūn, 2006/12/05. Mašālī, Sālī: "li-māḏā ṣamatat al-muʾassasāt ad-dīniyya fī azmat al-ḥiǧāb? wa-li-māḏā tabḥaṯ al-ʾān taḥrīm al-ḫitān."

al-iḫwān al-muslimūn, 2007/06/27. ʿIyād, ʿAlāʾ: "Laban yaḥḏir min al-fatāwā al-ḫilāfiyya al-muḍirra bi-waḥḍat al-umma al-islāmiyya."

al-iḫwān al-muslimūn, 2007/07/11. Dr. al-Qawāʿid, Ḥilmī Muḥammad: "taḥrīm al-ḫitān.. wa-stiqlāl al-umma!."

al-iḫwān al-muslimūn, 2007/07/25. al-Qāʿūd, Ḥilmī Muḥammad: "miḥnat al-ʿaṭš.. wa-naẓariyyat al-muʾāmara!!."

al-iḫwān al-muslimūn, 2007/08/21. ʿIyād, ʿAlāʾ: "ittihāmāt bi-tamwīl ad-daʿāya ḍidd al-ḫitān min ǧihāt tabšīriyya wa-yahūdiyya."

al-iḫwān al-muslimūn, 2007/09/04. Abū Zayd, Šīmā': "al-maǧlis al-qawmī li-l-mar'a.. dawr mašbūh wa-aǧinda ḫāriǧiyya."

al-iḫwān al-muslimūn, 2007/12/31. Ṣāliḥ, Aḥmad: "al-muwāfaqa ʿalā taʿdīlāt qānūn al-ʿuqūbāt bi-ǧawāz iǧhāḍ al-unṯā l-muġtaṣaba."

al-iḫwān al-muslimūn, 2008/02/25. Dr. Abū l-Ḥasan, Manāl: "al-baḥṯ ʿan Badūr!."

al-iḫwān al-muslimūn, 2008/03/26. Waǧdī, Duʿā': "taʿdīlāt qānūn aṭ-ṭifl.. alǧām li-tafǧīr al-muǧtamaʿ."

al-iḫwān al-muslimūn, 2008/08/01. Ramaḍān, Aḥmad: "fatwā iǧhāḍ al-muġtaṣaba ǧināyat al-iftā' bi-r-ra'y."

al-ǧazīra, 2006/05/31. "aš-šarīʿa wa-l-ḥayāt: al-iʿlām wa-fawḍā l-fatāwā."

al-maṣrī l-yawm, 2005/12/05. al-Ǧazzār, Aḥmad: "ḫitān al-ināṯ yuṭīr 'azma' fī mahraǧān al-qāhira.. wa-Šūbāšī yaqūl li-l-ǧamāhīr: 'ḫallīkum mutaḥaḍḍirīn'."

al-maṣrī l-yawm, 2006/02/18. Rašwān, Hudā: "rā'idāt mašrūʿ manʿ al-ḫitān yantaqidūn taqrīr at-tanmiya l-bašariyya."

al-maṣrī l-yawm, 2006/07/12. ʿAbd ar-Razzāq, Rāmī: "āḫir 'al-ʿašq'.. wa-rubbamā awwaluhu: bint fāšila muḥaṭṭama wa-šāb yabkī ʿalā d-dawwām."

al-maṣrī l-yawm, 2006/10/02. Šaraf al-Dīn, Nabīl: "qiṣṣat al-ġazw al-wahhābī li-miṣr."

al-maṣrī l-yawm, 2006/10/23. "aš-Šayḫ Yūsuf al-Badrī li-'l-maṣrī l-yawm': an-niqāb wāǧib šarʿī.. wa-70% fatāwā Suʿād Ṣāliḥ lā ʿalāqa lahā bi-d-dīn."

al-maṣrī l-yawm, 2006/11/20. Ḍiyā' Rašwān: "al-Ḥukūma wa-l-ḥiǧāb wa-l-iḫwān wa-t-taʿdīlāt al-dustūrīya."

al-maṣrī l-yawm, 2006/11/21. al-Buḥayrī, Aḥmad: "dār al-iftā' wa-mu'assasa almāniyya tunaẓẓimān mu'tamaran muštarikan li-manʿ ḫitān al-ināṯ."

al-maṣrī l-yawm, 2006/11/26. al-Buḥayrī, Aḥmad: "ḫalāf azharī ḥawl iṣdār qānūn yuǧrim ḫitān al-ināṯ."

al-maṣrī l-yawm, 2006/12/02. ʿAwāṭif ʿAbd ar-Raḥmān: "taʿālū ilā kalimat sawā'."

al-maṣrī l-yawm, 2006/12/04. al-Buḥayrī, Aḥmad: "al-muftī li-l-maṣrī l-yawm: ḫitān al-ināṯ lā ʿilāqa lahu bi-l-islām.. wa-bḥaṯ iṣdār fatwā bi-ʿadm šarʿiyyatihi."

al-maṣrī l-yawm, 2007/02/07. al-Bannā, Ǧamāl: "azmat al-fatwā aw iǧlāq bāb al-iǧtihād marratan uḫrā (1-2)."

al-maṣrī l-yawm, 2007/02/21. al-Bannā, Ǧamāl: "azmat al-fatwā aw iǧlāq bāb al-iǧtihād marratan uḫrā (2-2)."

al-maṣrī l-yawm, 2007/04/02. Hānī Rifʿat: "yumazziq šaqīqatahu bi-s-sikkīn bi-sabab zawāǧihā ʿurfiyan min ʿāmil."

al-maṣrī l-yawm, 2007/04/12. Farūq al-Ǧamāl: "kayfa tusayṭir Isrā'īl ʿalā ʿuqūl šabābinā."

al-maṣrī l-yawm, 2007/04/10. Rašwān, Hudā: "Mušīra Ḫaṭṭāb: 14 dawla fī l-minṭaqa 'āḫiruhā Irītriyā sabaqatnā bi-taǧrīm ḫitān al-ināṯ."

al-maṣrī l-yawm, 2007/05/12. Aḥmad Šalabī: "šurṭī yaqtul šaqīqatahu l-armila bi-sikkīn."

al-maṣrī l-yawm, 2007/05/16a. Muʿawwaḍ, Ibrāhīm: "intiqādāt li-kitāb 'al-fatāwā l-ʿaṣriyya' li-Ǧumaʿa wa-munāšadat al-Azhar iʿādat faḥṣihi wa-murāǧaʿatihi."

al-maṣrī l-yawm, 2007/05/16b. Rašwān, Hudā: "Šayḫ al-Azhar yuqirr mašrūʿ qānūn aṭ-ṭifl.. wa-yuftī bi-taǧrīm ḫitān al-ināṯ."

al-maṣrī l-yawm, 2007/05/18. Rašwān, Hudā: "Šayḫ al-Azhar yuwāfiq ʿalā taǧrīm ḫitān al-ināṯ.. wa-rafʿ sinn az-zawāǧ ilā 18 ʿāmman li-l-ǧinsayn."

al-maṣrī l-yawm, 2007/05/23. al-Buḥayrī, Aḥmad: "al-muftī: aṣ-ṣaḥāba kānū yatabarrakūn bi-kull šayʾ min an-nabī li-anna ẓāhirahu wa-bāṭinahu ṭāhir."

al-maṣrī l-yawm, 2007/06/22a. Nāfiʿ, Saʿīd: "aṭ-ṭifla 'Badūr' šahīdat 'al-ḫitān'.. mātat bi-ǧarʿa muḫaddir zāʾida."

al-maṣrī l-yawm, 2007/06/22b. Rašwān, Hudā: "ǧadl fī l-awsāṭ ad-dīniyya ḥawl al-ḫitān wa-nasab mawālīd al-ʿilāqāt ġayr aš-šarʿiyya fī taʿdīlāt 'qānūn aṭ-ṭifl'."

al-maṣrī l-yawm, 2007/06/23a. az-Zayāt, Yāsir: ""iḫtanū" ʿuqūlakum."

al-maṣrī l-yawm, 2007/06/23b. Rašwān, Hudā: "'al-qawmī li-l-umūma wa-ṭ-ṭufūla' yuʿlin musānadat usrat 'Badūr' ḍaḥīyat al-ḫitān.. wa-yuṭālib bi-tašdīd ʿuqūbat aṭ-ṭabība."

al-maṣrī l-yawm, 2007/06/24. Rašwān, Hudā: "niqābat al-aṭibbāʾ tuḥaqqiq fī wafāt 'Badūr'.. wa-maǧlis aṭ-ṭufūla yuṭālib usratahā bi-ʿadm at-tanāzul."

al-maṣrī l-yawm, 2007/06/25a. Fuʾād, Fīfiyān: "ad-duktūra Fīfiyān Fuʾād taktub: man qatal Badūr?.. ṭabībat al-Munyā laysat waḥdahā al-qātila.. kulliyyāt aṭ-ṭibb ṣanaʿat ẓāhirat 'taṭbīb al-ḫitān'.. wa-'ṣ-ṣiḥḥa' antaǧat qānūnan muʿīban."

al-maṣrī l-yawm, 2007/06/25b. Ǧāballāh, Ḫalīfa: "al-muftī: 'qulnāhā marra wa-tnēn wa-ʿašara ḫitān al-ināṯ ḥarām.. ḥarām.. ḥarām'."

al-maṣrī l-yawm, 2007/06/25c. as-Samkūrī, Muḥammad: "kūbrī Naǧaʿ Ḥamādī 'šarīk waṭanī' fī ṭuqūs ḫitān al-ināṯ."

al-maṣrī l-yawm, 2007/06/26a. Rašwān, Hudā: "Sūzān Mubārak tuṭālib bi-tašrīʿāt li-waqf al-ʿunf ḍidd al-aṭfāl.. wa-taqif "daqīqa ḥidādan" ʿalā rūḥ 'Badūr'."

al-maṣrī l-yawm, 2007/06/26b. Rašwān, Hudā: "Sūzān Mubārak: wafāt 'Badūr' bidāyat an-nihāya li-ḫitān al-ināṯ."

al-maṣrī l-yawm, 2007/06/26c. Ṯābit, Mamdūḥ: "mufaǧaʾa: 97% min az-zawǧāt al-miṣriyyāt 'muḫtatināt'."

al-maṣrī l-yawm, 2007/06/28a. "ḥamlat qawmiyya li-mukāfaḥat ḫitān al-ināṯ baʿd wafāt 'Badūr'."

al-maṣrī l-yawm, 2007/06/28b. ʿAbd al-Ḫāliq Musāhil, Muḥammad: "niqābat al-aṭibbāʾ tuḥaddir aʿḍāʾahā min ḫitān al-ināṯ."

al-maṣrī l-yawm, 2007/06/29. al-Buḥayrī, Aḥmad: "wizārat aṣ-ṣiḥḥa taḥẓur ǧirāḥāt ḫitān al-ināṯ nihāʾiyyan."

al-maṣrī l-yawm, 2007/07/02. Rašwān, Hudā: "masʿūla fī l-umam al-muttaḥida: ḫitān al-ināṯ yatarāǧaʿ bayn fatayāt al-madāris bi-nisbat 50%."

al-maṣrī l-yawm, 2007/07/03. Rašwān, Hudā: "al-Ǧabalī: tašrīʿ ǧadīd bi-taǧrīm ḫitān al-ināṯ fī d-dawra al-barlamāniyya al-muqbila."

al-maṣrī l-yawm, 2007/07/04. al-Buḥayrī, Aḥmad: "al-muftī yuḥarrim 'ḫitān al-ināṯ' rasmiyyan wa-yastanid fī qarārihi ilā arāʾ 'Ṭanṭāwī wa-l-Qaraḍāwī wa-l-ʿAwā'."

al-maṣrī l-yawm, 2007/07/06. Ṯābit, Mamdūḥ: "3000 muwāṭin yarfaʿūn ṣūrat 'aš-šahīda Badūr' fī masīra ḍidd ḫitān al-ināṯ bi-Asyūṭ."

al-maṣrī l-yawm, 2007/07/07a. az-Zayāt, Yāsir: "al-muftī 'l-muwāzī'."
al-maṣrī l-yawm, 2007/07/07b. Rašwān, Hudā: "ʿaraḍ masraḥī ḥawla wafāt 'Badūr' yantahī bi-šiʿār 'lā li-l-ḫitān'."
al-maṣrī l-yawm, 2007/07/11a. Ǧūda, Sulaymān: "ǧarīma ʿumruhā 13 sana!."
al-maṣrī l-yawm, 2007/07/11b. Ramaḍān, Raǧab: "Ṭanṭāwī: al-azhar lā yaḫḍaʿ li-irādat al-ḥākim wa-man yuḫālif al-ḥākim al-ʿādil ʿāṣin."
al-maṣrī l-yawm, 2007/07/11c. Ḫarsā, Rūla: "rifqan bi-n-nisā."
al-maṣrī l-yawm, 2007/07/12. Ḫāṭir, Manār: "fī masʾalat tašdīd ar-riqāba ʿalā l-ḫitān: awliyāʾ umūr sa-yaḏhabūn bi-banāthihim ilā l-mustašfayāt.. lakinnahum fī l-ḥaqīqa aṭibbāʾ min mudīriyyat aṣ-ṣiḥḥa."
al-maṣrī l-yawm, 2007/07/14. ʿAbd al-Ḫāliq Musāhil, Muḥammad: "ḥamla muštarika bayna l-maṣriyyīn fī ūrūbā wa-l-ḥukūma al-brīṭāniyya ḍidd al-ḫitān."
al-maṣrī l-yawm, 2007/07/19. Rašwān, Hudā: "5000 ṭifla fī masīrat taʾbīn 'Badūr' šahīdat al-ḫitān fī l-munyā."
al-maṣrī l-yawm, 2007/07/23. Amīn, Ṭāriq: "wizārat al-ʿadl tuʿidd qānūnan li-ḥaẓr ḫitān al-ināṯ."
al-maṣrī l-yawm, 2007/07/26. ʿAbd al-Ǧawwād, ʿAyd: "ḥamla li-munāhaḍat ḫitān al-ināṯ fī 4 muḥāfaẓāt bi-takallufat milyār dūlār."
al-maṣrī l-yawm, 2007/07/27. Amīn, Ṭāriq: "2007."
al-maṣrī l-yawm, 2007/07/29. Rašwān, Hudā: "Mušīra Ḫaṭṭāb: lā taʿāruḍ bayna qānūn aṭ-ṭifl li-taǧrīm al-ḫitān wa-mašrūʿ 'wizārat al-ʿadl'."
al-maṣrī l-yawm, 2007/08/04. ʿAbd al-Ǧawwād, ʿAyd: "muʾtamar as-sukkān fī l-Manūfiyya yadʿū li-iṣdār tašrīʿ li-yaǧrīm 'ḫitān al-banāt'."
al-maṣrī l-yawm, 2007/08/10. as-Saʿātī, Hudā: "al-Ǧabalī: ḫiṭṭa li-taḫfīḍ 'ḫitān al-ināṯ' bi-nisbat 20% ḫilāl ʿāmayn."
al-maṣrī l-yawm, 2007/08/11. Rašwān, Hudā: "'Karīma' ṯānī ḍaḥāyā ḫitān al-ināṯ ḫilāl šahrayn."
al-maṣrī l-yawm, 2007/08/13a. al-Buḥayrī, Aḥmad: "Zaqzūq li-l-aʾimma: qūlū fī ḫuṭ bat al-ǧumʿa inna 'ḫitān al-ināṯ' ʿāda qabīḥa wa-'mahbaṭ al-islām' lā tuṭabbiquhu."
al-maṣrī l-yawm, 2007/08/13b. Ḍurra, ʿĀdil: "an-niyāba lam yuwaǧǧih ayy ittihām li-ṭabīb 'ḍaḥīyat al-ḫitān'."
al-maṣrī l-yawm, 2007/08/13c. Rašwān, Hudā: "'al-qawmī li-ṭ-ṭufūla wa-l-umūma' yuḫaṣṣiṣ ḫubarāʾ li-r-radd ʿalā l-istifsārāt ḥawl al-ḫitān wa-yatalaqqā balāġāt al-muwāṭinīn ʿalā l-ḫaṭṭ as-sāḫin."
al-maṣrī l-yawm, 2007/08/14. Adwārd, Raymūn: "'fī l-mamnūʿ'.. Mušīra Ḫaṭṭāb: 102 alf ḥālat taḥarruš ǧinsī al-ʿām al-māḍī faqaṭ wa-arqām al-ḫitān 'ġayr daqīqa'."
al-maṣrī l-yawm, 2007/08/15. Amīn, Ṭāriq: "aṣ-ṣiḥḥa tatalaqqā balāġāt ʿan ʿamaliyyāt ḫitān fī 6 muḥāfaẓāt."
al-maṣrī l-yawm, 2007/08/16. Nāfiʿ, Saʿīd: "'Naǧlā'' tanǧū min al-mawt iṯnāʾ ʿamaliyyat ḫitān fī l-Munyā."
al-maṣrī l-yawm, 2007/08/17a. Fawda, Muḥammad: "niyābat al-Fayūm tuḥaqqiq maʿa ṭabība wa-'dāya' fī 4 waqāʾiʿ ḫitān."

al-maṣrī l-yawm, 2007/08/17b. ʿAbduh, ʿIzz ad-Dīn: "al-bayt baytak.. Mušīra Ḫaṭṭāb: ḥamalāt at-tawaʿʿiyya ḍidd al-ḫitān fī l-ġarbiyya miṯl ʿal-aḏān fī Mālṭā."

al-maṣrī l-yawm, 2007/08/20. Amīn, Ṭāriq: "ʿaṣ-ṣiḥḥaʾ takšif iğrāʾ ʿamaliyyāt ḫitān li-ṯalāṯ banāt fī l-Ġarbiyya."

al-maṣrī l-yawm, 2007/08/23. Amīn, Ṭāriq: "aṣ-ṣiḥḥa tuḥwil ṭabīban wa-dāya wa-ḥallāq ṣiḥḥa ilā n-niyāba li-iğrāʾihim ʿamaliyyāt ḫitān."

al-maṣrī l-yawm, 2007/08/26. Farġalī, Muḥammad: "iḥālat mumarriḍa ilā n-niyāba bi-tuhmat iğrāʾ 10 ʿamaliyyāt ḫitān fī yawm wāḥid."

al-maṣrī l-yawm, 2007/08/27. Muḥammad, Maḥmūd: "taškīl lağna min nuwwāb al-iḫwān wa-l-mustaqillīn li-muwāğahat al-aġlabiyya fī d-dawra al-barlamāniyya al-ğadīda."

al-maṣrī l-yawm, 2007/09/02. al-Ğundī, ʿAbd al-Ḥukm: "zawğ yuğbir zawğatahu ʿalā iğrāʾ ʿamaliyyat ʿḫitānʾ baʿd sana wa-niṣf."

al-maṣrī l-yawm, 2007/09/04a. al-Qaranšāwī, Šīmāʾ: "taʾğīl daʿwā wizārat aṣ-ṣiḥḥa ḍidd Yūsuf al-Badrī ḥawl manʿ al-ḫitān ilā 6 nūfimbir."

al-maṣrī l-yawm, 2007/09/04b. Rašwān, Hudā: "ʿaṣ-ṣiḥḥaʾ tablaġ an-niyāba ʿan dāyat ḫitān as-sayyida al-mutazawwiğa."

al-maṣrī l-yawm, 2007/09/07. Nāfiʿ, Saʿīd: "ḥaṣīlat aġusṭus: ḍabṭ 9 ḥālāt ḫitān ināṯ fī l-Minyā wa-iġlāq 4 ʿiyādāt."

al-maṣrī l-yawm, 2007/09/16. Rašwān, Hudā: "ʿYūnīsīfʾ: waḍʿ ḫitān al-ināṯ fī miṣr mubaššir wa-l-qaḍāʾ ʿalā ẓ-ẓāhira mumkin bi-ḥulūl ʿām 2015."

al-maṣrī l-yawm, 2007/10/11. al-Buḥayrī, Aḥmad: "ʿqaḍīyat raʾy ʿāmm.'"

al-maṣrī l-yawm, 2007/10/14. Nāfiʿ, Saʿīd: "manšūrāt fī l-Minyā: Ṭanṭāwī ḍidd Ṭanṭāwī fī fawāʾid al-bunūk wa-ḫitān al-ināṯ."

al-maṣrī l-yawm, 2007/10/19. al-Ğaʿāra, Saḥr: "ḥilmak yā Šayḫ ʿṬanṭāwī.'"

al-maṣrī l-yawm, 2007/10/28. Rašwān, Hudā: "Mušīra Ḫaṭṭāb: muʾtamar aṭ-ṭifl al-afrīqī yuṭliq ḥamla ğamāʿiyya li-munāhaḍat al-ḫitān fī l-qārra."

al-maṣrī l-yawm, 2007/11/19. Rašwān, Hudā: "wāqiʿat ḫitān drāmiyya fī l-Qalyūbiyya."

al-maṣrī l-yawm, 2007/11/20. Ḫalīl, Muḥammad Maḥmūd: "ad-dawla tuḥārib ḫitān al-ināṯ.. wa-lākinna 77,5% min ahālī al-Qalyūbiyya qālū ʿnaʿm li-l-ḫitān.'"

al-maṣrī l-yawm, 2007/12/13. ʿAlī, Wāʾil: "ḥamla li-daʿm qarār wazīr aṣ-ṣiḥḥa bi-manʿ ḫitān al-ināṯ."

al-maṣrī l-yawm, 2007/12/17. Rašwān, Hudā: ""al-ʿAwā": al-Islām barīʾ min ḫitān al-ināṯ.. wa-r-rasūl lam yaḫtin banātahu."

al-maṣrī l-yawm, 2007/12/19. Ṣalāḥ, Wafāʾ: "Ḫaṭṭāb: as-Saʿūdiyya mahd al-islām lā taʿrif ḫitān al-ināṯ.. wa-miṣr ʿalā qāʾimat al-mumārisīn."

al-maṣrī l-yawm, 2007/12/29. al-Buḥayrī, Aḥmad: "ḫilāf bayn šayḫ al-Azhar wa-mağmaʿ al-buḥūṯ bi-sabab fatwā ʿiğhāḍ al-muġtaṣaba.'"

al-maṣrī l-yawm, 2008/02/01. al-Malīğī, Saḥr: "fatwā iğhāḍ al-muġtaṣaba hal tanquḍuhā min anyāb naẓrat al-muğtamiʿ?."

al-maṣrī l-yawm, 2008/05/16. ʿAbd al-Qādir, Muḥammad: "al-lağna at-tašrīʿiyya bi-ʾš-šaʿbʾ tuwāfiq ʿalā tağrīm al-ḫitān wa-tarfuḍ nasab aṭ-ṭifl li-ummihi."

al-maṣrī l-yawm, 2008/06/08. ʿAbd al-Qādir, Muḥammad: "Surūr yaḥsim ḫilāf ʿal-waṭ anī - al-iḫwān' wa-yuḥīl māddat sinn az-zawāǧ ilā qānūn al-usra."

al-maṣrī l-yawm, 2008/06/13. Ǧumʿa, Maḥmūd: "ǧadl mustamirr bi-šaʾn qānūn aṭ-ṭifl al-ǧadīd bi-miṣr wa-ntiqād li-bunūdihi."

al-maṣrī l-yawm, 2008/06/18. Rašwān, Hudā, and as-Sāʿāʾī, Hudā: "Mubārak yaʿtamid qānūn aṭ-ṭifl al-ǧadīd wa-waraš ʿamal 'sirriyya' li-waḍʿ lāʾiḥatihi at-tanfīḏiyya."

aš-šarq al-awsaṭ, 2007/05/25. Walad Abāh, as-Sayyid: "azmat al-fatwā wa-maʾziq muʾassasat al-iftāʾ."

aš-šarq al-awsaṭ, 2007/07/19. Ḫalīl, Muḥammad: "ǧadal ḥawl mašrūʿiyyat ḫitān al-ināṯ fī miṣr."

aš-šarq al-awsaṭ, 2008/04/24. Ibrāhīm, ʿAbd as-Sattār: "miṣr: al-ǧamāʿa al-islāmiyya tuhāǧim taʿdīlāt qānūn aṭ-ṭifl wa-tuʿtabir ḥaẓr aḍ-ḍarb mustawrad min amrīkā wa-ʾūrūbā."

at-Taṣawwuf al-Islāmī, Rabī I 1428 / March 2007 (No. 339). Ḥasan Ḥusnī: "ʿUlamāʾ ad-dīn wa-ṭ-ṭibb yastankirūna fatwā tarqīʿ... Ratq ġašāʾ al-bakāra yušaǧǧiʿ ʿalā iḫtilāṭ al-ansāb wa-ntišār ar-raḏīla"

Atighetchi, Dariusch. *Islamic Bioethics. Problems and Perspectives*. N.p.: Springer, 2007.

baheyya, 2005/09/03. "Be It Resolved." #http://baheyya.blogspot.com/2005_09_01_archive.html

BBC News 2008, April 18. "Country Profile. Egypt". <http://news.bbc.co.uk/2/hi/middle_east/country_profiles/737642.stm >.

Dār al-Iftāʾ. "Fiqh al-Marʾa: Ḫitān al-Ināṯ" <http://www.dar-alifta.org/ViewWoman.aspx?ID=15 >.

Davis, Ronald M. et al. "Female Genital Mutilation. Council on Scientific Affairs, American Medical Association," *Journal of the American Medical Association*, (Vol. 274), 21 (1995): 1714–1716.

Eich, Thomas: "A tiny membrane defending 'us' against 'them': Arabic Internet debate about hymenorraphy in Sunni Islamic law," *Culture, Health & Sexuality* (Vol. 12), 7 (2010): 755–769.

Ercevik Amado, Liz: "Sexual and Bodily Rights as Human Rights in the Middle East and North Africa," *Reproductive Health Matters* (Vol. 12), 23 (2004): 125–128.

Ǧād al-Ḥaqq, Ǧād al-Ḥaqq ʿAlī. "Al-Mawḍūʿ (1202) Ḫitān Al-Ināṯ" Dār Al-Iftāʾ 29 January 1981. <http://www.dar-alifta.org/ViewFatwa.aspx?ID=709&CatID=118&Type=Ency >.

Gamble, A: "Stopping Female Genital Mutilation. An Update," *Freedom Review* (Vol. 26), 5 (1995): 22–23.

Hamdy, Sherine: *Our Bodies belong to God: Islam, Medical Science, and Ethical Reasoning in Egyptian Life*. Unpubl. PhD, New York University 2006.

Huntington, Dale: "Moving From Research to Program. the Egyptian Postabortion Care Initiative," *International Family Planning Perspectives* (Vol. 29), 3 (2003).

islamonline, 2006/11/17. Abū Bakr, Ḫālid: "wazīr aṯ-ṯaqāfa al-miṣrī: al-ḥiǧāb ʿawda li-l-warāʾ."

islamonline, 2007/08/08. "bi-masīhiyyatihi, miṣr murtadd ʿalā iʿtirāf rasmī."

Kienle, Eberhard: *A Grand Delusion. Democracy and Economic Reform in Egypt,* London, New York 2000.

Lee Bowen, Donna: "Abortion, Islam, and the 1994 Cairo Population Conference," *International Journal of Middle East Studies,* (Vol. 29), 2 (1997): 161–84.

ibidem: "Contemporary Muslim Ethics of Abortion." *Islamic Ethics of Life. Abortion, War, and Euthanasia.* Ed. Jonathan E Brockop. University of South Carolina, 2003. 51–80.

Lynch, Marc: "Blogging the New Arab Public," *Arab Media and Society* (2007). <http://www.arabmediasociety.com/?article=10>

MOHP 2007. "Mahāmm al-wizāra". <http://www.mohp.gov.eg/Sec/About/Mission.asp?x=1>.

Moustafa, Tamir: "Conflict and Cooperation Between State and Religious Institutions in Contemporary Egypt," *International Journal of Middle East Studies* (Vol. 32), 1 (2000): 3–22.

NCCM 2005a. "al-Haykal ar-raʾīsī". *al-mağlis al-qawmī li-ṭ-ṭufūla wa-l-umūma.* <http://www.nccm.org.eg/Default.aspx?culture=ar&tabId=91&key=view#magles1>.

NCCM 2005b. "al-Mağlis al-qawmī li-ṭ- ṭufūla wa-l-umūma." *al-mağlis al-qawmī li-ṭ-ṭufūla wa-l-umūma.* <http://www.nccm.org.eg/Default.aspx?TabID=51&culture=ar>.

NCCM 2005c. "Ahdāf al-mağlis." <#http://www.nccm.org.eg/Default.aspx?TabID=92&culture=ar>.

NZZ Online, 2008/07/04. "Zweijährige im Zürcher Oberland beschnitten. Eltern der Anstiftung zur schweren Körperverletzung angeklagt."

Pintak, Lawrence: "Reporting a revolution: the changing Arab media landscape." *Arab Media & Society* (2007). <http://www.arabmediasociety.com/?article=23>

Roberts, Hannah: "Reconstructing virginity in Guatemala," *The Lancet,* 2006 (Vol. 367), p. 1227f.

Rūz al-Yūsif, 2007/06/16 (No. 4123) a. Muğāhid, Ṣubḥī: "ḫarīṭat al-ittifāq wa-l-iḫtlāf bayna ṯālūṯ as-sulṭa ad-dīniyya.", pp. 25–27.

Rūz al-Yūsif, 2007/06/16 (No. 4123) b. Luṭfī, Wāʾil: "ṣirāʿ al-ʿulamāʾ wa-l-addʿiyāʾ wa-l-umarāʾ ʿalā ğumhūr al-fatāwā fī miṣr.", pp. 28–31.

Rūz al-Yūsif, 2007/06/16 (No. 4123) c. Bāšā, Aḥmad: "mağmaʿ tašrīd al-muslimīn", pp. 83–86.

Rūz al-Yūsif, 2007/11/16 (No. 4144). al-Miṣrī, Hudā / Asmā Naṣṣār: "yaḥduṯ fī z-Zaqāzīq wa-Kafr aš-Šaiḫ wa-ğamīʿ mudun ad-Diltā: mumarriḍāt yartadinna an-niqāb bi-š-šakl ğamāʿī.", pp. 18–25.

Rūz al-Yūsif, 2007/11/23 (No. 4145) a. al-Miṣrī, Hudā / Asmā Naṣṣār: „*Rūz al-Yūsif* tutābiʿ rudūd al-fiʿl fī š-Šarqīya wa Kafr aš-Šaiḫ. al-aṭibbāʾ multaḥūn wa-ṭ-ṭabībāt wa-l-mumarriḍāt ‚munaqqabāt' wa-ḥulmuhum: an nuṣbiḥ miṯl Īrān!!", pp. 22–27.

Rūz al-Yūsif, 2007/11/23 (No. 4145) b. Ḥamdī, Zainab: "qillat ʿadad al-mumarriḍāt al-muḍarribāt aqwā aurāq aḍ-ḍuġūṭ ʿalayhā – wizārat aṣ-ṣiḥḥa tantaẓir ġaṭāʾan dīnīyan li-taṭbīq al-qānūn!", pp. 28–31.

Rūz al-Yūsif, 2007/12/01 (No. 4147) a. "ḥamlat Rūz al-Yūsif taḥawwalat li-ʿāṣifa fikrīya wa siyāsīya – istiqālat wazīr... wa šuǧāʿat wazīr wa intihāziyyat naqīb.", pp. 20–24.

Rūz al-Yūsif, 2007/12/01 (No. 4147) b. Naṣṣār, Asmā: "Inna hazīmat al-Yahūd lan taʾtī illā bi-ntiqāb al-marʾa wa ǧulūsihā fī-l-bayt: al-Huwainī: al-liḥya wa-n-niqāb li-inqāḏ al-umma... wa taʿaddud az-zawǧāt wa-l-ḫitān farīda wāǧiba", pp. 28–31.

Seif El Dawla, Aida: "The Political and Legal Struggle Over Female Genital Mutilation in Egypt. Five Years Since the ICPD," *Reproductive Health Matters* (Vol. 7), 13 (1999): 128–136.

Skovgaard-Petersen, Jakob, *Defining Islam for the Egyptian State. Muftīs and Fatwas of the Dâr al-Iftâ*, Leiden et al. (Brill) 1997.

Walker, Christopher: "Abortions Are Illegal and Common in Egypt," *Women's Enews*, 4 December 2004.

WHO study group on female genital mutilation and obstetric outcome, et al: "Female Genital Mutilation and Obstetric Outcome: WHO Collaborative Prospective Study in Six African Countries," The Lancet (Vol. 367), 9525 (2006): 1835–1841.

IV

BIOETHICS AS A BATTLEGROUND FOR RELIGIOUS AND POLITICAL "CULTURE WARS"

The Politics of Bioethics

14 BIOETHICS IN AUSTRALIA

ON POLITICS, POWER, AND THE RISE OF THE CHRISTIAN RIGHT

Rob Irvine, Ian Kerridge, and Paul Komesaroff

Bioethics in Australia has an ambivalent genealogy that is steeped in controversy, conflict, and struggle in the social world. This chapter provides a brief analysis of bioethics as an effect of the collision of different and parallel processes of biotechnological innovation, power/knowledge, and resistance in a competition for influence in society. Our more specific aim is to examine critically the recent rise of a conservative religious formation, the Christian Right, and the marriage of religion, science, and critique in a politics of bioethics.

Our analysis draws from the sociological work of Sheila Jasanoff (2005) and Robert Entman (1993), who in turn have been influenced by Irving Goffman (1975) and his notion of the frame. Laying the foundations for our exploration, Entman provided the following definition of the frame: "[T]o frame is to select some aspects of a perceived reality and make them more salient in communicating text, in such a way as to promote a particular problem definition, causal interpretation, moral evaluation, and/or treatment recommendation" (Entman, 1993: 52). In other words, frames are hermeneutic devices that operate on existing discourses to enforce meanings, or narrow the range of available interpretations.

The Advent of Bioethics in Australia

The beginning of bioethics as a discipline in Australia is marked by two epistemological breaks away from well-established biomedical technologies and traditional approaches to ethics. The first break centered on biotechnological innovation. Of the multitude of developments that come into existence, some innovations are conferred special cultural and social significance. In 1980, the birth of the first child in Australia conceived by in vitro fertilization (IVF) was immediately caught up in a network of significations that set the terms for bioethics to be considered. In the politico-moral struggle that unfolded over "making life in a test tube," medicine's expanded power of intervention was represented in professional and popular media as a transgressive power that moved human life and society toward, and pushed it over, various limits (Charlesworth, 1985: 95; Khuse, 1982: 30–31; Kirby, 1980: 19; Singer & Wells, 1984; Waller, 1987). It was said that IVF threatened to reconstruct taken-for-granted ways of being, and how we interact as social and moral agents. It commodified human life and threatened to alter the constitution of societies (Connolly, 1982; Gunn, 1982; Overduin & Fleming, 1982).

Unlike some accounts that emphasize continuity between traditional medical ethics and the emergence of bioethics as an historical "event" (Jonsen, 1990; Pellegrino, 2000), the second break moved bioethics away from traditional ethics. From a critical philosophical perspective, conventional moral frameworks and vocabularies failed to come to terms with fast-changing biotechnological innovation. Max Charlesworth, a leading participant in the bioethics project, provides a succinct view of the two breaks:

> The new forms of biotechnology . . . all promise great human benefits. At the same time they raise formidable ethical and social problems of which there is no precedent. Our ordinary ethical and social and legal principles and categories simply can't cope with the novel issues raised by the manufacture of totally new living organisms by genetic engineering, the creation of live human embryos outside their mothers' bodies by in vitro fertilization . . .the new situations brought about by . . .the freezing of embryos, and so on, are difficult to fit under our ordinary ethical and legal principles. (Charlesworth, 1989: 15, 16).

In the first issue of the *Monash Bioethics Review,* published in 1981, Helga Khuse contended that advances in biomedicine challenged more or less fixed versions of ethics that were based on acculturation or in the command of God:

> [A] new field of philosophical inquiry born out of our being confronted by revolutionary developments in the biomedical sciences. These developments . . .present us with problems that challenge our traditional ethical frameworks and force us to rethink all the basic problems of morality (Kuhse, 1998, 1; also see Kuhse, 1982).

These reconfigured notions of biotechnology and morality opened a discursive space for alternative forms of inquiry, thought, and normative order-bioethics. Against a backdrop of deconstruction and rupture, the foundation of Monash Centre for Human Bioethics (MCHB) at Monash University in Melbourne, in 1980, marked the start of institutional bioethics in Australia (Arts Monash, 2005; Swan, 1983; Walters & Singer, 1982; Walters, 1991).

However, any account that explains the rise of bioethics as an adaptive response to the ethical issues raised by biotechnological innovation presents a picture that is misleadingly simple. The take-off of bioethics in Australia overlapped a period when the dominance of the medical profession was challenged, and medical scientists and their institutions were under significant stress. The central image narrative was of unrestrained and unregulated scientific objectification that threatened to plunge society into a frightening future (Connolly, 1982; Gunn, 1982:73; Hepburn, 1992; Overduin & Fleming, 1982).

While a host of local movements—feminist, patient's rights, consumerist—challenged the authority of medical science and the power of a male-dominated medical profession over patients (Bates, 1979; Bates & Lapsley, 1985; Taylor, 1979) it was the socio-moral criticism articulated by religious authorities that Australian philosophers and scientists seemed to take most seriously (Charlesworth, 1989; Kuhse & Singer, 1985; Singer & Wells, 1984:173–175; Singer & Kuhse, 2006:9). The opposition to IVF of the Victorian Catholic Bishops, and their sociopolitical cachet, acted as a key driver in setting up the MCHB (Kuhse & Singer, 1985; Kuhse, 1998; Singer & Dawson, 1992:76; Singer & Wells, 1984; Singer & Kuhse, 2006:9).

Bioethics seemed to offer a counterpoint to the normalizing forces that demanded the absolute prohibition of IVF (Charlesworth, 1989: 20, 131; Kuhse & Singer, 1985:65; Kuhse, 1998; Singer & Dawson, 1992:76; Singer & Wells, 1984; Singer & Kuhse, 2006:9). To arrive at solutions to the ethical questions posed by medicine and the biological sciences, the new discipline emphasized rational, clear, and "correct" reasoning rather than inherited custom. Its key social and epistemological functions included: introducing new patterns of reasoning to decision makers; examining the meanings of biotechnological change from a philosophical perspective; and clarifying the problems, risks, and moral effects of new biotechnologies and modern medical practice.

The establishment of MCHB as a center of excellence and prototypical research institution had a profound effect on the development of bioethics. It was regarded in some quarters as a direct threat to the moral leadership of the Christian churches in matters of social, cultural, and moral politics in health (Connolly, 1982:58; Hogan, 1987:257; Overduin & Fleming, 1982; Pell, 1995; Preece, 2002; Wierzbicka, 1997). Historically, Christian groups, especially the Catholic Church, occupied a strategic position in policy making and society. The provision and administration of services in the private and public health sectors by Christian groups provided them with a general source of power and influence in the marketplace of ideas and values. Federal and state governments also assisted religious thinkers and their institutions to secure privileged places on consultative committees, law reform commissions, and committees of inquiry concerned with the ethical aspects of medical practice and medical objects.

It is then unremarkable that throughout the 1980s and 1990s, centers of theological and religious bioethics were established. The Queensland Bioethics Centre was established in 1981. Continuing debates over IVF indirectly led to the establishment of the L.J. Goody Bioethics Centre in 1985, and the Southern Cross Bioethics Institute in 1987. Money and resources were concentrated at universities, speeding up the process of instantiating bioethics as an academic discipline. The growth of academic activity was fueled mostly by expenditures that provided fellowships, as well as research grants.

Bioethics Today

By the end of the second decade, bioethics in Australia was conspicuous as a discipline in academia and the public realm. Its centers offered courses and graduate programs on bioethics. Bioethics discourse covered a broad range of issues in healthcare organization, human experimentation and clinical practice, patient/practitioner interaction, patient expectations and choice, and responses to acute and chronic diseases. In the 1990s, the discourse expanded into patients' rights, new surgical techniques, the commodification of human life, and the organization and authority of relationships between healthcare professionals.

Initially, bioethics was framed as a specialization of philosophical, legal, and theological labor (Kirby, 1980; Kuhse & Singer, 1985). Today, these disciplinary frameworks must be viewed as partial elements in what has become a "multiperspectival" discipline. Its intellectually and professionally qualified staff is drawn from different knowledge cultures—medical, nursing, the humanities, social and behavioral sciences—informed by a range of theoretical frameworks, methods of inquiry, and value commitments alongside generalized standards of judgment.

Bioethics has been widely marketed throughout the academic and practitioner communities. Across the bioethical literature, in various expressions of bioethical theory and practice, bioethicists are posited as being both "interpreters" and "legislators" (Bauman, 1987). In a period where there are many competing value systems, beliefs, and cultural standards, bioethicists as interpreters examine the meaning of biotechnologies that reconstruct taken-for-granted ways of being from a cultural perspective, chiefly through discourse and applied theory. They generate public awareness of the ethical, legal, social, philosophical and other allied issues at stake in biotechnology, health care, medical practice and the biological sciences; develop and document areas of consensus; and assist experts and laypersons to reach ethical judgments that are rational, defensible, and politically acceptable to Australian society (Singer & Kuhse, 2006).

Bioethicists in their manifold contacts with the social body also act as "legislators." They pass judgments and make authoritative statements that arbitrate or mediate in controversies of opinions. They select those opinions which, "having been selected, [may] become correct and binding" (Bauman 1987:4). An eclectic and powerful enterprise, bioethics discourse often seeks to influence the way people and governments engage with, and speak about, biotechnologies and medicine. The act of legislating, particularly in the realm of public bioethics, may involve the active justification of a concrete set of demands, or articulating a concrete political or legal program with the aim of resolving difficult biotechnological and clinical issues. It may involve the mobilization or promotion of ideals and values to motivate action, and condition what is permitted and what is excluded technologically and behaviorally. It may also involve the discursive legitimation for standards of truth and law, goodness, and correct behavior.

Such views of bioethicists and the bioethical enterprise represent alternative outlooks, perspectives or emphases which co-exist and often compete in the complex system of bioethical belief and evaluation.

The Politics of Bioethics

We need to ask how bioethics in Australia might be different from other countries. For our purposes, three features are especially relevant. The first, as we have noted above, is the central fact of religious discourse in bioethical thought and practice. The second is the attention given in public affairs and academic discourse to "beginning of life" and reproduction issues and dilemmas. The third feature is the deep imbrication of bioethics in politics.

While bioethics discourse in Australia covers a broad range of topics, a number of Australian bioethicists have drawn attention to the intensity and consistency of debates over beginning-of-life and reproduction issues, to differentiate Australian bioethics from other countries (Ankeny, 2003:242; Singer & Wells, 1984; Lohan, 2005; Singer & Kuhse, 2006; Warhurst, 1983). In the 1990s, the regulation of the abortifacient RU486, late termination of pregnancy, and euthanasia legislation were the focus of national debate; at the start of the twenty-first century, human embryonic stem cell research (hESC) is a recent iteration of a key bioethical problematic. These issues reach beyond the realm of academic debate, to constitute an interface between academic and public bioethical discourse. Moreover, such issues are seldom finally resolved. Rather, they tend to form intractable public controversies that are lasting. For example, IVF reemerged at the beginning of the twenty-first century in political and public discourse, agitating public opinion and resisting any attempts to achieve normative consensus resolution. The preoccupation in recent debates in Victoria has been over who has access to the technology.

At no time in its history has bioethics been above the heat of political struggle, or outside the political field of power and influence. Many bioethical issues and dilemmas are manifestly political, and even those that are not may have political effects. The politics we have in mind is fourfold: First, following Weber (1970:94–99) bioethics is a "political mode of discourse" when one views politics as a public struggle for discursive hegemony. Bioethicists vie for dominance by securing support for their particular method of inquiry, theoretical orientation, or definition of reality as the best or most legitimate knowledge.

Second, contrary to the experience of countries like the United States, where bioethicists have expressed strong misgivings over the apparent "politicization" of bioethics (Kahn, 2006; Pelligrino, 2000), in Australia, some of its key institutions purposefully moved the bioethics discourse beyond philosophical or theological inquiry by connecting bioethics democratically to political activity. The Australasian Association of Bioethics & Health Law (formerly the Australasian Bioethics Association) purposefully encouraged its members to take up definite political projects and advance moral/political discourses within the organization (AABHL, 2010).

Third, bioethics functions socially and politically as a field or arena of intense conflict, struggle, and activity for certain "interests." With the support of some key institutions, Australian bioethicists have espoused overtly political preferences and positions of a critical type. For example, linking ethical awareness with political conviction and social activism, bioethicists in Australia—and New Zealand—formally and publicly challenged the Howard federal government's policies on the detention of refugees (Silove et al., 2001; Steel & Silove, 2004; Zion, 2007). These various characteristics make the tight interweaving of political and bioethical discourse understandable, if not inevitable.

The Changing Field of Bioethics

A recent development in bioethics as a political field is the expanding role of a loose alliance of conservative social groupings, which has become known as the "Christian Right" (CR; see Lohrey, 2006; Maddox, 2005; Warhurst, 2004). In academic and public bioethics, the CR has the resources and will to bear in upon and shape bioethical discussion in the marketplace of ideas. One of the major outcomes of the advent of the CR as a sociopolitical force has been the *amplification* of religious doctrines in bioethics discussions. How CR discourse has manifested itself at the level of the actual bioethics debates is the subject of the rest of this chapter. Persuaded that hESC is an exemplary case that is productive of knowledge, our aim is to provide an account of the range of discursive strategies that the CR employed to anathemize human embryonic stem cell research (hESC) and to vilify its advocates and secular bioethics. More specifically, using frame analysis, we examine the CR's appropriation and use of a selected stock of biomedical and biotechnological discursive materials, in a competition for political influence in bioethical discussion and debate.

The Australian Christian Right

Before proceeding further, some clarification of the term "Christian Right" is necessary. We define it here to refer to an assemblage of individuals, organizations, institutions, splinter and lobby groups, that independently or together engage in public debate and social and political activism in support of public policies they claim to be representative of an authentic Christian viewpoint. In Australia, the CR includes, among others, the Australian Christian Lobby, the Festival of Light, right-to-life organizations, and the Family First Party. There is considerable political support for the moral and sociopolitical agenda of the CR within state and federal governments in Australia (Bouma, 2006; Lohrey, 2006; Maddox, 2005; Warhurst, 2006:5–6). Its "leadership" is formed of a diverse range of prominent public intellectuals, academics, lawyers, theologians, religious leaders, politicians, and journalists—often vying with one another for resources, ideological authority, and influence, prestige, and power (Benford, 1993:681; Wiktorowicz, 2004; Zald & McCarthy, 1987).

The CR is loosely of "the right" in the sociocultural and political senses of the term, referring to a general conservatism both with respect to the prevailing political culture and contemporary Christian worldviews (see Pell, 1995). Views taken by members typically include: the defense and maintenance of "traditional Christian values"; the defense of the authority of the Bible in all areas of life; the necessity of faith in Jesus; and a general emphasis on moral absolutes and teaching. The concept of "sanctity of life" is amplified, elevated, and presumed basic, as one of the most idealized values. Importantly, the set of beliefs common to the CR are not promoted as something that applies only to persons of the Christian faith, but are prescribed as universally valid. As the Australian Christian Lobby (ACL), which often positions itself as centrist, states on its web page: "The vision of the ACL is to see Christian principles and ethics accepted and influencing the way we are governed, do business, and relate to each other as a community" (ACL, 2008).

From its emergence in the 1970s, the CR has argued that systematic social forces have successfully upset the established order, trivializing traditional values that properly warrant public reflection:

> Most Australians, and certainly all Christians, have simply had enough of the increasingly rapid erosion of traditional family values and ethics in Australia . . . [W]e see Australia failing to achieve that potential in the very values on which it is predicated are not upheld. We believe that our success as a nation and a community to date, is largely due to our strong Christian heritage (ACL, 2008; also see Pell, 1995).

The assemblage finds motivation in this embattled sense that religious values are under siege from both secular interests and liberal ideology:

> However, this heritage and or values are currently being eroded by self-serving interest groups who have achieved unwarranted political influence, largely because of our silence. The ACL aims to break that silence. After all, Christ calls us to be salt and light (ACL, 2008).

Protecting society and people against what they see as the arrogance of those who believe in the primacy of science, success is measured by its ability to obstruct or hold back the expansion of research norms at the national and state level. Confrontationalist in its methods, the CR is interested not simply in what is included on public policy agendas, but in what is not included in policy outcomes to restore social (Christian) order.

Framing Bioethical Politics in Australian Culture

The CR often adopts a standpoint of overview, and presents itself as speaking for the public interest when it asserts some generalized sense of the wrongness of some biotechnology, medical procedure, or patient–health professional relationship. Yet, to have any impact on society and biopolitics, it must be cognizant of the public perspectives regarding biotechnology, medicine, and science. In this regard, it is important to note the public attitude studies conducted since 1999 by Biotechnology Australia into the way Australian publics view health and medical applications of biotechnology. Over this period, public support for the use of embryonic stem cells to conduct medical research has risen, from 53% in 2002 to 59% in 2003. In 2005, the moral acceptability of using stem cells, including embryonic stem cells, to conduct medical research was accepted by 80%. By 2007, support for these applications had increased to 92%. In 2005, 60%

of respondents felt that biotechnology would improve our way of life in the future. By 2007, this figure had risen to 68% (Biotechnology Australia, 2007).

In pluralist Australia, deeply held religious beliefs may be of great importance for both individuals and communities, but allegiance to such beliefs does not necessarily grant the discourse power and legitimacy. In bioethical politics, oppositional discourses that are framed in the language of pre-given religious injunctions, and then applied to publics that do not share or accept similar beliefs and values, might be denied the support of the community at large (ABC Radio National, 2006c; Brennon, 2006:2; Coady, 2002; Oakley, 2002; Perry, 2000). Bioethical frameworks and policies have to be "sold" to have a political effect in a specific political context (Finlayson, 2004:535). Adroit handling and control of public meaning, through the use of suitably legitimate vocabularies, is politically important to success in bioethical conflicts.

In apparent recognition that it stood in need of some other authority besides its own testimony, between 2002 and 2007 the CR shifted the register of its rhetoric away from finite constructions exclusively grounded on religious discourse, as it is commonly represented in the "culture wars" literature, toward a more ontologically mobile rhetoric. Science and biotechnology provided the CR with the authoritative language needed to negotiate the marketplace of ideas. In the following sections, we trace the enrollment of science and biotechnology into religious discourses in the struggle for supremacy in public communication and public policy.

We identified two basic framing strategies relevant to the reordering of scientific discourse. The first relates to a substantive biological science frame. To reach the widest possible audience within what was a continuously developing politico-moral project, the CR drew heavily from adult stem cell research and other nondestructive methods. The scientific discourse used by the CR framed nondestructive techniques as providing universally beneficial outcomes that embodied all of the "potential" benefits of hESC research. The second strategy may be called the "science/moral consequences frame." This frame was formed in public discourse from a complex of religious, scientific, and cultural ideas about hESC research and its underlying objectives.

Substantive Science Frames

While the aim of science is to extend knowledge and understanding of the sorts of things that are possible in the world, and how and why they are, the "truth" of biotechnological innovation often remains fragile, unstable, and contingent. In his book, *French DNA: trouble in purgatory*, Paul Rabinow (1999:9) argues that while biotechnology introduces new, concrete practices and ideas into social life, it actually occupies a space of profound epistemological, ontological, and biopolitical uncertainty. Biotechnologies are too complex, the variables too many, and the outcomes too uncertain for social actors to know with certainty what they should do. He labels this dimension the "purgatory zone": a space between heaven and hell where biotechnologies—ambiguous and transitional—are constitutively open and subject to contestation (Rabinow, 1999; Rabinow & Dan-Cohen, 2005; also see Jasanoff, 2005).

Now, as a form of human knowledge, biotechnologies are plastic enough to be adapted to wide-ranging appropriations, translations, attributions, and reconfigurations of meaning that fit the local needs of the parties employing it.

Recognizing the underdetermined character of stem cell research generally, the CR seized upon the comparative uncertainly and ambiguity that surrounded hESC, and created a new interpretive frame with which to conceive of, represent, think about, and ask questions about hESC. In the public discourse, the uncertainty that surrounded hESC research was reframed as evidence of its failure as science, and as a field of medical endeavor (Australian Catholic Bishops Conference, 2006; Australian Federation of Right to Life Associations, 2006; Caroline Chisholm Centre for Ethics Inc, 2006; Southern Cross Bioethics Centre, 2006). For example, in its submission to the Lockhart Review (2006), the Coalition for the Defence of Human Life wrote:

> Claims of imminent cures have been sharply moderated. Words such as *hype*, used in 2002 only by opponents of embryonic research, are in 2005 increasingly used by supporters (Lord Winston, reported on September 5, 2005, is only the most recent to warn against inflated claims). We are now being told that developing clinical applications may take ten years (which, in a field like this, is equivalent to saying that no one knows how long it will take). (Coalition for the Defence of Human Life, 2006)

CR discourses also appropriated and played off one scientific power against another, to construct a particular conception of hESC. In direct contrast to approaches taken by hESC advocates and supporters, who consistently recognized both the validity of adult stem cell research and the important uncertainties regarding the biological and therapeutic characteristics of different types of stem cells, the CR consistently drew an important distinction between adult stem cells derived from blood, bone marrow, fat, and other tissues, and embryonic stem cells derived from discarded IVF cultures, aborted fetuses, or embryos created in a laboratory. Purported positive empirical results from the work undertaken by reputable adult stem cell researchers was counterpoised to the lack of success of hESC research; particularly its apparent failure to satisfy basic requirements of science (such as "proof of concept"), or provide evidence of therapeutic benefit.

These frames took the form of a "dividing practice" (Foucault, 1980). Distinctions were drawn between the supposedly productive nature of nondestructive stem cell research, and the unproductive results from hESC research. This provided opponents with a vehicle for opposition that framed hESC as simultaneously unnecessary on empirical grounds, and contrary to accepted research principles—and, therefore, impossible to justify.

Frames also have the important quality of closing down discursive space by setting limits on what it is possible to debate, to think, to believe, or to see. Various protagonists attempted to stop debate before it began. Or, they interceded to bring debate to a halt after it had started. For example, the West Australian Bishop threatened Catholic Parliamentarians who voted in favor of hESC with excommunication. Within the federal government, the campaign against hESC research was led by Tony Abbott, then Minister for Health. At an early stage in the process, Abbott attempted to close down debate over hESC and pre-commit Australia irrevocably to a binding set of rules that would prohibit such research. Exaggerating the already elastic adult stem cell research, Abbott observed:

> [If] you actually look at what's been happening, in terms of research leading to medical advances, it seems that adult stem cell research is very much more effective in giving us potential cures, than embryonic stem-cell research and these new human cloning possibilities that people suddenly seem to be wanting us to explore (ABC, 2006a and 2006b).

Similarly, in its submission to the Tasmanian Government's review of the Human Embryonic Research Regulation Act 2003 and the Human Cloning and Other Prohibited Practices Act 2003, the Australian Christian Lobby argued:

> Given that overwhelming numbers of scientific breakthroughs are coming from adult stem cells, it could be argued that it seems pointless for the research on excess embryos to continue. This is especially true considering that there are large hurdles that need to be overcome before embryonic stem cell therapy will actually benefit patients. For instance, researchers have only recently noted that embryonic "stem cells cultured for long periods in the lab develop genetic changes in areas known to be involved in human cancers."

While the clinical benefits of adult stem cell research outside of the haemato-oncology setting were largely unproven, this did not stop the CR from integrating this technology into policy discourses that justified prohibition of hESC research. The ACL concluded:

> Adult stem cell research should continue to be supported, pursued, and funded by the Tasmanian government. All the Lockhart review recommendations regarding further liberalization of the current laws concerning embryonic stem cell research, such as therapeutic cloning, creation of embryos by any means for the purposes of research and experimentation, etc., should be opposed (Australian Christian Lobby, 2006b).

These discourses set the parameters within which the decision is to be: nothing outside the frame of adult stem cell research was to be considered morally legitimate now or in the future:

Furthermore, given recent developments, a strong case could be mounted that even the clauses permitting use of excess ART embryos should be repealed (Australian Christian Lobby, 2006b).

The mobilization of the science discourse was positive and productive on a number of levels. The CR's position was framed so that it appeared as neither anti-science nor anti-progress. Drawing attention to the strengths of biotechnology also created space to make connections with a wider constituency on the basis not of morality, but of a common interest in curing disease. For example, in a media statement, Archbishop Pell stated:

> All of us wish to find cures and treatments for disease or genetic conditions. Many Australians are afflicted by terrible suffering and we share their hope for effective treatments. The Catholic Church of NSW, through grants and through its hospitals and research institutes, is a promoter of ethical stem-cell research on adult and umbilical stem cells (Pell, 4/06/07).

Two features of the Archbishop's rhetoric deserve comment. First, the social and political distance between selected components of religious doctrine are aligned with the practices of biological sciences. Second, a connection is made between anti-hESC rhetoric and the immediate life situations of those who live with disability. Critics of the CR's exclusionary discourse, including Christian critics, have observed that it seems to ask those who live with acquired and inherited disability to forgo what, in the long run, may be in their own best interests for the sake of principles they do not hold (Brock, 2006 and 2007). The text therefore demonstrates concern for the living, rather than indifference to the suffering of others for the sake of principle, as critics had charged (Brock, 2007).

Examination of the texts and utterances of the CR further demonstrate the way in which the CR carefully selected, appropriated, and reworked scientific data so that they could be safely integrated within a conservative Christian worldview and doctrinal interests (ABC, 2006b; Australian Catholic Bishops Conference, 2006; Australian Christian Lobby, 2006 and 2006a; Caroline Chisholm Centre for Health Ethics Inc, 2006; Do No Harm, 2006; Festival of Light, 2006:3–4; Family Life International, 2006; Pro-Life Victoria, 2006; Pell, 2007; Right to Life Australia Inc, 2006; Santamaria, 2006; Shanahan, 2006:41; Southern Cross Bioethics Centre, 2006).

To summarize, in opposing hESC, the CR appealed to the "persuasible" evidence of science to advance the cause of opposition. References to adult stem cell research conveyed to potential supporters, other members of the CR, and adversaries, the reasonableness and well-foundedness of its claims, actions, and practices against hESC research (Weber, 1967). This potent master frame did not replace older moral discourses based on religious faith. Rather, it served to strengthen them. The rhetorics of science and medicine were reworked as a rhetoric of faith, and the authority of science reframed as supporting the authority of the "church."

The Science/Moral Consequences Frame

Of course, the oppositional rhetoric of the CR contained overt public moral components. For example, the CR directly attacked the moral foundation of "rival" hESC research, and questioned whether it is right or just or ethically defensible to use hESC in pursuit of scientific knowledge, biomedical technique, or medical benefit. The reasoning processes and personal histories of individual researchers formed a central part of this attack. In his address upon receiving the "Mysterium Vitae" Grand Prix Award from the Archdiocese of Seoul for his pro-life work, Cardinal Pell observed:

> I am encouraged by the work of the Japanese scientist Shinya Yamanaka, which involves the reprogramming of human skin cells back to pluripotent stem cells. These cells have all the therapeutic and research potential of pluripotent stem cells derived from human embryos without any of the ethical problems associated with the cloning and killing of human embryos (Pell, 2008).

In this passage, the commitment of the research scientist in the laboratory is invoked as raw material to resolve both conceptual and moral problems. Later in his address, Pell observed:

> But what interested me most about Dr. Yamanaka was the revelation that it was ethical qualms about destructive embryo research that moved him to work on reprogramming, and how these developed in the first place. In an interview with the *New York Times*, Dr. Yamanaka, a father of two,

> recalled a day eight years ago when he peered through a microscope at a friend's IVF clinic. 'When I saw the embryo', he said, 'I suddenly realized there was such a small difference between it and my daughters.... I thought, we can't keep destroying embryos for our research. There must be another way' (Pell, 2008).

There are two patterns of orientation in this discussion that are important. First, the tacit, taken-for-granted knowledge within which hESC researchers routinely comprehend or assimilate the phenomenal world of research is rendered problematic and in need of repair. Second, there is a powerful endorsement of rational self-inspection as a source of dependable moral and technical evaluation, knowledge, and understanding. As a working scientist, Shinya Yamanaka conferred legitimacy to anti-hESC rhetoric. He is brought into the frame as a moral exemplar: the "good scientists" as self-conscious carriers of "good science" and family life. Through the personage of the "good scientist," science and values were framed not in opposition to religious values, but deeply consistent with them. The scientist monitored and conducted "himself" according to accepted cultural norms. This discourse closed the gap between a scientific worldview grounded upon reason, and a putative moral responsibility to the embryo.

Culture Wars

Science is often set against religion in bioethical accounts of resistance (Dodds & Ankeny, 2006:104; Kasimba & Singer, 1989; Oakley, 2002; Siebers, 2003; Skene & Parker, 2002; Savulescu, 2000). This dualism is especially marked in debates that are configured as the "culture wars" (Callaghan 2005:424–425). Such dualist structures may not be adequate to an understanding of the strategies that the CR used to construct opposition to hESC and medical practice. Nor do they help us appreciate the ways in which discourses and ideas move from one domain (the laboratory, the clinic) into politics.

While religious belief sustained and drove the social and political commitments of the CR (Brennan, 2007:3; Hall, 2004), it is important to note that in the majority of documents we reviewed there was no evidence that religious discourses, techniques, and practices alone provided the sole public vehicle for its resistance to hESC. Nor was scientific discourse ranged directly against religion. Notwithstanding the CRs unforgiving view of hESC, the CR appropriated the critical tools of scientific discourse and research, making them an instrument of power. In a series of strategic maneuvers, science and religion dissolved into one another to form new frames that superseded earlier religious critiques of biotechnology, without disregarding its own foundational position.

There are many other frames that served the rhetorical hermeneutics of the CR in its strategic attempts to motivate political opposition to hESC. We identified three lines of attack: "frame debunking"—casting doubt on the validity or accuracy of competing hESC discourses by making them appear untrustworthy or wrong; "frame discrediting"—attacking the honesty and integrity of rivals and vilifying opponents; and "frame transgression"—framing hESC research as a threat to human identity and social relations. Each of these frames sought to subvert the authority,both social and moral, of hESC advocates in the eyes of fellow activists and publics. Given the scope of the issues at hand, and the limitations of space, we are preempted from doing more than drawing attention to these additional frames that are relevant here.

Conclusion

What general conclusions about the present condition of bioethics in Australia can be drawn from this analysis? We understand bioethics in Australia to be a dynamic and conflicted historical object. The discipline came into existence during a period of sociocultural transformation, when social and moral issues related to biomedicine and biotechnology were becoming increasingly prominent in public discourse. We suggest that the general picture that emerges from the study of bioethics today is a field of ongoing politico-moral contestation and struggle, where discourses, people, institutions, and organizations collide, and where science is often used in political communication as a tool to persuade publics of the moral necessity of a particular course of action, and to win their consent.

Yet, it must be said that the situation in Australia is not devoid of attempts by bioethics to bridge conflicting interests. However, so long as bioethical debates are framed by the participants as conflicts from which only one victor may emerge, bioethics in Australia will remain an arena where opposition, explosive encounters, and protracted conflicts, strategic alliances, and competition are an ordinary part of the discipline.

Glossary

Australasian Association of Bioethics & Health Law (formerly the Australasian Bioethics Association) An organization formed in 1991 designed to promote the study of bioethics and legitimate the field and practice of bioethics, and improve its performance.

Biopolitics A programme of direct political and cultural intervention in the body. The politicization of the body.

Epistemological Break In the realm of ideas, it describes a leap in knowledge from the past. An historical "event" that involves a radical break with a pattern or frame of reference and the construction of a new pattern of ideas or the recasting of knowledge.

Field An arena or social space which has been socially instituted. It is "made-up" of strategic and non-strategic action, purposeful behavior in competitive circumstances.

Frame Analysis There is not yet a formal set of analytic indicators that can be used to reliably identify common frames (Koenig, 2004; Maher, 2001; Semetcko & Valkenberg, 2000:94). Nor is there an algorithm for researchers to specify how frames may be identified (Jasanoff, 2005; Tesh, 2000). Accordingly, it may be useful to sketch out in a schematic way our approach to identifying frames. To gain insight into the framing strategies that the CR used to fix meanings and communicate them to various publics and audiences, we interrogated actual texts occurring in real contexts. In 2005, the Lockhart Committee was appointed to conduct an independent review of the federal legislation, *Prohibition of Human Cloning Act 2002* and *Research Involving Human Embryos Act 2002*. The review was a "critical juncture" and key theatre of biopolitical activity. We analyzed submissions of participants to the Committee. Electronic and written media, media releases from individual leaders and organizations, and official web sites provided additional testimonies regarding significant reactions to hESC.

After reviewing past work on framing, we chose to use an "issue development" approach (Gray, 2003) to frame identification. We began by reading the assembled material with reference to the following questions: How were topics organized? What aspects of hESC research appeared to be most salient in the communication? In what way(s) was hESC research/researchers problematized? How were hESC researchers represented? Was hESC subject to moral/religious evaluation? Does the text challenge or affirm restrictive policy values? The purpose of this initial analysis was to form general impressions of the broad "rhetorical thrust" of anti-hESC discourse.

The next step was to identify the specific resources and tropes that the CR deployed. Here we drew upon existing work that provided preexisting categories for frame analysis. Frames are discursive constructions that describe and delineate the basic elements of objects—for example, events, conditions, ideas, thoughts, situations, and experiences (Jasanoff, 2005:25; Jordanova, 1989). Collected and structured in discourse, frames were identified by general discursive attributes, including specialized vocabularies, phrases, images, numerical and non-numerical conceptual and notational devices, metaphors, analogies, taxonomies, typologies, and scales of measurement that make them salient in text (Entman, 1993:52; Gray, 2003). Following our initial reading, a line-by-line reading was then conducted, asking the question: What are the core terminologies used to represent hESC research? Topics included justification, cause, and consequences of hESC research.

We also paid particular attention to how different frames played against each other in the text.

As identification of the people who oppose and support biotechnologies and their relationship to others is an important aspect of frame analysis (Entman, 1993: 52; Jasanoff, 2005), we also established frames from the vantage point of the thoughts, utterances, or dialogue of Christian activists, noting whether specific frames were used across multiple texts. We also focused on the relations between subjects appearing in each of the frame categories: the persons and institutions that were mobilized to make connections between discourses critical of hESC research and hESC researchers. Below, we cite examples from texts to clarify each frame and their related rhetorical strategies.

Hermeneutics The theory and method of interpreting meaningful human action.

Human embryonic stem cell (hESC) Self-replicating cells derived from human embryos or human fetal tissue.

In vitro fertilization (IVF) The process of fertilization accomplished outside the body.

National Health and Medical Research Council Australia's peak body for supporting health and medical research, for developing health advice for the Australian community, health professionals, and governments, and for providing advice on ethics in health care and in health and medical research.

Social practice Routinized interconnected action consisting of bodily and mental activities, background knowledge, know-how, shared understandings, emotions, standards, motivations, performances, and equipment and other apparatus and their use.

References

Ankeny, R.A. (2003). A view of bioethics from down under. *Cambridge Quarterly of Healthcare Ethics*, Vol. 12, pp. 242–246.

Arts Monash. See http://arts.monash.edu.au/bioethics/history/index.php. Accessed 19/09/08.

Australian Association of Bioethics & Health Law (2010). Engaging with the political-a policy document. Available at: http://aabhl.org/page/about_us.html. Accessed 20/12/10.

Australian Broadcasting Corporation. (2006a).Tony Abbott on the stem cell debate. *Insiders*, Broadcast 20/08/2006. Available at: http://www.abc.net.au/insiders/content/2006/s1719258.htm. Accessed 10/04/08.

Australian Broadcasting Corporation On Line (2006b). Stem cell bills unnecessary says Abbott. Available at: http://www.abc.net.au/news/stories/2006/08/25/1724293.htm Accessed 02/04/08.

Australian Broadcasting Corporation. (2006c). Stem cell research. *Health Report*, Broadcast 3/04/06. Available at: www.abc.net.au/rn/healthreport/default.htm. Accessed 22/01/08.

Australian Broadcasting Corporation. (2007).When you are going to die: making treatment decisions with the help of religion. *Encounter*, Broadcast 19/08/07. Available at: http:www.abc.net.au/rn/encounter/stories/2007/2003837.htm. Accessed 20/09/08.

Australian Catholic Bishops Conference. (2006). *Senate Inquiry into the Legislative Responses to Recommendations of the Lockhart Review*. Available at: www.aph.gov.au/Senate/Committee/clac_ctte/completed_inquiries/2004-07/leg_response_lockhart_review/. Accessed 07/04/08.

Australian Christian Lobby. (2006). *Public Submission: Legislative Review of Australia's Prohibition of Human Cloning Act 2002 and Research Involving Human Embryos Act 20*. Available at:http://www.aph.gov.au/Senate/committee/clac_ctte/completed_inquiries/2004-2007/leg_response_lockhart_review/submissions/sub90.pdf Accessed 07/04/08.

Australian Christian Lobby (2006a). *Re: Inquiry into the Legislative Responses to the Lockhart Review*. Available at: www.aph.gov.au/Senate/Committee/clac_ctte/completed_inquiries/2004-07/leg_response_lockhart_review/. Accessed 07/04/08.

Australian Christian Lobby. (2006b). *Submission: Review of the Tasmanian Human Embryonic Research Act 2003 and the Human Cloning and Other Prohibited Practices Act 2003*. Available at:http://australianchristianlobby.org.au/wp-content/uploads/060810-ACL-Tas-cloning-submission.pdf Accessed 2/05/08.

Australian Christian Lobby. (2008). *National Home Page*. Available at: www.acl.org.au. Accessed 7/19/08.

Australian Federation of Right to Life Associations. (2006). Submission tot the Senate Community Affairs Committee on the Legislative responses to the Recommendations of the Lockhart Review. Available at: http://www.aph.gov.au/Senate/committee/clac_ctte/completed_inquiries/2004-2007/leg_response_lockhart_review/submissions/sub37.pdf Accessed 07/04/08.

Australian Government. (2010). Bioethics Portal. Canberra. http://www.bioethics.gov.au. Accessed 14/12/10.

Bates, E. (1979). Decision making in critical illness. *The Australian and New Zealand Journal of Sociology*, Vol. 15 No. 3, pp. 45–54.

Bates, E. and Lapsley, H. (1985). *The Health Machine: The Impact of Medical Technology*, Penguin, Ringwood Victoria.

Bauman, Z. (1987). *Legislators and Interpreters*, Polity Press, Cambridge.

Benford, R.D. (1993). Frame Disputes within the nuclear disarmament movement. *Social Forces*, Vol. 71, pp. 677–701.

Biotechnology Australia. (2007). Strong public support for health and medical use of biotechnology, Media Release, August 1, 2007. Available at: www.biotechnology.gov.au. Accessed 08/06/08.

Bouma, G. (2006). *Australian Soul: religion, and spirituality in the twenty-first century*, Cambridge University Press, Port Melbourne.

Brennan, F. (2006) Public ethics in bioethics-a response to the Lockhart Review. Thomas Moore Lecture. 22nd July, 2006. Canberra. Available at: http://cathnews.acy.edu/606/doc/23Brennan.htm. Accessed 12/12/10.

Brock, P. (2006). Submission to the Senate Standing Committee on Community Affairs in Support of the Exposure Draft Somatic Cell nuclear Transfer and Related Research Amendment Bill, 2006, Available at: www.aph.gov.au/Senate/Committee/clac_ctte/completed_inquiries/2004-07/leg_response_lockhart_review/Accessed 07/04/08.

Brock, P. (2007). The Christian thing to do? *Daily Telegraph*, 07/06/07. Available at: http://www.dailytelegraph.com.au/news/opinion/the-christian-thing-to-do/story-e6frezz0-1111113692622. Accessed 08/01/08.

Callahan, D. (2005). Bioethics and the Culture Wars. *Cambridge Quarterly of Healthcare Ethics*, Vol. 14, pp. 424–431.

Caroline Chisholm Centre for Ethics, (2006). Submission of the Caroline Chisholm Centre for Health Ethics to the Senate Community Affairs Committee on Legislative Responses to Recommendations of the Lockhart Review. Available at: http://www.aph.gov.au/Senate/committee/clac_ctte/completed_inquiries/2004-2007/leg_response_lockhart_review/submissions/sub68.pdf Accessed 07/04/08.

Catholic Women's League of Tasmania Inc. (2006). Submission to the Senate Community Affairs Committee: Inquiry into the Legislative responses to Recommendations of the Lockhart Review. Available at: http://www.aph.gov.au/Senate/committee/clac_ctte/completed_inquiries/2004-2007/leg_response_lockhart_review/submissions/sub91.pdf Accessed 07/04/08.

Catholic Women's League of Victoria & Wagga Wagga Inc. (2006). Submission on the Inquiry into the Legislative responses to Recommendations of the Lockhart Review. Available at: http://www.aph.gov.au?Senate/committee/clac_ctte/completed_inquiries/2004-2007/leg_response_lockhart_review/submissions/sub33.pdf Accessed 03/01/10.

Charlesworth, M. (1985). Medical ethics: principles and practice. *The Medical Journal of Australia*, Vol. 143 August 5, pp. 95–96.

Charlesworth, M. (1989). *Life, Death, Genes and Ethics: Biotechnology and Bioethics*. ABC Enterprises, Crows Nest.

Coady, C.A.J. (2002). Religious meddling: a comment on Skene and Parker. *Journal of Medical Ethics*, Vol. 28 No. 4, pp. 221–222.

Coalition for the Defence of Human Life. (2006). Submission on the Prohibition of Human Cloning for Reproduction and Regulation of Human Embryo Research Amendment Bill 2006. Available at: http://www.aph.gov.au/Senate/committee/clac_ctte/completed_inquiries/2004-2007/leg_response_lockhart_review/submissions/sub23.pdf Accessed 07/04/08.

Connolly T.J. (1982). The scientists as priest. In T.J. Connolly (Ed), *Health Care in Crisis: A Bioethical Perspective*, Laurdel Bioethics Foundation, Catholic Institute of Sydney, Sydney, pp. 52–64.

Do No Harm/Australians for Ethical Stem Cell Research. (2006). The Case Against Cloning. Available at: www.cloning.org.au/ Accessed 18/02/08.

Dodds, S. & Ankeny, R. (2006). Regulation of hESC research in Australia: promises and pitfalls for deliberative democratic approaches. *Journal of Bioethical Inquiry*, Vol. 3, pp. 95–107.

Endeavour Forum. (2006). *Submission on Review of Human Cloning Act 2002 and Research Involving Human Embryos Act 2002, 2005*, Available at: www.aph.gov.au/Senate/Committee/clac_ctte/completed_inquiries/2004-07/leg_response_lockhart_review/. Accessed 07/04/08.

Entman, R. (1993). Framing: Toward Clarification of a Fractured Paradigm. *Journal of Communication*, Vol. 43 No. 4, pp. 51–8.

Family Life International Australia. (2006). Submission to the Inquiry into the Legislative responses to Recommendations of the Lockhart Review, Available at: http://www.aph.gov.au/Senate/committee/clac_ctte/completed_inquiries/2004-2007/leg_response_lockhart_review/submissions/sub86.pdf Accessed 07/04/08.

Festival of Light. (2006). Submission on the Inquiry into the Legislative Responses to the Recommendations of the Lockhart Review to the Senate Community Affairs Committee, Available at: http://www.aph.gov.au/Senate/committee/clac_ctte/completed_inquiries/2004-2007/leg_response_lockhart_review/submissions/sub34.pdf Accessed 07/04/08.

Foucault, M. (1980). *Power/knowledge: Selected interviews and writings*. Pantheon Books, New York.

Goffman, E. (1975). *Frame analysis: an essay on the organization of experience*. Penguin, Harmondsworth.

Gray, B. (2002). Framing environmental disputes. In R.Lewicki, B. Gray and M. Elliot (eds.), *Making Sense of Intractable Environmental Conflicts: Concepts and Cases*, Island Press, Washington D.C. pp. 11–34.

Gunn, C. (1982). Health care and reductionist scientific materialism: progress of dehumanisation. In T.J. Connolly (ed.), *Health Care in Crisis: A Bioethical Perspective*, Laurdel Bioethics Foundation, Catholic Institute of Sydney, Sydney, pp. 66–82.

Hall, W. (2004). The Australian policy debate about human embryonic stem cell research. *Health Law Review*, Vol. 12 No. 2, pp. 27–33.

Hepburn, L. (1992). *Ova-dose*. Allen & Unwin, Sydney.

Hogan, M. (1987). *The Sectarian Strand: Religion in Australian History*, Penguin Books, Ringwood Victoria.

Jasanoff, S. (2005). *Designs on Nature*. Princeton University Press, Princeton, NJ.

Jonsen, A. (1990). *The New Medicine and the Old Ethics*. Harvard University Press, Cambridge, Mass.

Jordanova, L.J. (1989). *Sexual Visions: Images of Gender in Science and Medicine between the Eighteenth and Twentieth Centuries*, Harvester Wheatsheaf, Hemel Hempsted.

Kahn, J. (2006). What happens when bioethics discovers politics? *Hastings Center Report*, Vol. 36, No. 3, p. 10.

Kasimba, P. & Singer, P. (1989). Australian commissions and committees on issues in bioethics. *Journal of Medicine and Philosophy*, Vol. 14 No. 4, pp. 403–424.

Kirby, M. (1980). New dilemmas for law and medicine. *Malcolm Gillies Oration*, Royal North Shore Medical Association, Sydney, September 22, 1980.

Koenig, T. (2004). Frame Analysis., Available at: http://www.restore/lboro/resources/links/frames_primer.php. Accessed 04/03/08.

Kuhse, H. (1982). An ethical approach to IVF and ET: what ethics is all about. In W. Walters and P. Singer (eds.), *Test-tube babies: a guide to moral questions, present techniques, and future possibilities*, Oxford University Press, Melbourne.

Kuhse, H. (1998). Editorial. *Monash Bioethics Review*, Vol 17, No. 4, p. 1.

Kuhse, H. & Singer, P. (1985). *Should the Baby Live: The problem of Handicapped Infants*. Oxford University Press, Oxford.

Lockhart, J.S. (2005). Legislative Review Committee. Issues Paper: outline of existing legislation and issues. For public consultation [Legislation Review of Australia's Prohibition of Human Cloning Act 2002 and Research Involving Human Embryos Act 2002], Biotext, Canberra.

Lohan, K. (2005). Going Public. *Meanjin*, Vol. 64 No. 3, pp. 83–90.

Lohrey, A. (2006). Vote of Jesus: Christianity and Politics. *Quarterly Essay*, Vol. 22, pp. 1–79.

Maddox, M. (2005). *God under Howard: The Rise of the Religious Right in Australian Politics*. Allen & Unwin, Sydney.

Maher, T.M. (2001). Framing: an emerging paradigm or a phase of agenda setting. In S.D. Reese, O.H. Gandy & A.E. Grant (eds.), *Framing Public Life: Perspectives on Media and Our Understanding of the Social World*, Lawrence Erlbaum Associates, Mahwah, NJ.

Oakley, J. (2002). Democracy, embryonic stem cell research, and the Roman Catholic Church. *Journal of Medical Ethics*, Vol. 28 No. 4, p. 228.

Overduin, D.C., and Fleming, J.I. (1982). *Life in a Test-tube: Medical and Ethical Issues Facing Society Today*, Lutherine Publishing House, Adelaide.

Pell, G. (1995). Evangelium Vitae-Catholicism, the media and the "culture of death. *AD2000*, Vol. 8 No. 10, p. 3.

Pell, G. (2007). No Catholic could in good conscience vote for Cloning bill—NSW Bishops Media Statement, Polding Centre, Sydney, 4/06/07.

Pell, G. (2008). Being in awe of life. Available at: http://www.zenit.org/article-21581?1=english. Accessed 20/03/08.

Pellegrino, E.D. (2000). Bioethics at Century's Turn: Can normative ethics be retrieved? *Journal of Medicine and Philosophy*, Vol. 25, No. 6, pp. 655–675.

Perry, D. (2000). Patient's voices: the powerful sound in the stem cell debate. *Science*, Vol. 287, No. 5457, p. 1423.

Preece, G. (ed.). (2002). *Rethinking Peter Singer*. InterVarsity Press, Illinois.

Pro-Life Victoria. (2006). Submission by Pro-Life Victoria to Review of Legislative responses to recommendations of the reports of the Legislation Review Committee on the Prohibition of Human Cloning Act 2002 and the Research Involving Human Embryos Act 2002 (the Lockhart review). Available at: http://www.aph.gov.au/Senate/committee/clac_ctte/completed_inquiries/2004-2007/leg_response_lockhart_review/submissions/sub 43.pdf Accessed 07/04/08.

Rabinow, P. (1999). *French DNA: Trouble in purgatory*. University of Chicago Press, Chicago.

Rabinow, P. & Dan-Cohen, T. (2005). *Biotech Chronicles: a machine to make the future*. Princeton University Press. Princeton and London.

Right to Life Australia. (2006). Submission to the Senate Community Affairs Committee on Legislative Responses to recommendations of the Lockhart Review In particular the bill sponsored by Senator Kay Patterson. Available at: www.aph.gov.au/Senate/Committee/clac_ctte/completed_inquiries/2004-07/leg_response_lockhart_review/. Accessed 07/04/08.

Santamaria, J. (2006). Submission to the Lockhart Inquiry on the Regulation of Stem Cell Research. Available at: http://www.aph.gov.au/Senate/committee/clac_ctte/completed_inquiries/2004-2007/leg_response_lockhart_review/submissions/sub25.pdf Accessed 07/04/08.

Savulescu, J. (2000). The ethics of cloning and creating embryonic stem cells as a source of tissue for transplantation: time to change the law in Australia. *Australian & New Zealand Journal of Medicine*, Vol 30, p. 492.

Semetco, H.A. & Valkenberg, P.M. (2000). Framing European Politics: A Content Analysis of Press and Television News. *Journal of Communication*. Vol. 50 No. 2, pp. 93–109.

Shanahan, A. (2006). Cloning by any other name. *Quadrant*, October, Vol. 50 No. 10, pp. 40–43.

Siebers, T. (2003). What can disability studies learn from the culture wars? *Cultural Critique*, Autumn, No. 55, pp. 182–216.

Silove D, Steel Z. & Mollica R. (2001). Detention of asylum seekers: assault of health, human rights, and social development. *Lancet*, Vol. 357 No. 9266, pp. 1436–1437.

Singer, P. & Dawson, K. (1992). IVF technology and the argument from potential. In P. Singer, H. Kuhse, S. Buckle, K. Dawson and P, Kasimba (eds.). *Embryo Experimentation: Ethical, Legal and Social Issues*, Cambridge University Press, Cambridge, pp. 76–89.

Singer, P. & Kuhse, H. (2006). 1980-2005: Bioethics then and now. *Monash Bioethics Review*, Vol. 25 No. 1, 9–14.

Singer, P. & Wells, D. (1984). *The Reproductive Revolution; New Ways of Making Babies*. Oxford University Press, Oxford.

Skene, L. & Parker, M. (2002). The role of the church in developing the law. *Journal of Medical Ethics*, Vol. 28, pp. 215–218.

Southern Cross Bioethics Centre, (2006). Submission to Australian Senate Community Affairs Legislative Committee Re Legislative Responses to recommendations of the Lockhart Review., Available at: www.aph.gov.au/Senate/Committee/clac_ctte/completed_inquiries/2004-07/leg_response_lockhart_review/. Accessed 07/04/08.

Steel, Z. & Silove, D. (2004). Science and common good: indefinite detention, non-renewable mandatory detention of asylum seekers and the research imperative. *Monash Bioethics Review*, Vol. 23, No. 4, pp. 510–522.

Swan, J.M. (1983). Introduction. Proceedings of a Conference: Ethical Implications in the Use of Donor Sperm, Eggs and Embryos in the treatment of Human Fertility. Monash Centre for Human Bioethics, Melbourne, 4th March, 1983.

Taylor, R. (1979). *Medicine Out of Control*. Sun Books, Melbourne.

Tesh, S.N. (2000). *Uncertain Hazards: Environmental Activists and Scientific Profession*. Cornell University Press. Ithica, NY.

Waller, L. (1987). In Australia, the debate moves to embryo experimentation. *The Hastings Centre Report*, June, pp. 21–22.

Walters, W. & Singer, P. (eds.). (1982). *Test-tube babies: a guide to moral questions, present techniques, and future possibilities*. Oxford University Press. Melbourne, Oxford.

Walters, W. Forward. (1991). In K.R. Mitchell and T.J. Lovat. *Bioethics for Medical and Health Professionals. Social Science Press*, Wentworth Falls.

Warhurst, J. (1983). Single-issue politics: the impact of conservation and anti-abortion groups. *Current Affairs Bulletin*, Vol. 60 No. 2, pp. 19–31.

Warhurst, J. (2004). The Catholic Lobby: religious networks and public policy. *The Public Policy Network Summer Conference*. Adelaide, South Australia, Feb 1–2, 2004.

Warhurst, J. (2006). Religion in 21st Century Australian National Politics. *Australian Senate Occasional Lecture Series*. Parliament House, Canberra, May 5, 2006.

Weber M. (1970/1919). Politics as a Vocation. In H.H. Gerth and C. Wright Mills (trans. and ed) *From Max Weber: Essays in Sociology*. Routledge & Kegan Paul. London. 1970/1919, pp. 77–128.

Weber, M. (1967). *From Max Weber: essays in sociology*. H.H. Gerth & C. Wright Mills (trans. and ed.). Routledge and Kegan Paul, London.

Wierzbicka, A. (1997). Peter Singer and Christian Ethics. *Quadrant*. April, pp. 27–31.

Wiktorowicz, Q. (2004). Framing Jihad: intramovement framing contests and al-Qaeda's struggle for sacred authority. *International Review of Social History*. Vol. 49, pp. 159–177.

Zald, M.N. & McCarthy, J.D. (1987). Social Movement Industries: competition and conflict Among SMOs. In M.N. Zald & J.D. McCarthy (eds.). *Social Movements in an Organizational Society*. Transaction Publishers, New Brunswick, NJ, pp. 161–184.

Zion D. (2007). Caring for detained asylum seekers, human rights and bioethics. *Australian and New Zealand Journal of Public Health*, Vol. 28, No. 6, pp. 510–512.

15 BIOETHICS IN THE UNITED STATES

CONTESTED TERRAIN FOR COMPETING VISIONS OF AMERICAN LIBERALISM

Bruce Jennings and Jonathan D. Moreno

The Nazi doctors trial at Nuremberg in 1947 marks the modern revival of biomedical ethics. The spirit and principles that grew out of the postwar examination of Nazi atrocities have been periodically renewed in bioethics during the ensuing decades, and have been extended to cover not only medical research with human beings, but also clinical medicine, the use of biomedical technologies and their social implications, and public policy regarding the governance of science and the financing and delivery of medical care.[1]

Hence, bioethics was born at the zenith of twentieth-century liberalism—the "American century," as Henry Luce triumphantly called it—and it has shared the fate of that public philosophy, at least in the United States, ever since. This is what makes bioethics a sociologically and historically important object of study. Bioethics has grown out of—and is unimaginable in the absence of—the moral triumph and vindication of an open society: that is, a society respectful of individual rights and interests; dedicated to a moral style of reasonable moderation, compromise, and mutual accommodation; and optimistic about the possibility of creating and sustaining a system of individual privacy, freedom of choice, equality of opportunity, and ordered liberty under law. The United States believes in moral progress, and American bioethics takes itself to be an agent of such progress.

The Founding Context of American Bioethics

This moral sensibility was particularly well-suited to the new liberalism, progressive and consumer oriented, of the late 1960s and 1970s. Within that context, the authoritarianism and paternalism of mainstream

---

1. For a broader historical perspective, see Fox, 1987; Fox & Swazey, 2008; Jonsen, 2000; and Rothman, 1992.

medicine (particularly in the areas of research, psychiatry, and obstetrics) came under attack. The dehumanizing effects of biomedical technology also came under scrutiny. To many, advances in medical technology seemed to offer compelling ethical dilemmas and value conflicts that neither prevailing social norms nor legal precedents were adequately prepared to resolve.

U.S. bioethicists normally trace the birth of the field to the late 1960s, when a handful of physicians, theologians, and philosophers become concerned about the implications of a series of scientific and medical breakthroughs. The decoding of the human genome, recombinant DNA technologies, organ transplants, artificial organs, life-extending technologies, controversial human experiments, and the growing costs of healthcare were among the stimuli for these early conversations. For example, a significant philosophical difference between traditional medical ethics and the new bioethics was an emphasis on the proposition that doctors should tell patients the truth, even at the risk of emotional upset, because truth-telling is considered to be a necessary element of valid informed consent, which in turn is required by the principle of "autonomy" or "respect for persons." Nothing in medicine should be done to an individual without his or her free, informed consent. Contained in that credo is the kernel of both the great strength, and the curious blindness, of American bioethics.

At the core of the concerns of bioethics with the new biomedical technologies was the possibility that they could lead to fundamental, not wholly foreseeable, and perhaps undesirable, changes in what it is to be human. Some saw a slippery slope and worried about the inevitability of a degradation of dignity. Others believed it possible to introduce ethically justified guidelines, regulation, or even law to shape trends. Thus began a tension in American bioethics between radical and reformist—prophetic versus regulatory—bioethics that persists today.

Several incidents in the 1970s seemed to have such compelling social implications that they moved the still-emerging field in the direction of a legal or quasi-legal approach to the issues. One such incident was the scandal surrounding the U.S. Public Health Service syphilis study in Tuskegee, Alabama, out of which grew the creation of a federal research ethics commission and, subsequently, much more clearly articulated rules for human experiments. Another turning point was the scientific community's self-imposed moratorium on recombinant DNA research, followed by the creation of a federal government advisory committee to scrutinize research involving genetic manipulation. Yet another important event for the development of U.S. bioethics was the New Jersey Supreme Court's ruling in the Karen Ann Quinlan case that recognized her parents' authority to withdraw ventilator support, and also recommended the creation of "ethics committees" for such tragic circumstances rather than resort to the courts.

By the early 1980s a noticeable shift was underway from the "prophetic" bioethics of the early period to a "regulatory" bioethics that enlisted more lawyers, policy-oriented health professionals, and even some social scientists, albeit more from sociology and anthropology than from economics.[2] Clinical ethicists cropped up in hospitals; their expertise included local institutional protocols, as well as state law and regulation, particularly on end-of-life decision making. Research ethicists were authorities on the interpretation and application of federal rules governing human experiments.

In addition to controlling the societal effects on biomedical technology, a long-term focus of U.S. bioethics has been distributive justice, and securing access to more universal access to such technology and health services. Yet, strikingly absent from the achievements of U.S. bioethics in the first decade or so was a societal consensus on providing health care for all. A presidential bioethics commission appointed by President Jimmy Carter prepared a report that, in staff draft, appeared to support the concept of a "right" to health care. However, as new commissioners appointed by President Ronald Reagan cycled onto the panel, objections to this formulation were raised, evidently having to do with concerns about "socialized" medicine. According to one account, the document that resulted backed off from the strong position in earlier drafts.[3] The struggle to rationalize the U.S. healthcare system has continued without this basic philosophical agreement ever since. Of the four often-cited bioethical principles articulated in canonical form by Tom Beauchamp and James Childress, justice has been less central to the U.S. conversation than autonomy, beneficence, and nonmaleficence.[4] As U.S. bioethics looks more toward global health issues and public health ethics, that may change.

Bioethics has become a new discipline and a new profession rapidly and successfully in the United States because it has performed an essential ideological service to the public philosophy of postwar American liberalism.[5] It has fashioned a moral identity, a style of acting in the life world of high-technology medicine, and an intellectually rigorous discourse of conceptual analysis, each centered around the notion of individual autonomy. This accommodation of mainstream liberalism, and hence of what has become mainstream bioethics, involves a modus vivendi between the structures of power in capitalist medicine and biotechnology (which progressive liberalism wishes to control but not to

2. Bulger et al., eds., 1995; Danis, Clancy, & Churchill, eds., 2002. Cf. Callahan, 1995.

3. Bayer, 1984.

4. Beauchamp & Childress, 2008. For further discussion of this point, see Jennings, 2007.

5. Cf. Jennings, 1998. For an acute discussion of the ideological role of bioethics discourse in the area of genetic engineering, see Evans, 2002. See also Eckenwiler & Cohen, eds., 2007.

challenge fundamentally) on the one hand, and the social ideal of the competent, self-sovereign, and unencumbered individual, on the other.[6]

Bioethics and the New Liberalism

American bioethics took shape at a time when social action and individual choice in relation to health were in flux. It was driven by a perception of a cultural lag between normative and scientific knowledge, the so-called "biological revolution."[7] What the new biology and the new medicine enabled people to do was beginning to change faster than the capacity of the traditional means of guiding and governing the use of technology or the direction of personal choice: ethics, cultural mores, religion, and the law. Safe medical and surgical techniques of abortion and effective hormonal contraception for women were two cases in point, as was the advent of in vitro fertilization (IVF). Physicians were facilitating (or hindering) these new powers and choices. Investors sought to profit from them, governments strove to regulate them. But all were acting without a legal roadmap or an ethical compass. A new discourse, which came to be known as "biomedical ethics" or "bioethics," was needed to alleviate the danger inherent in this cultural and normative lag.

But this was not merely a situation limited to technology and social morality in the sphere of medicine and the life sciences. It was a manifestation of a much more pervasive ideological shift taking place in the United States at the time. This was a flowering of individualism, libertarianism, personal autonomy, and authenticity that would bring about an important realignment of American liberalism in the Vietnam War era.

This realignment was about social fluidity and diversity, not about the class-based politics of nineteenth- and early twentieth-century liberalism. This was the politics of respect, recognition, and ethnic or gender identification, not the politics of right versus left, laissez faire economics versus the welfare state, or liberty and private property rights versus equality and social justice.[8]

Autonomy and Identity Liberalisms

How can we best make sense of the contested terrain of liberalisms that dominate our normative discourse today? For the purposes of placing American bioethics

6. Rose, 2007.

7. Callahan, 1995; Jonsen, 1990 and 2003.

8. Taylor, 1991; see also Fraser & Honneth, 2003.

in its broader ideological context, we propose to focus on two main theoretical constellations that we call *autonomy liberalism* and *identity liberalism*. We shall stress the differences between them, even while recognizing that in the work of individual theorists they tend to overlap and to blend together.[9] Various works and schools of thought in American bioethics (e.g., foundationalism, principlism, feminism, casuistry, and the like) track these divisions and tensions rather faithfully.[10]

Autonomy liberalism takes individual autonomy to be the overriding value in political and in private morality. No single concept has been more important in the contemporary development of bioethics, and the revival of medical ethics, than the concept of autonomy. Autonomy in bioethics means freedom from outside restraint, and the freedom to live one's own life in one's own way. To be autonomous is to live according to your own values and principles, as these are refined in the light of informed, rational deliberation and settled convictions—your own convictions, or convictions and beliefs that you have embraced and accepted as your own. It is to be self-sovereign. It is to be the author of your life, your self, and your actions.

Autonomy liberalism defines autonomy not only as a moral right but as the fundamental universal feature of humankind. Autonomy conveys human identity sui generis. It is essentially the same in all lives, and in anyone, anywhere.

In contrast, the central concept of identity liberalism is respect for—and the interpersonal and cultural validation of—identity that adheres precisely in difference rather than universality. The core is on the surface and the surface is the core of the self.

Identity liberalism has developed in response to social scientific, feminist, and ethnic critiques of individualism. It searches for a liberal society comprising second-order rules of social cooperation, toleration, and mutual respect, under which flourish a variety of different communities of belief and practice. In its

9. Compare Galston, 1995. Among thinkers who may be characterized as autonomy liberals are the early John Rawls, Robert Paul Wolff, Ronald Dworkin, Judith Thompson, Joel Feinberg, Robert Dahl, and Richard Flathman. Regarding identity liberalism, one can mention Isaiah Berlin, Stuart Hampshire, the later Rawls, Bernard Williams, George Kateb, Michael Walzer, John Kekes, Charles Anderson, Nancy Rosenblum, William Connolly, Martha Nussbaum, Iris Marion Young, Joseph Raz, Donald Moon, William Galston, Will Kymlicka, and John Gray. Excellent overviews of the contested terrain of liberalism in the United States today are found in White, 2000, and Mulhall & Swift, 1996. Some of these themes are brought into contact with areas of bioethics by Emanuel, 1991, and in the various contributions to Kleinman, Fox, & Brandt, eds., 1999.

10. On these schools of bioethics, see Gert, Culver, & Clouser, 2006; Beauchamp & Childress, 2008; Wolf, ed., 1996; and Jonsen & Toulmin, 1990.

public realm, the society posited by identity liberalism is pluralistic—although this is more a pluralism of groups than of values—while the private sphere of the society is comprised of communities that may be internally monistic and even nonliberal.

Some versions of this theory reject individualism and border on being nonliberal forms of communitarianism; other versions remain closer to the liberal tradition by arguing that true individualism (autonomy or self-identity) can only be found by affirming one's membership in communities and relationships of substantive belief and practice. For the unencumbered or "thin" self—the self as author of its own identity and agency—of autonomy liberalism, identity liberalism turns to embedded or "thick" selfhood of persons leading lives of substantive membership in communities of shared meaning, tradition, and purpose.

Most discussions of American bioethics have noted, as we did above, the predominant influence of the concept of autonomy and autonomy liberalism. However, that is only part of the story of bioethics in the United States. Identity liberalism, particularly beginning in the 1990s, has also come to have a very significant influence on work in American bioethics. This has moved the disciplinary center of gravity in American bioethics away from the tradition of analytic moral philosophy and mainstream biomedical science, and toward critical theory in the law, feminism, postmodern versions of social science, disability studies, and cognate orientations in the humanities.

Moreover, the culture wars type of backlash against bioethics, among conservative thinkers and on the American religious right, has been directed largely against the substantive positions and the cultural ethos of autonomy liberalism in bioethics. This can be seen in issues such as end-of-life decision making and assisted dying, civil liberties and privacy orientations in the use of medically assisted reproduction, genetic testing, policies for coping with HIV/AIDS, and the like.[11] We will discuss this further below.

Because its influence in bioethics has been relatively neglected, therefore, somewhat more explication of identity liberalism is appropriate here. Three somewhat different orientations and emphases may be distinguished in identity liberalism: (1) anti-essentialism, (2) recognition and social justice, and (3) the social basis of self-identity.

Anti-essentialism. This position leans heavily on epistemological skepticism or relativism, and this view is widely congenial to many in the ethnographic social science disciplines today.[12] It holds that the universal understanding of humanity integral to autonomy liberalism is an illusion. Philosophy and reason will never

---

11. Smith, 2000; Satel, 2000; and Meilaender, 1995.

12. Rorty, 1989.

discover the truth about our humanity (either because they lack the capacity to do so, or because there is no final truth to be found). Moreover, philosophical worldviews such as Enlightenment rationalism and universalism (so deeply embedded in autonomy liberalism and much of mainstream bioethics) are viewed by identity liberalism (and by postmodernism generally) as a "totalizing" discourse that historically has functioned as a means of imposing power used by privileged groups to dominate more vulnerable groups. The discourse of Enlightenment, in other words, turns out to be a betrayal of liberalism because it leads to domination rather than liberation.

Recognition as justice. A second version of identity liberalism takes its bearings from a moral rather than an epistemological perspective.[13] It holds that genuine liberal justice requires respect for difference and treating persons as equals, with equal dignity and respect, *not in spite of their differences but precisely because of them.* It is no moral achievement to live with and to respect those whom we regard as fundamentally the same as ourselves. But to respect the rights and freedoms of those whom we find to be strangers is an admirable and just mode of relationship in both political and professional life.

Difference as self-identity. Finally, identity liberalism offers a critique of the abstract individualism inherent in the liberal notion of autonomy—perhaps not the Kantian notion, but in the version of autonomy that has been predominant in American bioethics.[14] This argument is based on the notion that human self-realization comes in and through life lived in culturally meaningful practices, not by abstraction or escape from those practices. It follows, then, that it is ethically and philosophically incoherent to require individuals to shed their culturally, ethnically, or religiously specific skin and to adopt a universal mode of reasoning, decision making, and a universal code of behavioral norms as the price of entry into the liberal society. When a person becomes an autonomous liberal self in this sense, he or she is not just shedding superficial wrapping, but eviscerating the very things that give us identity and make us human in the first place.

Moreover, the formalism implicit in the tradition of autonomy liberalism works to its own disadvantage when we appreciate the emptiness of freedom of choice, or even the exercise of human rights, sheerly for their own sake.[15] What makes choice or the protection of rights meaningful to the self who has them, is the culturally specific and thick traditions, practices, institutions, and forms

---

13. Young, 1990.

14. Jennings, 2007. See also Kymlicka, 1989; Taylor, 1991 and 1994; Moon, 1993.

15. Taylor, 1991.

of life that constitute the object of choice, or the context of protected interests and freedoms. If the self granted freedom of choice must first be a thin or culturally unencumbered self, then freedom of choice will have little moral value, because such a self will have little or nothing of independent worth or value to choose.

The New Right Critique of Bioethics

This new liberalism and the politics of recognition spawned a new left and, somewhat later, a new right. It was offshoots of the new left that mainly affected and shaped bioethics in the 1970s and 1980s, and informed the autonomy and identity liberalisms that we have reviewed above. In the last two decades, however, the new right has taken up the domain of bioethics and has created a more obvious and more politicized division into contending camps. Progressive liberalism still remains predominant in mainstream bioethics, but at least since 2000 it has been on the defensive. Disagreements are sharper both for philosophical reasons and because bioethics in the United States now has more direct linkages to the policymaking process than ever before. Moreover, in the years 2001 through 2008, the Bush administration, the religious right, and the disability community have made several bioethics issues the center of their attention, including end-of-life care and human stem cell research. Let us consider these two examples in turn.

The influence of the new right on American bioethics was clearly illustrated in the Schiavo case. Never in American bioethics, and rarely in American politics, have we witnessed such an extraordinary intervention by the state in the medical treatment of an individual. In 2005, Terri Schiavo was a young woman in persistent vegetative state (PVS), whose family was in conflict concerning the discontinuation of artificial nutrition and hydration. Under the guise of saving Ms. Schiavo, the Bush administration and the Republican-controlled Congress led a frontal assault on the ethical and legal position developed over two decades by mainstream American bioethics and jurisprudence. However, the judiciary balked and put down the revolt. It embraced once again the perspective of autonomy bioethics and liberalism, that it is the right of an individual such as Ms. Schiavo to refuse medical treatment via advance directive, and it is appropriate for her husband, as proxy decision-maker, to honor her wishes.

Consider now human stem cell research. Although mammalian reproductive cloning (more properly called *somatic cell nuclear transfer*) had been predicted, few expected it to mark a turning point in the politics of bioethics. The birth of Dolly the sheep in 1996 excited fears that human cloning was now within technical reach. President Clinton's ethics commission declared that there should be a moratorium on any such efforts. The controversy intensified when, in 1998, two teams of American scientists nearly simultaneously announced that they had successfully derived early stem cells from human embryos. The significance of this achievement, combined with mammalian cloning, was immediately appreciated by those who had for years theorized about such a conjunction of events: The day might not be far away when significant medical benefits could be gained by using cloned human embryos to obtain potentially healing stem cells with DNA compatible with a patient's immune system.

The prospect of routine creation and destruction of human embryos finally opened up a long-simmering divide. While most in the academic bioethics establishment preferred not to enter into abortion-related discussions if they could avoid them, it now became nearly impossible to work in the field and not declare oneself on the question of the embryo's moral status. By the 2000 presidential election, even those whose work did not directly involve reproductive issues found themselves pressed to take a position. Not since Roe v. Wade had a bioethical issue been swept up in national partisan politics, but at that time the field of bioethics had not yet become a self-conscious profession. In 2000 it was.

A few months before the Bush–Gore election, the Clinton administration authorized rules under which the National Institutes of Health could fund research involving human embryonic stem cells, so long as federal funds had not been used in the process of deriving the stem cells from embryos that would thereby be destroyed. The latter rule was a consequence of an amendment to the NIH reauthorization budget bill that was tacked on every year since 1995. Other rules were conventional, including that the donating couple had to provide informed consent. But time ran out before any such projects were actually funded, setting up a decision for the next president. President Bush determined on August 9, 2001 that Federal funds could only be used for research in which human embryos had been destroyed before that date.

Although neither side was delighted with the policy, opponents of stem cell research appreciated that federal funds would not be used to destroy "nascent human life" for what they regarded as highly speculative research on problems that could be addressed by other means. Proponents told themselves that the president had at least made some federally funded research possible, and that he had left the door open for a more permissive policy. But scientists' hopes dimmed as a result of various developments over the next 6 years, including the fact that far fewer stem cell lines were available under the policy than previously thought, the federally eligible lines suffered from technical limitations, and that there was no sign that the president would expand the policy. Instead, many have turned to a number of states, especially California, which have made unprecedented commitments to step into the breach left by the federal standard.

A striking feature of the way that President Bush arrived at his policy was a concerted effort to make the public point that it was based on ethical advice from various scholarly sources. Indeed, several bioethicists were in fact invited to meet with the president to discuss the arguments and options. One of them was Leon Kass, a University of Chicago professor and among the early bioethicists, who was subsequently given the task of chairing the bioethics council with a specific mandate to examine the ethics of stem cell research.

Kass was among those who expressed early misgivings about reproductive technologies like in vitro fertilization. Kass's writings were, and continue to be, heavily influenced by Martin Heidegger, who saw technology as the root of human beings' existential crisis, a deep distraction from our ability to dwell authentically within "Being."[16] A few other conservative theologians with loose ties to the bioethics establishment, such as Gilbert Meilaender, held similar views but seemed to have a limited audience, at least in academia.[17] These figures hewed more closely to the prophetic style of the early days, preferring to raise large philosophical questions that suggested caution rather a management approach to ethics.

Under Kass's leadership, the tone of the council was much more academic and scholarly than is normally the case for presidential commissions, and perspectives from the humanities were more prominent in the council's various reports. More Socratically oriented than previous bioethics council chairs, Kass was more interested in giving public voice to certain kinds of reflection than to achieving consensus, or at least the kind of agreement that often comes from narrowing the scope of the issue. Sessions of the council often focused on the disquieting implications of biotechnology as undermining human dignity.

Press coverage of the council focused on Kass's high-academic demeanor and the fact that the panel's membership included some very conservative commentators. News was made when two more liberal members were not renewed at the end of their terms, including one distinguished biologist (thus reducing the scientist members by one-third), and were replaced with conservatives who were not widely recognized in the academic world. This incident combined with accusations that the administration had tried to "pack" science advisory committees and squelch views that were incompatible with its policies.

What many observers missed, however, were some aspects of the larger context of the president's council. First, though it's common to focus on members of federal commissions, often the staff members are just as important, as they normally draft the reports and therefore can drive the process. American bioethics

16. Kass, 2002.

17. Meilaender, 1995.

commissions in the late 1970s and early 1980s drafted highly influential reports that still frame national policy on human research and informed consent to medical care, for example. The drafters were skilled academic philosophers and lawyers, who in many cases went on to become senior leaders in the field.

In the case of the Bush bioethics council, several senior staff members and consultants were associated with the Ethics and Public Policy Center, a Washington, DC think tank which, since the latter 1990s, has had an interest in bioethics and publishes the journal, *The New Atlantis*. What distinguished these individuals from the staff of previous presidential bioethics commissions was not only their quite public identification with conservative or neoconservative politics and policies, but also their previous experience and training. Some had been staff to Newt Gingrich, for example, and none held degrees from established graduate programs in bioethics, or held positions at established bioethics centers. While some of those programs and centers might have been dismissed as liberal hotbeds that would have been allergic to conservative views, that was by no means true in all cases. In any event, it is clear that the professional pathway for the president's council staffers was different from that of previous bioethics commissions.

From Critique to Appropriation

The unique intellectual background of the president's council staff was only one indication of a cultural divide that had taken root in bioethics. The second major contextual difference for this commission was the growing interest among conservative religious groups in claiming the mantle of bioethics as their own. In some cases, existing pro-life organizations expanded their activities to embrace the stem cell debate; in other instances, new centers were created. The energetic leaders of these efforts have been skillful in the use of Web-based media like blogs to spread their message. These evangelical Christian groups found sympathetic ears on the president's council, and have surely been effective at the grass roots, stirring up a portion of the Bush political base on issues like stem cells and the withdrawal of artificial nutrition and hydration from persons in PVS.

Yet, though the neoconservative council members and staff shared some ultimate concerns with the conservative Christian bioethics groups, the neoconservatives are mainly secularists who often appeal to religious principles, among other authoritative moral sources—but not as their sole or principal source of moral guidance, as is generally the case for conservative Christians. It will therefore be interesting to see if this alliance can be sustained. For example, neoconservatives tend to base their concerns about biotechnology on what are finally empirical questions: Will novel reproductive techniques actually lead to less respectful treatment of some groups of human beings? Many of these writers have not wholly ruled out even embryo research, for instance, but express grave doubts about what they regard as the moral dilemma it creates. They see stem cell research as part of a larger problem with the life sciences and human dignity. Conservative Christian bioethicists are more likely to take principled positions that rule out embryo-destructive research a priori, regardless of the outcomes for science or society. Thus, Francis Fukuyama (a member of the president's council), has emerged as a stronger advocate of regulation of certain technologies than his neoconservative colleagues, but this position puts him outside the range of acceptable views among many conservative Christians.[18]

Neither the new right bioethicists nor their Christian allies are in good standing with traditional market conservatives. Like the larger political scene, while traditional conservatives tout their commitment to moral values, neoconservatives and religious conservatives are suspicious of the market. Capitalists should be no more comfortable with religious and neoconservatives than they are with progressives. Both seek to impose external moral constraints on the marketplace. As yet, this basic difference in worldviews has not caused the deep rift that would surely emerge if these movements were pressured to take a clearer stand on market freedom.

Since the President's Council changed leadership in 2005, it assumed a much lower profile. The council published no white papers or reports from September 2005 to December 2008.

Bioethics in the Next Decade: A Progressive Response?

Progressive thinkers have been slow to grasp the right's embrace of bioethics. In 2005, the Women's Bioethics Project produced a detailed analysis of conservative institutions' engagement in bioethics, as compared to progressive foundations and think tanks.[19] Not surprisingly, the results illustrated the same sort of discrepancy that has frequently been noted in the intellectual competition between the right and the left in recent years: Conservative organizations have been systematically developing a research and communications infrastructure, supported by significant investment, intended to drive the country's social conversation about ethics and biotechnology. Both the Women's Bioethics Project, and the Progressive Bioethics Initiative at the Center for American Progress, have taken some first steps to address this weakness on the left.[20]

18. Fukuyama, 2002.

19. Cf., www.womensbioethics.org.

20. www.americanprogress.org.

What advantages and disadvantages characterize a progressive bioethical view of biotechnology? In one respect, neoconservative and conservative Christian bioethics tap into a deep well of cultural anxiety about science, reaching at least as far back as Mary Shelley's *Frankenstein* and continuing with Aldous Huxley's *Brave New World*. Science fiction images are frequently cited by new right critics of biotech, rather than the science itself. But for all the popularity of "mad scientist" media, Americans also strongly identify themselves with innovation, appreciating not only the excitement of the new but also what science and technology have meant for the American economy, not to mention the growing need to compete with emerging innovative rivals, especially China.

Whatever the future of neoconservative bioethics (mainly practiced by a tiny elite), that movement should not be conflated with a more explicit, religiously inspired, conservative bioethics. Theirs is a substantial constituency joined together by a unifying cultural perspective. Though perhaps never close to a majority of either political party, as a consequence of their organization and solidarity their influence is familiar and impressive. If history is any guide, religious values will not vanish from the contest of ideas in the American public square, or in U.S. bioethics.

References

Bayer, R. 1984. Ethics, politics and access to health care: A critical analysis of the President's Commission. *Cardozo Law Review 6*: 303–320.

Beauchamp, T., and Childress, J. (2008). *Principles of Biomedical Ethics*. 6th ed. New York: Oxford University Press.

Bulger, R.E., Boddy, E.M., and Fineberg, H.V. (eds.). (1995). *Society's Choices: Social and ethical decision making in biomedicine*. Washington, DC: National Academy Press.

Callahan, D. (1995). "Bioethics," in W. Reich, ed. *Encyclopedia of Bioethics*, New York: Macmillan.

Danis, M., Clancy, C., and L. R. Churchill, L.R. (eds.). (2002). *Ethical Dimensions of Health Policy*. New York: Oxford University Press.

Eckenwiler, L.A. and Cohn, F.G. (eds.). (2007). *The Ethics of Bioethics: Mapping the moral landscape*. Baltimore: Johns Hopkins University Press.

Emanuel, E. (1991). *The Ends of Human Life: Medical Ethics in a Liberal Polity*. Cambridge, MA: Harvard University Press.

Evans, J.H. (2002). *Playing God? Human genetic engineering and the rationalization of public bioethical debate*. Chicago: University of Chicago Press.

Fox, R.C. (1987). *Essays in Medical Sociology*. 2nd enlarged ed. New Brunswick: Transaction Books.

Fox, R.C. and Swazey, J. (2008). *Observing Bioethics*. New York: Oxford.

Fraser, N. and Honneth, A. 2003. *Redistribution or Recognition? A political-philosophical exchange*. London: Verso.

Fukuyama, F. (2002). *Our Posthuman Future: Consequences of the biotechnology revolution*. New York: Farrar, Straus and Giroux.

Galston, W.A. (1995). Two concepts of liberalism. *Ethics 105*:(3)516–534.

Gert, B.C., Culver, C.M., and Clouser, K.D. (2006). *Bioethics: A systematic approach*. 2nd ed. New York: Oxford University Press.

Jennings, B. (1998). Autonomy and difference: The travails of liberalism in bioethics. In R. DeVries and J. Subedi, eds. *Bioethics and Society*. (pp. 258–269). Upper Saddle River, NJ: Prentice Hall.

Jennings, B. (2007). Autonomy. In B. Steinbock, ed. *The Oxford Handbook of Bioethics*. (pp. 72–89). New York: Oxford University Press.

Jonsen, A.R. (1990). *The New Medicine and the Old Ethics*. Cambridge, MA: Harvard University Press.

Jonsen, A.R. (2000). *A Short History of Medical Ethics*. New York: Oxford University Press.

Jonsen, A.R. (2003). *The Birth of Bioethics*. New York: Oxford University Press.

Jonsen, A.R. and Toulmin, S. (1990). *The Abuse of Casuistry: A history of moral reasoning*. Berkeley, CA: University of California Press.

Kass, L.R. (2002). *Life, Liberty and the Defense of Dignity: The challenge for bioethics*. San Francisco: Encounter Books.

Kleinman, A., Fox, R.C., and Brandt, A. (eds.). (1999). Bioethics and beyond. *Daedalus 128*:4 (Special Issue).

Kymlicka, W. (1989). *Liberalism, Community, and Culture*. New York: Oxford University Press.

Meilaender, G.C. (1995). *Body, Soul, and Bioethics*. Notre Dame, IN: University of Notre Dame Press.

Moon, D.J. (1993). *Constructing Community: Moral Pluralism and Tragic Conflicts*. Princeton, NJ: Princeton University Press.

Mulhall, S., and Swift, A. (1996). *Liberals and Communitarians*. 2nd ed. Oxford: Blackwell.

Rothman, D.J. (1992). *Strangers at the Bedside: A history of how law and bioethics transformed medical decision making*. New York: Basic Books.

Rorty, R. (1989). *Contingency, Irony, and Solidarity*. Cambridge: Cambridge University Press.

Rose, N. (2007). *The Politics of Life Itself: Biomedicine, power, and subjectivity in the twenty-first century*. Princeton: Princeton University Press.

Satel, S. (2000). *PC, MD: How Political Correctness is Corrupting Medicine*. New York: Basic Books.

Smith, W.J. (2000). *Culture of Death: The Assault on Medical Ethics in America*. San Francisco: Encounter Books.

Taylor, C. (1991). *The Ethics of Authenticity.* Cambridge, MA: Harvard University Press.

Taylor, C., et. al. (1994). *Multiculturalism: Examining the politics of recognition.* Princeton, NJ: Princeton University Press.

White, S.K. (2000). *Sustaining Affirmation: The strengths of weak ontology in political theory.* Princeton, NJ: Princeton University Press.

Wolf, S.W. (ed.). (1996). *Feminism and Bioethics: Beyond reproduction.* New York: Oxford University Press.

Young, I.M. (1990). *Justice and the Politics of Difference.* Princeton, NJ: Princeton University Press.

INDEX

Note: All page numbers in bold refer to glossary definitions